Home Health Financial Management

Tad McKeon, MBA, CPA
Consultant
Jeffersonville, Pennsylvania

AN ASPEN PUBLICATION®
Aspen Publishers, Inc.
Gaithersburg, Maryland
1996

Library of Congress Cataloging-in-Publication Data

McKeon, Tad.
Home health financial management/by Tad McKeon.
p.   cm.
Includes bibliographical references and index.
ISBN: 0-8342-0729-X
1. Home care services—United States—Business management.
2. Home care services—United States—Accounting.   I. Title.
RA645.35.M39 1995
362.1'4'0681—dc20
95-21945
CIP

Editorial Resources: Bonnie Lawhorn

Library of Congress Catalog Card Number: 95-21945
ISBN: 0-8342-0729-X

Printed in the United States of America

1   2   3   4   5

To my wife Leslie and daughter Victoria

Table of Contents

Introduction

My objective in writing this book was to develop a text that integrates the disciplines of financial management, quality, and process improvement and that is understandable to both financial and nonfinancial managers. The text covers six primary areas that managers need to incorporate into their decision-making processes. These are financial reporting, prospective and retrospective payment systems, cost accounting, management accounting, financial management, and strategic management. To my knowledge, there is no other book that addresses these issues together.

Throughout the book, I attempt to stress the importance of teamwork among all levels and across the organization. Regardless of changes in payment systems, referral sources, and service delivery procedures, home health providers will need to demonstrate quality, low-cost solutions and transition to proactive outcome management systems. Outcome management systems will blend clinical and financial realities.

It is my personal belief that everyone within an agency must work toward customer service and develop outcome management systems that honor clients, coworkers, and innovation and that balance clinical and financial organizational requirements. It is hoped that the tools and concepts outlined in this book will provide a new way of looking at managing agency operations to ensure long-term financial viability and realization of organizational vision.

Acknowledgment

Thanks to **Donna A. Peters**, PhD, RN, FAAN, CNAA, for words of encouragement, new insights, and many thought-provoking conversations.

Part I

Financial Accounting

1

Chapter 1

Financial Statements

Financial statements are used for myriad purposes. Statements are developed for internal and external users. Internal users are the management staff of the home health agency (HHA). Typically, this would be administrators, department heads, the controller or chief financial officer (CFO), the chief executive officer (CEO), director of nursing (DON), and chief operating officer (COO). External users are basically unlimited, but the typical users are banks, leasing companies, the board of directors, and the fiscal intermediary. A full set of financial statements consists of an income statement, balance sheet, statement of cash flow, and statement of retained earnings or fund balance. These statements can be produced internally or by an external accounting firm. Notes and supplemental schedules are attached to increase the users' ability to understand the financial statements.

Statements are produced on a monthly, quarterly, semiannual, and annual basis. The frequency of reporting is determined by who is using the reports and who is preparing the reports. Report preparation is a time-consuming process that requires preparation by an individual with accounting knowledge. Depending on the size of the HHA, this person may not be on staff, thus requiring an outside firm to prepare statements. Agencies that have internally prepared statements often produce them on a monthly basis and ignore everything except the income statement and balance sheet.

The concept of timeliness is a critical issue affecting the value of financial statements. Financial statements that are not available in a timely fashion will provide less value for timely decision making. Internal uses for financial statements include monitoring operational results, assisting in decision making, and providing the basis for future plans. *Results of operations* is a term used to summarize how well the entity did for the reporting period. An entity is determined by its legal structure. Examples of a structure are a voluntary nonprofit organization, partnership, or corporation.

3

MONITORING OF OPERATIONS

Income statements normally report the current period with a year-to-date amount. Internal and external users can determine how profitable the HHA was for the reporting period. Results can be monitored in comparison to prior month activity or budget or to prior year. Evaluation of results against a standard or benchmark assists in the decision-making process. The decision-making process is assisted by the timely and accurate preparation of financial statements. Once the decision maker has had an opportunity to review the financial statements, he or she can choose to act or to gather additional information concerning the results of operation.

Operational results can be monitored for efficiency and effectiveness. Often, supplementary schedules will be presented in conjunction with the financial statements. Supplementary statements help the reader to understand the correlation between activities for the period and the results of operation. For instance, a schedule that supports an HHA's financial statement could be one that lists visit activity by payor, aged accounts receivable, or visits by field employee.

Review of supplemental schedules in conjunction with financial statements reveals how changes in the payor mix or worker productivity affect financial results. A change in payor mix from a payor who pays for services at a rate greater than the cost of providing care to a payor who reimburses at less than the cost of providing care will have a detrimental effect on the organization. Worker productivity becomes an issue when a field employee is paid a salary but performs only a few visits on a weekly basis.

Illustrated below are several examples of changes in payor mix. The first example, Table 1–1, is the current period and illustrates total activity of 3,615 visits with a payor mix of 34.6% private-pay visits, 13.8% health maintenance organization

Table 1–1 Visit Summary by Discipline and Payor: Current Period

Discipline	Private	HMO	Medicaid	Medicare	Total
Skilled nursing	700	350	50	500	1,600
Physical therapy	200			100	300
Occupational therapy	100			80	180
Speech therapy				70	70
Medical social services				50	50
Home health aide	250	150	15	1,000	1,415
Total	1,250	500	65	1,800	3,615
Percentage	(34.6)	(13.8)	(1.8)	(49.8)	(100.0)

(HMO) visits, 1.8% Medicaid visits, and 49.8% Medicare visits. The subsequent period, Table 1–2, has the same total visit volume but a much different payor mix.

The payor mix for the subsequent period is significantly different from the current period. This change in payor mix will have a substantial impact on the agency. Tables 1–3 and 1–4 illustrate how revenue can be affected by a change in payor mix. The following example assumes a payor mix change similar to the shift in business demonstrated above. An additional assumption, for illustrative purposes, is the reimbursement rate per discipline for each discipline and payor.

Monitoring of operations is not limited solely to internal management, albeit management has a responsibility to make decisions that ensure the entity will remain profitable and solvent. Management is responsible to the employees who work for it, banks, other creditors, suppliers, and the patient population that it serves.

Profit is a realistic component of doing business because it demonstrates financial viability. Without profit, there would not be money to buy equipment, pay salaries, and continue operations. This concept applies to both proprietary and nonprofit agencies. The most significant difference is that nonprofit agencies have other funding sources available to them, such as United Way, and fundraising activities. For-profit entities are dependent on profitable operations, bank loans, and loans from the owners.

Operations are also monitored by external organizations, such as unions, creditors, and third-party payors. External organizations such as creditors are concerned about the agency's ability to meet its obligations and will monitor organizational results for compliance. They want to verify that sufficient profit is being generated to repay any loans that they may have made. The fiscal intermediary uses an agency's financial statements as a tool to reconcile reported costs and to monitor the financial health of the agency. Board members review results in an attempt to assist management if there is a problem developing.

Table 1–2 Visit Summary by Discipline and Payor: Subsequent Period

Discipline	Private	HMO	Medicaid	Medicare	Total
Skilled nursing	100	350	50	900	1,400
Physical therapy	25			100	125
Occupational therapy	10			80	90
Speech therapy				70	70
Medical social services				50	50
Home health aide	115	150	15	1,600	1,880
Total	250	500	65	2,800	3,615
Percentage	(6.9)	(13.8)	(1.8)	(77.5)	(100.0)

Table 1–3 Visit, Rate, and Revenue Analysis by Discipline and Payor: Current Period

	Private	HMO	Medicaid	Medicare	Total
Visits by discipline					
Skilled nursing	700	350	50	500	1,600
Physical therapy	200			100	300
Occupational therapy	100			80	180
Speech therapy				70	70
Medical social services				50	50
Home health aide	250	150	15	1,000	1,415
Total	1,250	500	65	1,800	3,615
Percentage	(34.6)	(13.8)	(1.8)	(49.8)	(100.0)
Rate by payor ($)					
Skilled nursing	$ 95	$75	$55	$70	
Physical therapy	95	75	55	70	
Occupational therapy	95	75	55	70	
Speech therapy	75	75	55	70	
Medical social services	140	50	55	70	
Home health aide	50	35	25	70	
Revenue by payor ($)					
Skilled nursing	$ 66,500	$26,250	$2,750	$ 35,000	$130,500
Physical therapy	19,000			7,000	26,000
Occupational therapy	9,500			5,600	15,100
Speech therapy				4,900	4,900
Medical social services				3,500	3,500
Home health aide	12,500	5,250	375	70,000	88,125
Total (%)	$107,500	$31,500	$3,125	$126,000	$268,125
Percentage	(40.1)	(11.7)	(1.2)	(47.0)	(100.0)

BASIC PRINCIPLES OF FINANCIAL REPORTING

Internal and external users of an HHA financial statement depend on several of the inherent principles behind financial reporting. This concept allows external users to evaluate an agency's financial statements and make educated decisions from the reports that are supplied by management. These principles transcend all industries and are not specific to home health.

Generally Accepted Accounting Principles

Generally accepted accounting principles (GAAP) represent the principles, tenets, and practices utilized in preparing financial statements. These guidelines were

Table 1–4 Visit, Rate, and Revenue Analysis by Discipline and Payor: Subsequent Period

	Private	*HMO*	*Medicaid*	*Medicare*	*Total*
Visits by discipline					
Skilled nursing	100	350	50	900	1,400
Physical therapy	25			100	125
Occupational therapy	10			80	90
Speech therapy				70	70
Medical social services				50	50
Home health aide	115	150	15	1,600	1,880
Total	250	500	65	2,800	3,615
Percentage	(6.9)	(13.8)	(1.8)	(77.5)	(100.0)
Rate by payor ($)					
Skilled nursing	$ 95	$75	$55	$70	
Physical therapy	95	75	55	70	
Occupational therapy	95	75	55	70	
Speech therapy	75	75	55	70	
Medical social services	140	50	55	70	
Home health aide	50	35	25	70	
Revenue by payor ($)					
Skilled nursing	$ 9,500	$26,250	$2,750	$ 63,000	$101,500
Physical therapy	2,375			7,000	9,375
Occupational therapy	950			5,600	6,550
Speech therapy				4,900	4,900
Medical social services				3,500	3,500
Home health aide	5,750	5,250	375	112,000	123,375
Total	$18,575	$31,500	$3,125	$196,000	$249,200
Percentage	(7.5)	(12.6)	(1.2)	(78.7)	(100.0)

developed, and continue to be developed, to provide a standard for presentation. In other words, GAAP represent a consistent application of practices, concepts, and principles. Public or governmental agencies must follow the rules established by the Governmental Accounting Standards Board (GASB) versus proprietary agencies that follow the rules established by the Financial Accounting Standards Board (FASB).

The concept of matching revenue and expenses to the period that the service was provided is one of the objectives of financial reporting and is an example of cause and effect. It is assumed that expenses must be incurred to generate revenue. Therefore, you cannot have a billable visit without having the direct cost of providing that visit and the administrative cost that made that visit possible.

A second concept is matching expenses of long-lived assets such as equipment to the accounting periods that will benefit from the acquisition. In this example, there is no cause-and-effect relationship between the purchase of a computer and its benefit in future periods, so accounting theory dictates that the acquisition cost of the computer be depreciated in a rational and systematic fashion to spread the cost into future periods.

A third concept is immediate recognition of revenue and costs. This concept applies to revenue and costs for which there is no cause-and-effect relationship, so accounting theory dictates that the cost be recognized in the current period. An example would be the recognition of the CEO's salary, where the CEO's salary was incurred, regardless of whether there was any revenue generated in the period.

Going Concern

The theory behind the *going concern* concept is that an agency will be able to continue to operate indefinitely and is involved with continuous and ongoing activities. The organization has sufficient resources to meet all of its obligations and to satisfy its creditors. This principle supports accounting methodology such as depreciation and amortization of assets. The inherent assumption is that the agency will continue to operate into the future, so assets that are purchased today will have a future useful life. Therefore, their expense can be spread to future periods.

Accounting Period

An accounting period is determined by the frequency of reporting. Accounting periods are normally monthly; however, they can be quarterly, semiannually, and annually. The difficulty with accounting periods of long duration is that they do not provide adequate information to the users of financial statements for making informed decisions. Additionally, consistent accounting periods lend validity to the financial statements.

Conservatism

Conservatism is another accounting principle that lends validity to the financial statements by attempting to measure uncertainty. Conservatism is a guiding principle when an accountant is unable to quantify risk or a potential liability. The concept is to err on the side of conservatism by recognizing potential losses and ignoring anticipated gains. This is generally used when estimating allowances for uncollectible receivables, potential lawsuit settlements, or annual settlements from the Medicare program.

Consistency

Accounting principles need to be applied consistently. This concept helps readers in evaluating results of operation. Once an organization adopts an accounting convention, it is assumed by the reader that the chosen convention will be applied every time the financial statements are produced. An example of an accounting convention that requires consistency is the selection of depreciation methods. Accounting methodology that is changed will require reporting the facts related to the change and the dollar value of the change.

Material

The *material* concept suggests that if an event or activity could change the reader's interpretation (the reader is assumed to be a reasonable person) of the financial statements that he or she is reviewing, then the event or activity needs to be included in the financial statements.

Double-entry Accounting

Double-entry accounting is one of the foundations of accounting. Accounting transactions consist of two components: (1) debit and (2) credit. Debits and credits must be equal; otherwise, the financial statements would be out of balance, causing inaccurate information to be reported due to missing information. The concept of double-entry accounting is similar to "for every action, there is a reaction." For instance, when a patient is visited, an entry is required to record the billable visit from a financial statement perspective. This creates revenue for the agency and a receivable due from the patient's insurance carrier. Recognition of this event would require a double-sided entry and is illustrated by recording a debit to accounts receivable and a credit to revenue. Every entry to the books of an HHA utilizes the double-entry accounting approach.

Accrual Accounting

Accrual accounting is the process that recognizes and reports all revenues and gains when earned and expenses and losses when incurred. Accrual accounting is a requirement for the Medicare Cost Report. Accrual accounting is the best way to measure the cost of providing care, management performance, earnings, and stewardship.

An example of accrual accounting would be when a field employee performs a visit at the end of the month but is not paid for that visit until the next time payroll checks are issued. Payroll will not be issued again until the following month. Accrual accounting recognizes the agency's liability to pay the field employee for that visit in the month in which it was performed. Another example of accrual accounting is when an insurance policy is paid. The premium for the entire year is paid in one installment. Accrual accounting requires that this cost be spread across the 12 months that benefit by the coverage instead of being included in the month in which the premium is paid.

Cash Basis Accounting

Cash basis accounting does not offer the reader an accurate understanding of the true performance of an organization. Cash basis accounting is nothing more than recording the total cash received for the period and the total amount of payments made during the period. There is no attempt to match expenses that will be paid in subsequent months (unpaid bills) and record the expense in the month in which the visit is performed. Revenues are recorded when received and not when they are earned.

Modified Accrual

Modified accrual is a method of accounting used primarily by governmental or public HHAs. They will maintain their records using the cash basis of accounting during the year, then for year-end reporting, accrue costs that belong in the year in which they are reporting.

Historical Cost

Historical cost is commonly used when acquiring assets such as buildings, equipment, furniture, and fixtures. This is often referred to as an *exchange price*. Assets are recorded at historical cost unless they have been donated or gifted to the agency. Donated assets are recorded at their fair market value at the time the gift was made.

FINANCIAL STATEMENTS

Financial statements consist of four main statements and the footnotes that inform the reader of significant accounting transactions and events. The balance sheet is a record of all activity from inception to the balance sheet's date. The balance sheet can also be referred to as the *statement of financial position*. The income statement can be for one month or several months, but will never exceed a one-year period. The statement of cash flow is the third primary statement. This statement summarizes how the agency's cash was used for the reporting period and separates cash between operations, financing, and investing. The last statement indicates the increases or decreases in earnings or fund balance for a stated period of time and is referred to as the *statement of retained earnings* or *fund balance*. This statement is typically included as part of the income statement. The objectives of financial reporting are defined by the Financial Accounting Standards Board in Exhibit 1–1.

Figure 1–1 illustrates the interrelatedness of the balance sheet, income statement, and cash-flow statement. Results of operation for the current period are re-

---

Exhibit 1–1 Objectives of Financial Reporting as Defined by the Financial Accounting Standards Board

- Financial reporting should provide information that is useful to present and potential investors and creditors and other users in making rational investment, credit, and similar decisions. The information should be comprehensive to those who have a reasonable understanding of business and economic activities and are willing to study the information with reasonable diligence.

- Financial reporting should provide information to help present and potential investors and creditors and other users in assessing the amounts, timing, and uncertainty of prospective cash receipts from dividends or interest and the proceeds from the sale, redemption, or maturity of securities or loans. Since investors' and creditors' cash flows are related to enterprise cash flows, financial reporting should provide information to help investors, creditors, and others assess the amounts, timing, and uncertainty of prospective net cash inflows to the related enterprise.

- Financial reporting should provide information about the economic resources of an enterprise, the claims to those resources of an enterprise (obligations of the enterprise to transfer resources to other entities and owners' equity), and the effects of transactions, events, and circumstances that change its resources and claims to those resources.

  The primary focus of financial reporting is ordinarily considered to be information about earnings and its components. Earnings analysis gives clues to (a) management's performance, (b) long-term earning capabilities, (c) future earnings, and (d) risks associated with lending to and investing in the enterprise.

  Financial reporting should also provide information about how management has discharged its stewardship function to stockholders for the use of the enterprise's resources entrusted to it. Management is responsible not only for the custody and safekeeping of enterprise resources but also for their efficient and profitable use.

  Management through financial reporting can provide significant financial information to users by identifying events and circumstances and explaining their financial effects on the enterprise. However, investors, creditors, and others who rely on financial reporting must do their own evaluating, estimating, predicting, and assessing and not rely exclusively on management's presentations.

Source: Woelfel, Charles J., *Financial Statement Analysis: The Investor's Self Study Guide to Interpreting and Analyzing Financial Statements*, Probus Publishing, Chicago, Illinois, 1994.

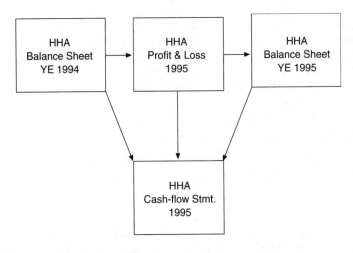

Figure 1–1 Financial Statement Flow

flected on the profit-and-loss statement. The corresponding effects of operations are also reflected on the balance sheet. The difference between the prior year and current balance sheet, and the current year profit and loss, is reflected on the statement of cash flow.

Balance Sheet

The balance sheet consists of assets, liabilities, and equity. Agencies who have elected a nonprofit status would substitute the term *fund* for *equity balance*. Listed below is a description of the various components of the balance sheet and typical transactions that would be categorized in each of these sections. (Sample comparative HHA balance sheets are shown in Exhibit 1–2.)

Assets

Assets refer to organizational resources.

Current Assets. *Current assets* represent anything that can be converted to cash or consumed in the normal operating cycle or within a year. Typical accounts in this classification include cash, petty cash, patient accounts receivable, allowances against patient receivables, investments, other receivables, and prepaid expenses. Account classification is sequenced based on its nearness to cash. Each of these accounts will be explained in detail below.

- *Cash*—Cash represents monies that have been deposited into a savings or checking account or have the ability to be deposited. Examples of cash in-

Exhibit 1–2 Comparative Balance Sheets

Sample Home Health Agency
Balance Sheets
December 31, 1995 and 1994

	1995	1994
Assets		
Current assets		
Cash and cash equivalents	$ 74,000	$ 41,000
Investments	112,000	102,000
Accounts receivable		
(net of estimated uncollectibles of $61,000 in 1995 and $30,000 in 1994)	752,000	476,000
Other receivables	27,000	22,000
Total current assets	965,000	641,000
Assets whose use is limited		
Cash	35,000	35,000
Bank certificates of deposit	100,000	100,000
	135,000	135,000
Equipment		
Medical & office equipment	56,000	39,000
Vehicles	50,000	37,000
	106,000	76,000
Less accumulated depreciation	(45,000)	(24,000)
Net equipment	61,000	52,000
Deferred finance charges		
(Net of accumulated amortization of $15,000 in 1995 and $10,000 in 1994)	20,000	25,000
	$1,181,000	$853,000
Liabilities and fund balances		
Current liabilities		
Current maturities of long-term debt	$ 13,000	$ 13,000
Accounts payable	40,000	21,000
Accrued payroll and vacation costs	496,000	352,000
Estimated third-party payor settlements	28,000	31,000
Advances from third-party payors	70,000	66,000
Total current liabilities	647,000	483,000
Long-term debt less current maturities	105,000	118,000
Fund balance	429,000	252,000
	$1,181,000	$853,000

Source: Reprinted from *Audits of Providers of Health Care Services*, p. 165, with permission of the American Institute of Certified Public Accountants, © 1994.

clude cash, coins, checks, money orders, bank drafts, and petty cash. The petty cash fund, or cash on hand, is intended for those items that require immediate payment and not as a source of money instead of going through accounts payable. An agency will establish petty cash funds to pay for daily operating expenses that may require immediate payment. An example of this would be postage expenses, coffee, or a minor office supply.

Typically, agencies have three accounts. One account is usually interest bearing and is used as a general depository. The other two accounts are for payroll and accounts payable activities. Additionally, the general classification of cash and cash equivalents can also include money market accounts, certificates of deposit (CDs), or time deposits.

- *Investments*—Investments are stocks and bonds owned by the HHA. These securities can be converted into cash within one year and are reflected on the balance sheet at the lower of cost or market. The nontechnical explanation of the lower of cost or market concept is to reduce the cost of the asset to reflect current market conditions.

- *Accounts Receivable*—Patient receivables represent money owed to an HHA for services that have been provided to patients. HHAs should set up separate accounts by payor. Most HHAs set up their largest payors and group their smaller commercial payors into one category. This assumes that an agency has a supporting or subsidiary schedule to manage its accounts receivable.

Accounting procedures require that accounts receivable be reflected net of allowances. This is to identify to the reader that the agency will collect something less than its gross charges or a net realizable amount where the net realizable amount is gross charges less allowances for uncollectible receivables. This is true for cost-reimbursed payors and for any payor for whom the agency has agreed to accept an amount less than its standard charges as payment for the services provided. This is referred to as a *contractual adjustment*. Additional reductions would be reflected on the books of an HHA to estimate an agency's inability to collect all of its accounts receivable. This is referred to as an *allowance* or *reserve* for uncollectible receivables.

The *allowance account* for cost-reimbursed providers represents the difference between the providers' charges and their cost. Allowances for payors whose reimbursement is known are the difference between charges and anticipated reimbursement. Allowance accounts are generally set up by payor for easy reconciliation of outstanding balances. Allowances can also include an estimate for uncollectible receivables. The older a receivable becomes, the less likely that the agency will be able to collect it.

Other receivables is a classification used for money owed to the agency from employees, related parties, or any nonpatient-related activity, such as rental activity.

Notes receivable are an unconditional promise to pay the agency. Notes are in writing, are for a specific dollar value, and include a stated interest rate, and the terms of the repayment include definite and definable terms and dates.

- *Prepaid Expenses*—Prepaid expenses are expenses that will benefit a future period. An example of a prepaid expense is the annual payment for malpractice insurance. The cost of the policy is paid at one time; however, the policy coverage period is for an entire year. The portion of the policy that covers future periods is treated as a prepaid expense. Other examples include prepaid rent, advertising, and equipment maintenance contracts.

- *Inventory*—Most agencies record supply cost as a current period cost on their income statements instead of recording the purchase of supplies as an increase to inventory. Agency supply cost consists of two types of supply cost: (1) supply cost related to soft supplies, such as bandages and wound dressings, and (2) resale supplies and equipment that are billable to the patient.

The concept of inventory records the cost of supplies and equipment as an asset instead of an expense. Supplies purchased for an agency would be delivered and placed in a central repository, and when a nurse needs to take supplies to a patient or replenish his or her bag, inventory would be decreased, thus representing an expense. Inventories are normally valued at cost or at the lower of cost or market value. Cost can be determined by the following methods: specific identification; average cost; first in, first out (FIFO); or last in, first out (LIFO). Each method will have a different effect on the agency's cost.

Assets Whose Use Is Limited. Assets that are not available for general use have restrictions placed on them. Cash usage can be restricted or dedicated for specific types of expenditures—for instance, replacement of fixed assets—and is referred to as a *restricted fund*. Restrictions can also be due to donation or grant requirements. Use of these funds is only permitted when the agency has satisfied the conditions of the donation or grant requirements.

The Statement of Financial Accounting Standards No. 117, *Financial Statements of Not-for-Profit Organizations (SFAS No. 117)*

requires that organizations report three classes of net assets in the statement of financial position: unrestricted net assets, temporarily restricted net assets, and permanently restricted net assets. Information about the nature and amounts of restrictions should be disclosed by reporting their amounts on the face of the statement or by including a description in the notes. Separate line items may be used to distinguish permanent restrictions for holding of assets donated with stipulations that (1) they be used for a specified purpose, be preserved and not be sold, or (2) they be invested to provide a permanent source of income (endowment funds). Similarly, separate lines may be reported within temporarily restricted net assets to distinguish between temporary restrictions for support for a particular activity, investment for a specified term, use in a specified future period, and acquisition of long lived assets.[1]

Property, Plant, and Equipment. Property, plant, and equipment represents buildings, furniture, computer equipment, automobiles, and other machinery and equipment purchased to support agency operations. Acquisitions are reflected on the agency's books at the cost of acquisition. Cost of acquisition can include freight and sales tax. The agency will group assets by category. Common categories are land and building, leasehold improvements, capital improvements, equipment, and automobiles. Each asset except for land is depreciated. Depreciation reflects normal usage and attempts to match each asset's useful life to the future period that will benefit by it.

Assets are normally reflected net of depreciation. *Accumulated depreciation* is the term used to reflect the total amount of depreciation expense taken by asset category. Once the asset has been totally depreciated, depreciation expense will cease to be recorded.

Book value of an asset is the historical cost of the asset less the accumulated depreciation for that asset. Book value does not necessarily represent the true value of the asset.

Intangible Assets. Intangible assets are long-lived assets that reflect costs not associated with the current operations and have a future benefit to the entity. Intangible assets generally include goodwill, start-up costs, patents, trademarks, customer lists, company name, franchise fees, and convenants not to compete.

- *Goodwill*—This is a cost related to the acquisition of an agency. The purchase price that is not definitely assignable to assets is referred to as *goodwill*. Goodwill is an intangible cost that is amortized.
- *Start-up Cost*—This is the cost of setting up the new operation. It is predominantly labor, legal fees, and office costs related to starting a new company. From Medicare's perspective, this is the cost associated with documentation of policies and procedures for licensure or application for a certificate of need. Start-up costs are amortized over five years.

Liabilities

Liabilities are obligations of the HHA from prior events that will be paid some time in the future. Liabilities are classed according to the timeframe in which they will be paid, with the most current maturities listed first.

Current Liabilities. Current liabilities are expenses and obligations of the HHA that are expected to be paid within the year. This definition differentiates short-term creditors from long-term creditors. Short-term creditors are employees, independent contractors, and suppliers. Long-term creditors are banks, leasing companies, and bond holders.

- *Short-term obligations*—Short-term obligations represent the current portion of notes, bonds, mortgages, and capital lease obligations. Short-term obligations are due and payable within the 12-month period. Short-term debt can also include credit card debt.

- *Accounts Payable*—Accounts payable represent monies owed to vendors who have provided services and supplies to the HHA. Typical activities that generate accounts payable are medical supplies, office supplies, repair services, maintenance services, phone bills, utility bills, equipment purchases, and legal and accounting fees.

- *Accrued Expenses*—Accrued expenses represent obligations that the agency anticipates incurring within the year. Typical expenses that an agency would accrue could be the cost of their annual audit, workers' compensation liabilities, malpractice claims, interest, property and local taxes, or any large expense for which the cost is representative of a larger period than the month in which it is paid. Fees owed to independent contractors or staffing agencies could be included here or under accrued fees.

- *Accrued Payroll*—Accrued payroll is money that is owed to employees for services provided but not yet paid. Included in this category would be bonuses, payroll taxes, paid time-off (PTO) accruals, pension liability, and salaries and wages to be paid. Agencies normally have separate accounts for each category to increase the ease of reconciliation.

- *Overpayments*—Overpayments are monies that have been paid to the agency in error. These amounts represent a liability to the agency and are generally returned to the payor who made the overpayment. Medicare utilizes a Credit Balance Report to report any overpayments that the agency may have received.

- *Estimated third-party settlements*—This category reflects any money that is owed to a third-party payor because of pending cost reporting adjustments.

Long-term Obligations. Long-term obligations are the portion of notes, bonds, mortgages, and capital leases that exceed 12 months.

Equity or Fund Balance

This is commonly referred to as *retained earnings*. This follows the accounting formula of "assets less liabilities equal equity." Equity is the excess of revenues over expenses that remains in the entity. Equity for a nonprofit entity would be represented by a positive fund balance.

Contributions made by owners to the entity are referred to as *additional paid in capital*. The initial capital structure of a proprietary agency is determined when the entity is incorporated. The owner of each entity is issued stock that represents the ownership of the entity.

Income Statement

An income statement is commonly referred to as a *profit and loss statement*. The income statement reports the agency's revenues, expenses, and the resultant profit or loss from the agency's activities. Revenues and expenses can be identified as operating and nonoperating. Operating revenues and expenses would pertain to patient care, or the primary mission of the HHA, whereas nonoperating would be incidental revenues and expenses, such as rental income or vending machine receipts. (Sample HHA statements of revenue and expenses and changes in fund balance are found in Exhibit 1–3.)

Revenues

Revenue represents billable activity that will be reimbursed by a patient, his or her insurance carrier, state, or federal program. Revenues are identified by discipline, such as skilled nursing, physical therapy, occupational therapy, speech therapy, medical social service, home health aide, private-duty nursing by type, medical supplies, or whatever service the agency is providing. Revenue can also be identified by payor, service line, or other means of classification important to management.

Traditional revenue has been either cost-reimbursed or fee-for-service. Under a cost-reimbursed payment system, such as Medicare, revenue is determined by the lower of cost, charges, or limits. The interim rate is a function of cost as defined by Medicare's lower of cost, charges, or limits formula and then divided by total visits. Each of the six disciplines (nursing, physical therapy, occupational therapy, speech therapy, medical social services, and home health aide) would have the same interim rate. Supply cost is included in the interim rate.

Fee-for-service revenue would have a different rate by discipline or a common rate for skilled services and a lower rate for aide services. Calculation of revenue is straightforward when the reimbursement rate is known. Revenue equals number of visits multiplied by the reimbursement rate for those visits.

The managed care movement and health care reform are introducing episodic payment and capitated payment mechanisms. An episodic payment would be one flat rate paid to a provider, and it would be up to the agency to provide all services from admission through discharge. This type of payment mechanism is utilized within hospice.

Exhibit 1–3 Comparative Statements or Revenue and Expenses and Changes in Fund Balance

Sample Home Health Agency
Statements of Revenue and Expenses and Changes in Fund Balance
December 31, 1995 and 1994

	1995	1994
Net patient service revenue	$4,042,000	$2,687,000
Other revenue	27,000	32,000
Total revenue	4,069,000	2,719,000
Expenses		
Professional care of patients	2,714,000	1,835,000
General and administrative	1,042,000	675,000
Occupancy	90,000	83,000
Provision for bad debts	46,000	21,000
Depreciation	21,000	15,000
Interest	16,000	19,000
Total expenses	3,929,000	2,648,000
Income from operations	140,000	71,000
Nonoperating gains		
Contributions	19,000	15,000
Investment income	18,000	12,000
Total nonoperating gains	37,000	27,000
Revenue and gains in excess of expenses	177,000	98,000
Fund balance at beginning of year	252,000	154,000
Fund balance at end of year	$ 429,000	$ 252,000

Source: Reprinted from *Audits of Providers of Health Care Services*, p. 166, with permission of the American Institute of Certified Public Accountants, © 1994.

A capitated payment would pay agencies based on the number of patients in the population for which they are responsible. The agency would receive a monthly payment based on the number of members within the population that it is serving. The amount of service provided is left to the discretion of the agency; however, quality of care and maximization of outcomes are still valid concerns of the payor and provider.

Patient service revenue is comprised of three components: (1) gross revenue, (2) contractual allowances, and (3) net revenue.

Gross Revenue. Gross revenue represents charges for activities based on the agency's stated or published rate. A stated rate is a fixed rate by discipline and type of service and can be per visit or hourly. Gross revenue represents an activity multiplied by the agency's stated rate. For example, if the agency's published rate is $100 for every skilled nursing visit, and the agency performs three visits, then the gross revenue for skilled nursing is $300. Gross revenue is also recorded for medical supplies. Medical supplies may be billable to payors or included in the per-visit reimbursement. Medical supplies are normally marked up over cost.

Contractual Allowances. Contractual allowances are the difference between gross charges and the anticipated reimbursement, or net revenue. Some contractual allowances are known at the time services are provided. An example of this would be when care is provided to a patient who has insurance that pays less than the agency's gross charges. When the anticipated reimbursement is known, the contractual allowance can be recognized at the time of revenue recognition.

Contractual allowances for services provided to the Medicare and Medicaid cost-reimbursed programs will change throughout the year because of changes in the agency's cost and volume of services provided. Contractual adjustments are made during the recognition of revenue and adjusted as circumstances change.

Contractual allowances can also occur when payment for services is received. A typical example is when the agency bills a patient who has commercial insurance, and his or her policy pays less than the agency's gross, or stated charge. This may be due to the patient's policy paying 80 percent of charges, and the patient is responsible for the difference of 20 percent. If the agency does not bill patients for the 20 percent balance, then the agency will recognize the 20 percent as an adjustment to revenue. This is referred to as a *write-off.*

Charity Allowances. Charity allowances arise when a client of the agency has insufficient funds to pay for services provided. Often the agency will work out a discounted fee arrangement with the patient. Recognition of revenue should be at gross with an offset to charity allowances to arrive at the net amount due the agency.

According to the Healthcare Financial Management Associations (HFMA) Principles and Practices Board,

> Each provider of healthcare services must establish criteria for charity service consistent with the organization's mission and financial ability. Some providers have financial resources designated for the provision of charity service while other providers must recover the cost of charity service from the amounts paid by or for other patients. Some communities provide financial support to specific organizations to ensure that charity service is available, while other communities prefer that each provider arrange for charity service based on demand. For these reasons, no single set of criteria is universally applicable and each provider must develop and administer its own criteria.

Criteria for determining the amount of charity service for which a patient is eligible for an occasion of service could include the following factors[2]:

- individual or family income,
- individual or family net worth,
- employment status and earning capacity,
- family size,
- other financial obligations,
- the amount and frequency of bills for health care services, and
- other sources of payment for services rendered.

Discounts and Other Allowances. Discounts are adjustments to gross revenue. Discounts could be attributable to contract negotiation, volume, or incentive for prompt payment. As home health transitions into prospective payment, discounts from gross revenue will have less meaning.

Net Revenue. Net revenue is the result of subtracting allowances from gross revenue. Net revenue is the actual amount of money an agency will receive for providing services. The concepts of net revenue and net realizable receivables are synonymous in that both revenues and receivables need to be recorded to reflect anticipated collections.

Payors can be grouped into two categories: (1) retrospective and (2) prospective. Retrospective payors such as Medicare and some Medicaid programs are cost-reimbursed. The true receivable will not be known until the intermediary settles the cost report. This process could take up to two years. Upon settlement, the actual contractual allowance and net receivable will be known. Conversely, contractual allowance and net revenue are known for prospective payors.

Other Revenue. Other revenue represents revenue to an agency that is not the direct result of providing services to patients. Examples of types of other revenue can include the gain on sale of equipment, grants, investment income, contributions from funding sources such as the United Way, municipal funding sources, donations, and fundraising activities.

Expenses

Expenses are costs incurred in the direct provision of patient care and the related support activities. Support activities include general and administrative expenses for staff and supplies, facility cost, depreciation of equipment, interest expense, and bad-debt expense.

Professional Care of Patients. The cost of providing care to patients includes payment of field staff, field staff benefits, travel expenses, medical supplies, and equipment. This is one of the largest costs that an agency incurs, and it is important to understand the relationship between costs and revenues. Simply stated, costs in this section should include all costs related to the direct provision of care.

Costs will vary by the type of service provided and the type of field staff utilized by the agency to provide services. For instance, an agency may choose to employ registered nurses (RNs) and home health aides and subcontract for all of its therapy requirements. Another agency may not subcontract and instead employs therapists to meet its operational requirements. Staffing strategies will affect cost of services.

Payment strategies will also affect cost of service. Agencies may choose to pay field staff per visit, per hour, per diem, or salary. Differences in payment strategies could affect agency profitability. This concept is known as *productivity*. The following is an example of how cost of service will be affected by productivity. If an agency pays an RN a salary of $38,000 to provide field visits, and he or she does 1,000 visits, the average cost per visit is $38. If the RN performs only 800 visits during the year, then his or her average cost per visit has risen to $47.50. This represents a 25 percent increase in cost per visit. Historically, cost-reimbursed providers were not too concerned about productivity; however, prospective payment and managed care will change this.

The cost of providing professional care to patients includes *fringe benefits* for field staff. Fringe benefits are vacation time, sick time, and personal time, commonly referred to as *paid time off*. Fringe benefits can also include health insur-

Table 1–5 Nurse Employee: Cost per Visit Calculation

	RN A (800 visits/yr)	RN B (1,000 visits/yr)	RN C (1,200 visits/yr)
Salary	$38,000	$38,000	$38,000
Benefits			
Health insurance	2,000	2,000	2,000
Pension contribution	1,000	1,000	1,000
Continuing education	500	500	500
Employer expenses			
FICA*	2,850	2,850	2,850
Unemployment	600	600	600
Workers' compensation	380	380	380
Malpractice insurance	500	500	500
Total benefits	7,830	7,830	7,830
Total compensation	$45,830	$45,830	$45,830
Average cost per visit	$57.29	$45.83	$38.19

*Federal Insurance Contributions Act.

ance, pension contributions, deferred compensation plans, and continuing education. In addition to fringe benefits, an agency will pay employer payroll taxes, malpractice insurance, and workers' compensation on behalf of its employees.

Fringe benefits and employer taxes substantially increase the cost of providing care. When productivity of salaried employees is not taken into consideration, the financial impact to the agency could be detrimental in a prospective reimbursement environment. Table 1–5 illustrates estimated benefit cost for a salaried field employee and the resultant increase to the average cost per visit for an RN who does 1,000 and 800 annual visits. The average cost per visit for the RN who does 1,000 visits increased from $38.00 per visit to $45.83. The average cost per visit for the RN who did 800 visits increased from $47.50 per visit to $57.29.

Another consideration is the concept of replacement cost. Replacement cost comes into play when employees take time off. It does not matter whether they take sick, vacation, or personal time, or they are unable to perform visits due to in-services or poor scheduling. Replacement cost is an incremental cost of providing care.

The cost of providing professional care to patients includes cost incurred for transportation to the patients' homes. *Transportation expense* has two components. The first component is the actual cost of transportation. This could be mileage, use of an agency vehicle, or public transportation costs. The second component of transportation cost is the time spent commuting between patients' homes. Commute time can be aggravated by the geographic area an agency covers, scheduling difficulties, and resource availability.

Medical supplies cost is also included in the cost of providing professional care to patients. Medical supply cost includes soft supplies such as bandages, tape, and gloves required as part of the nursing visit. Supply cost also includes supplies that have been sold to the patient, intravenous (IV) therapies, and durable or home medical equipment (DME or HME).

General and Administrative Expenses. Administrative expenses are costs incurred by an agency to provide patient care. These costs include the indirect costs of providing care, such as clerical support staff, agency management, professional fees, insurance cost, and office supplies. Listed below are several major classification categories for administrative expenses. Expense categories are normally maintained by type of expense and combined for reporting purposes.

- *Salaries and Benefits*—Support staff are required for the provision of patient care. Support staff include managers, executive management, billers, schedulers, file clerks, accounting personnel, information system personnel, data-entry staff, intake and referral staff, human resource personnel, secretaries, and receptionists. Staffing requirements will vary based on the size and complexity of the HHA. Included in this category are wages for hourly and salary employees, overtime, employer payroll taxes, workers' compensation, health insurance, bonuses, pension payments, employer's contribution toward 401K plans, and other employee benefits.

- *Professional Fees*—Professional fees are costs incurred by an agency for legal expenses, accounting and reimbursement services, union arbitration, administration of pension plans, and consulting costs associated with training and development. These expenses are incurred because it is usually cost-prohibitive to hire professionals in these areas as full-time employees. Therefore, costs can be incurred on an as-needed basis. For instance, legal expenses may be incurred when negotiating contracts and purchase arrangements, lease review, and conducting employee negotiations.

- *Insurance Expense*—Insurance expense represents costs to protect the agency from wrongful and negligent acts that may have been caused by its employees. Typical types of insurance include malpractice, directors and officers, office contents, employee dishonesty, and automobile. Malpractice insurance coverage can be purchased using a claims-made policy or an occurrence policy. Claims-made policies provide coverage for claims made during the policy period. Occurrence policies provide coverage for the policy period and for claims submitted subsequent to the policy period that apply to the policy period. Whenever possible, attempts should be made to purchase tail coverage for claims-made policies.

- *Office Expense and Supplies*—This category captures the cost of supporting operations and the employees of those operations. Examples of office expense include equipment maintenance, paper and stationery supplies, computer maintenance and supplies, copy machine expense and supplies, telephone expense, and technical reference materials.

- *Marketing Expense*—Marketing expenditures include telephone directory advertisements, radio and television advertising, billboard rental, and advertisements in trade journals or local publications. Marketing expenditures can be viewed as expenses incurred for survival and are often incurred regardless of whether they will be reimbursed by Medicare.

Facility Cost. Costs commonly associated with this category are incurred for the occupancy, operation, and maintenance of the office. Expenses include rental expense, building repairs and maintenance, cleaning services, utilities, restroom supplies, snow removal, and landscaping. Costs for mortgage interest and building depreciation are classified as part of facility cost for internally produced financial statements. However, for purposes of external reporting, these costs are reported in their respective categories.

Bad-debt Expense. "The basic distinction between bad debts and charity service in the healthcare setting is adequately described in the literature by differentiating between the unwillingness of the patient to pay and the demonstrated inability of the patient to pay."[3]

Bad-debt expense consists of estimates against the collectibility of receivables and write-offs. Estimates regarding the inability to collect receivables are referred to as a *provision against doubtful accounts.* Provision for bad debt can be based on the relative age of patient receivables, third-party regulations, payor history, or a combination of actual history and age. The concept is that the older a receivable becomes, the more difficult collection will be.

Write-offs occur because the debt is uncollectible or because of agency policy. Bad debts can be due to a denial by the payor to pay for services provided, incomplete billing information, or the inability of the responsible party to satisfy his or her obligation. Write-offs can also occur because of agency policy, administrative courtesy to a preferential customer, or administrative decision to ignore outstanding balances. An example of an agency policy would be the writing off of a patient's 20 percent copayment responsibility.

Depreciation. Depreciation expense represents the cost of buildings and fixtures, automobiles, furniture, and equipment spread over the asset's useful life. Depreciation methods differ for Medicare versus financial reporting. Medicare requires the use of the straight-line method of depreciation. Depreciation methods for financial reporting include straight-line and several accelerated methods of depreciation.

Interest. Interest expense is a cost incurred for external financing. External financing includes funding by owners, banks, and other creditors. Interest paid to owners and related parties is not reimbursable from Medicare's perspective; however, it is a requirement for financial reporting unless waived. Financing can be for working capital, mortgages, automobile and equipment leases, credit card interest, and late payments.

Revenues and Gains in Excess of Expenses. This is profit or net income. Without operational profits, an organization will be totally dependent on contributions and donations to fund its operations. Operational profits are necessary for investment in equipment, research and development, and operational shortfalls.

Statement of Retained Earnings or Fund Balance

The statement of retained earnings or fund balance will reflect the following information:

* *Beginning Balance*—The dollar value of an organization's retained earnings, or fund balance, as of the close of the previous fiscal year.
* *Net Income or Revenues and Gains in Excess of Expenses*—Represents the current fiscal year results. Profits will increase the retained earnings or fund balances.
* *Contributions*—Capital contributed during the course of the year.

- *Ending Balance*—A mathematical calculation adding net income, capital contributions, and the beginning balance.

See Exhibit 1–3.

Statement of Cash Flows

The statement of cash flow utilizes information from the income statement and the balance sheet. (See Exhibit 1–4.) This statement provides readers with another level of detail about operations, specifically about cash flow and funding activities. Cash is the second half of every transaction, and by understanding how an agency manages its financial operations, creditors and other external agencies are better able to evaluate their risk when extending credit to an organization.

There are two acceptable formats for presenting the statement of cash flows: the (1) direct and (2) indirect methods. The direct method requires no reconciling of noncash activities, such as depreciation and amortization. The direct method begins by listing all cash receipts collected from customers and interest income and then lists payments to arrive at net cash provided by operations. In contrast, the indirect method begins with net income, adjusts for noncash expenditures, and identifies the net change in current assets and liabilities in arriving at net cash provided by operations

Use of the direct method requires a reconciliation of net income to cash flows from operating activities. Thus, the direct method of reporting requires reporting in both the direct and indirect methods. Additionally, the direct method offers the reader a better understanding of how cash was used for operations and provides a better analytical format. However, the indirect method is usually the format of choice because of its ease in preparation.

The cash flow statement consists of five sections. The following is the content using the direct reporting method.

Net Cash Provided by (Used by) Operating Activities

This section contains net income from operations and adjustments to net income. Adjustments to net income include an add-back for depreciation, gain or loss in the sale of equipment, and changes in current assets and liabilities. Changes in current assets are listed in a subsection for current assets. The heading for each major current asset category begins with (Increase) or Decrease. Increases are in brackets to represent the use of an organization's cash. Conversely, when assets decrease (e.g., collection of receivables), this generates cash for the organization. For example, an increase in business will increase accounts receivable. Increases in accounts receivable use an organization's cash. If collection efforts are slow, it will require that an organization invest more money into its receivables.

Changes in current liabilities are listed below current assets. The heading for each major current liability category begins with Increase or (Decrease). Increases

Exhibit 1–4 Comparative Cash Flow Statements

Sample Home Health Agency
Statements of Cash Flow
December 31, 1995 and 1994

	1995	1994
Cash flow from operating activities and nonoperating gains		
Cash received form patients and third-party payors	$ 3,721,000	$ 2,542,000
Other receipts from operations	22,000	32,000
Cash paid to employees and suppliers	(3,683,000)	(2,540,000)
Interest paid	(11,000)	(14,000)
Nonoperating gains	37,000	27,000
Net cash provided by operating activities and nonoperating gains	86,000	47,000
Cash flows from investing activities		
Purchase of equipment	(30,000)	(19,000)
Purchase of investments	(10,000)	(15,000)
Net cash used by investing activities	(40,000)	(34,000)
Cash flows from financing activities		
Payments of long-term debt	(13,000)	
Net cash used by financing activities	(13,000)	
Net increase in cash	33,000	13,000
Cash at beginning of year	41,000	28,000
Cash at end of year	74,000	41,000
Reconciliation of revenue and gains in excess of expenses to net cash provided by operating activities and nonoperating gains		
Revenues and gains in excess of expenses	177,000	98,000
Adjustments to reconcile revenue and gains in excess of expenses to net cash provided by operating activities and nonoperating gains		
Provision for bad debts	46,000	21,000
Depreciation and amortization	26,000	20,000
Increase in accounts receivable	(322,000)	(150,000)
Increase in other receivables	(5,000)	(2,000)
Increase in accounts payable and accrued expenses	163,000	50,000
(Decrease) increase in estimated third-party receivables	(3,000)	3,000
Increase in advances from third-party payors	4,000	7,000
Net cash provided by operating activities and nonoperating gains	$ 86,000	$ 47,000

Source: Reprinted from *Audits of Providers of Health Care Services*, p. 167, with permission of the American Institute of Certified Public Accountants, © 1994.

to current liabilities indicate a source of cash and, therefore, are reflected positively. Decreases to current liabilities are reflected with brackets denoting that the decrease of current liabilities is using the organization's cash. Examples of an increase is the accruing of expenses. The expense is accrued and recognized on the financial statement but will be paid at a later date. Conversely, when the expense is paid, liabilities will decrease. In essence, this section is converting an accrual-based statement to a cash-basis statement by identifying increases and decreases in working capital for the reporting period.

Net Cash Provided by (Used by) Investing Activities

This section contains sources and uses of cash from cash contributions, purchases of equipment that were and were not debt financed, proceeds from the sale of equipment, and changes in notes receivable.

Net Cash Provided by (Used by) Financing Activities

This section identifies cash inflow and outflow from external financing activities. Included in this section are bank borrowings and repayments, bond issuances and related costs, principle payments on long-term obligations, and increases and decreases in long-term obligations.

The Statement of Financial Accounting Standards No. 117, *Financial Statements of Not-for-Profit Organizations (SFAS No. 117)* requires that

> financing activities include the receipt of donor-restricted resources that must be used for long-term purposes, contributions and investments income that are restricted by the donor for the purposes of acquiring long-lived assets or establishing or increasing a permanent or term endowment, and interest and dividends that are donor restricted for long-term purposes. Not-for-profit organizations should include information about the contribution of a building or investment in non-cash investing and financing activities.[4]

Net Change in Cash during the Period

This section is composed of three pieces. The first component is the net increase in cash and cash equivalents. This is the mathematical sum of the operational, investment, and financing cash flows. The second section is the beginning cash balance for the fiscal year or the ending cash balance from the prior year. This number is also the cash balance reported on the balance sheet for the prior year. The third section is the ending cash balance for the reporting period. This is the mathematical sum of cash and cash equivalents at the beginning of the year and the net increase in cash and cash equivalents from the current year. This is the cash balance number reported on the balance sheet.

Supplemental Disclosure of Noncash Investing and Financing Activities
This section lists all interest and income tax payments.

NOTES

1. L.A. Gioia and R.B. Steinberg, A Look at the New Financial Rules for Non-Profits, *Pennsylvania CPA Journal* (August 1994), 17.
2. Healthcare Financial Management Association Principles and Practices Board. 1991. *Charity Service-Exposure Draft*, Westchester, Illinois.
3. Ernst & Young, *Implementing the New Health Care Audit Guide* (October 1990), 8.
4. Gioia and Steinberg, A Look at the New Financial Rules for Non-Profits, 36.

Chapter 2

Collection and Maintenance of Financial Data

The preceding chapter identified some of the primary principles, concepts, and theories that go into the presentation of a home health agency's (HHA's) financial statements. This chapter looks at the transactions that produce accounting data, the steps necessary to record data, and the processes used to transform data into accounting information.

Perhaps the best way to begin is to look at a typical patient transaction cycle that would take place in an HHA. Figure 2–1 illustrates a simple episode of care. A referral is accepted, and a patient visit is scheduled. How quickly the potential patient is seen depends on the availability of staff and agency policy. The agency's policy may dictate that all patients are seen within 12 hours of receipt of referral 7 days a week including holidays.

The initial visit assesses the needs of the patient, and the visiting nurse codevelops a plan of care with the patient and physician. The plan of care will determine the type of services that the patient will receive (i.e., the frequency of visits, medical supply and equipment requirements, outcomes to be achieved on each visit, and discharge criteria). From this point, subsequent visits are scheduled and made, progress is monitored and charted, and the plan of care is updated to reflect changes from the original nursing diagnosis. Once goals have been met, the patient is discharged.

Table 2–1 illustrates the plan of care that was developed during the initial assessment. Additionally, the patient was admitted to the agency midmonth, remained on service for six weeks, had supplies delivered the first week, then was discharged at the completion of the sixth week. The first three weeks of service will fall into the month of admission, and weeks four through six will fall into the following month.

The simple admission in Table 2–1 created several accounting transactions. Revenue is created for the agency when billable services are provided. However,

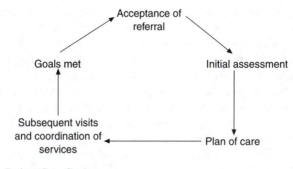

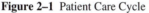

Figure 2–1 Patient Care Cycle

revenue is different by payor source, and each payor will have different payment practices and billing requirements. Concurrently, the agency incurs an obligation to pay for the services of the field employee or independent contractor who provided the services. The agency also incurs the cost of the support staff from admission through discharge of the patient, supply cost, and agency overhead.

Revenue is created every time a billable activity takes place (assumes a noncapitated or episodic payment environment). In the above example, if this patient has Medicare coverage, the agency would bill every 30 days. The first month (represented by weeks 1 through 3), the agency would bill for 8 nursing visits, 6 physical therapy visits, and 13 home health aide visits. The agency would also include charges for the medical supplies delivered to the patient's home. The second month, the agency would bill for 4 nursing visits, 1 physical therapy visit, and 5 home health aide visits. If this patient had commercial insurance, the agency could choose to use a different billing cycle, such as weekly or biweekly, to enhance cash flow instead of waiting for the month to close.

Table 2–1 Illustrative Plan of Care: On Service for 45 Days

Week	Nursing visits/week	Physical therapy visits/week	Home health aide visits/week
Week 1	3	2	5
Week 2	3	2	5
Week 3	2	2	3
Week 4	2	1	3
Week 5	1		2
Week 6	1		

Note: Majority of supplies were delivered the first week. The balance of supplies came from the registered nurse's bag. Weeks 1, 2, and 3 represent Month 1. Weeks 4, 5, and 6 represent Month 2.

The differences in billing practices can have a significant effect on an agency's cash flow. Cash flow is always a consideration for any business but especially for an HHA. An agency that is able to generate bills quickly and efficiently and get them paid in a short amount of time will be better off than an agency that is unable to bill and collect in a timely fashion. This is because an agency needs to pay the employees who performed the visits, support staff, and agency overhead. If the agency does not have sufficient cash coming in to satisfy its obligations, it will need to borrow money. Borrowing money will cause the agency to incur interest charges, thereby increasing its monthly payments.

Expenses associated with the above transaction include payroll costs for the employees who provided the visits; supply cost; and the cost of support staff employees to take care of billing, data entry, collection, scheduling, records, quality improvement, nursing supervision, and so forth. Overhead expenses would include a list of operating expenses identified in Chapter 1. Additionally, employees, suppliers, landlords, and bankers are not interested in waiting until money is collected so they can be paid.

This is the concept of working capital. Working capital enables an HHA to pay its short-term obligations, such as employees and their benefits, employer payroll taxes, vendors, landlords, suppliers, and the bank. Working capital is generated from business profits, prompt collections, owner capital contributions, donations, fundraising activities, and loans from banking institutions. It is important to understand how working capital is consumed, how patient transactions affect working capital, and how the accounting systems help to manage it. Additionally, an understanding of the accounting systems and the reports that are produced by the system will assist in the management of financial operations.

BILLING AND ACCOUNTS RECEIVABLE

Billing is the process that collects and summarizes all billable activity for an HHA. Billing is a two-part transaction. The first part is the revenue that a transaction creates. A transaction could be a unit of service such as a visit, an hour of care, the rental of a walker, or the delivery of a wound kit. The second part of the transaction is the identification of the responsible party or account receivable. As explained in Chapter 1, there is not a one-to-one correlation between revenue and accounts receivable for all payors. For instance, an agency's charge may not always equal the amount receivable for a service or transaction. This could be due to contractual arrangements made with different payors or nuances of a cost-reimbursement system.

This is one of the functions of a billing and accounts receivable system. The system is set up and maintained by the accounting group to allow for different billing rates by discipline, by type of service provided by the agency, and by payor requirements. The billing system also tracks patient demographics and clinical activity that can be used for billing and satisfaction of agency regulatory requirements. The billing system becomes a database of all the patients who were admitted, were discharged, and are currently on service with the agency. Furthermore, the database tracks statistics about those patients, such as the number of visits and hours by type, payor, referral source, employee, and discipline.

The billing system's primary purpose is to generate bills and manage accounts receivable. Without adequate cash flow, an agency will not remain financially viable. Bills can be generated manually and mailed to payors or generated electronically and sent via modem. The latter method is a way to enhance cash flow, reduce data entry errors at the payor, and increase productivity in the HHA.

Source of Billing Information

Data used in the billing process begin to be collected at the time of referral. Patient information is provided to the agency via fax or telephone. This information is entered into the billing system and the patient's chart, providing initial information prior to the assessment visit. Once the assessment is completed, additional information will be available regarding the patient. Every time there is visit activity with that patient, communications with his or her physician, or case conferences, the results will be entered into the patient's chart and the billing system.

Information is generally forwarded by the nurse, therapist, or aide for entry into the system. Entry of data into the system can depend on how the agency has set up its collection processes. For instance, an agency may choose to have its field staff come into the office and complete required paperwork when all of their field visits have been completed. Completed documentation would provide the source for entry of data into the billing system. Another agency may choose to have its nurses submit all documentation using a tape-recorded message, then have information transcribed for the patient's records. The transcription process would also trigger the entry of data into the billing system.

Agencies are now looking at giving their field staff lap-top computers that will load information directly into the billing system, thus eliminating a data entry requirement. As advances in technology become more affordable, there will be more options available to agencies for the collection of patient data.

Patient Data

There is an old saying about systems that says that garbage into the system will produce garbage from the system. This is true of the billing and accounts receivable system. Information collected or entered into the system incorrectly will create numerous problems in the collection of accounts receivable. Verification of insurance information prior to admission or immediately after the first visit is one of the key elements to a successful billing operation. Insurance information that is incorrect can cause denials, wasting time and energy correcting billing information and rebilling. Billing problems can occur as a result of transpositions when recording patient information. Additionally, it is a good practice to identify secondary and tertiary payors in the event that a service is partially paid or not covered by a primary carrier.

Patient detail goes beyond the collection of insurance information. Patient detail includes patient demographics such as name, address, social security number, age, sex, referral source, physician, and clinical information. Clinical information can include medical diagnosis, ICD-9 code, primary and secondary nursing diagnosis, difficulties with activities of daily living, and the availability of another caregiver in the house. Additional clinical information would include status at the time of admission, previous admissions, outcome identification at the time of discharge, reason for discharge, and discharge date. Understanding how clinical detail and outcomes relate to financial activity will provide agencies with an extremely powerful competitive advantage when negotiating with managed care providers.

Charge Structure

An agency's charge structure is dependent on several factors. Agencies that are licensed to provide services to the Medicare program establish their charge structure so that they do not have any back-end problems with reimbursement. The Medicare program currently reimburses at the lower of cost, limits, or charges. Therefore, it is in the agency's best interest to set its charges greater than the current Medicare limits.

Some charges, or the reimbursement methodology, will be established by the payor. The Medicaid program is different by state. Some states prospectively reimburse their providers; that is, the rate is known prior to providing the service. Other states follow the Medicare program and reimburse their providers at cost. Additionally, many states have waiver programs that have different reimbursement methodologies.

Another factor influencing charges is the marketplace. An agency must determine what the market will bear for its services. If an agency's charge structure is excessive, it may not get a great deal of business, or if it is too low, the agency may get a lot of business but not make any money. The pricing of services is often done arbitrarily; however, results of operations should be reviewed on a regular basis to understand how well the agency is doing as a result of its pricing decisions. Pricing is an art.

Managed care organizations (MCOs) and other payors are beginning to dictate what they will pay for services. Prices are determined by volume estimates, estimated service requirements of specific patient populations, and the market. Prices are often severely discounted from the agency's posted charges. MCOs typically have three types of payment vehicles: (1) per visit, (2) episodic, and (3) capitated.

The actual charge structure will depend on the type of services that an agency offers. The traditional pricing structure uses the six disciplines of (1) nursing, (2) physical therapy, (3) occupational therapy, (4) speech therapy, (5) medical social services, and (6) home health aide. Unfortunately, a singular pricing structure does not recognize the differences in the type of visit, duration of the visit, and specialty requirements. This has caused an expansion in the charge structure. For instance, a high-tech nursing visit should be priced greater than a routine nursing visit because of the additional technical expertise required; an admission visit should be priced greater than a routine visit because of an increased time element; a pediatric nursing visit should be priced differently than an intermittent adult nursing visit because of different requirements; and so forth. Agencies will also charge for services by the hour, fraction of the hour, shift, per diem, and per episode. An additional consideration is what services or supplies are included or excluded from an agency's charges.

Payor Information

Once patient charges have been entered into the system, the system will be able to match charges for services, supplies, and equipment to the predetermined reimbursement rates that have been defined for each payor. Reimbursement rates are known for all payors who the agency has a contract with and that utilize a prospective payment methodology. Reimbursement rates for cost-reimbursed providers are not known until the cost report is settled. This process could take up to two years.

During data entry, a service code is identified that matches the agency's charge to a particular service. The system identifies the patient's payor and identifies the anticipated reimbursement or receivable for that service, then calculates the contractual allowance. The contractual allowance is the difference between the charge and the anticipated reimbursement. Table 2–2 identifies the different contractual allowance computations that would occur when a nursing visit is billed to five different payors.

When an agency bills a commercial carrier, the agency could receive less than the sum of its charges. This may be due to the patient's insurance policy only paying for 80 percent of charges, and the balance is the responsibility of the patient, or the insurance company reducing the charge amount to what it deems to be reasonable and customary for that type of service. In this example, the agency will

Table 2–2 Payor Rate Schedule and Corresponding Allowance Requirements (Agency Charge for a Nursing Visit = $100)

Payors	Charge ($)	Payment ($)	Allowance ($)
Medicare	100	80	20
HMO	100	70	30
AAA	100	65	35
Medicaid	100	80	20
Commercial	100	100	0

Note: HMO = health maintenance organization; AAA = area agency on aging.

recognize an adjustment to revenue after the fact. This type of adjustment is normally considered a write-off but has the same effect as the contractual allowance did when revenue was initially recognized by reflecting the receivable at the net realizable amount.

Typical payor information that an agency will require consists of a provider number or identifier; the payor's name and address; and a service agreement that details what services will be paid by the payor, what services will be excluded, and billing requirements. It is helpful if all of an agency's managers are knowledgeable about the billing requirements by payor so that potential problems can be avoided.

Billing

Billing occurs when all the data for the current period have been accumulated, entered into the system, and reviewed. Review of preliminary billing information is useful to verify that all information is in for the current period and that the information that is in the system is consistent with care plans or other billing criteria. Once the preliminary data have been confirmed, it is possible to begin printing bills.

Some payors request bills in a specific format, such as the UB-92, or a customized format. The billing system needs the ability to handle many different billing formats and to update these formats as customer expectations or regulations change. Additionally, the system needs to be able to accommodate multiple billing cycles. A billing cycle is the length of time that activity will be held prior to submission to a payor. Medicare utilizes a 30-day billing cycle. Commercial payors can be billed on a weekly cycle.

Advances in technology have made electronic billing an option. Electronic billing will reduce the amount of time in getting the invoice out of the door and to the payor. Additionally, electronic billing has the potential to enhance payor turnaround and speed up remittances. Unfortunately, payors have cash-flow issues, too, and telephone follow-up may still be required.

Reporting

Information contained in the billing system is used for an assortment of management, financial, and cost-reporting purposes. Reports can consist of pure statistics such as the number of visits for the month, visits by discipline, or visits by discipline within a payor classification. Reports can include patient names, clinical information regarding patients currently on service, visit activity by referral source, outcomes by patient problem, and any combination of clinical and financial information. Reports can be produced in a detail or summary fashion and are dependent on the users' needs.

One of the primary purposes of the billing system is to summarize all activity for the current period for the financial records. The billing system needs to be able to summarize total visit activity by discipline, hours by discipline or service, medical supply and equipment sales, and all other forms of revenue for categorization on the financial statements. The billing system also needs to summarize total receivables by payor, contractual adjustments, and cash receipts.

Cash remittances are posted to the system to relieve an agency's receivables. Cash is posted to outstanding balances with a posting date that corresponds to the date the check was deposited. It should be a primary goal of every agency to deposit its checks the same day that they are received. Agencies generally will receive remittance advice along with a check. The remittance advice is used to identify the appropriate patients and payors to apply the cash posting. Some Medicare providers have elected to participate in the periodic interim payment (PIP) program. Providers participating in this program will receive a check every two weeks regardless of when they receive their remittance advice. Accounting considerations for PIP providers will be addressed in Chapter 3.

A billing system will also produce an aged accounts receivable. An aged accounts receivable is an extremely useful tool to evaluate an agency's collection efforts. The aged accounts receivable report can be used by internal management, by external creditors, and as a supplemental schedule for an agency's balance sheet. The primary function of this report is to identify total outstanding balances by payor classification and to age the outstanding balance. The process of aging looks at the current date or report date and determines the approximate age of the receivable. Age is calculated as the difference between the report date and the date the receivables are processed. Commonly, the period end date or the mailing date is used to represent the processing date. Once the age of the receivable is known, the system will place the amount in a column representing the average number of days the receivable has been outstanding. Aged receivables reports generally use 30-day increments for purposes of aging.

The age of a receivable signifies several things to the reader of the report. First, the older that the receivable gets, the more difficult it will be to collect. Therefore, as the likelihood of collection diminishes, accountants calculate a reserve against the probability that the account will not be collected. The amount of the reserve is increased as the age of the receivable increases.

The aged receivable report will visually represent billing problems. If there is a gap between the normal range of open claims and the oldest claim on the report, there may be other problems associated with that particular claim. For instance, the payor may never have received the claim, may have lost the claim, or may have determined that there are problems with the claim and therefore would not process it. A proactive agency will call the payor and determine what needs to happen in order to get the claim paid. Additionally, the report can signify when different follow-up steps need to be implemented by the agency, such as rebilling, telephone follow-up, or use of a collection agency.

Cash flow is integral to an agency's survival, and efforts should be made to collect monies that are due to the agency in the least amount of time possible. Collection of cash receipts enables an agency to pay its employees on time and to satisfy all of its monetary obligations.

PAYROLL

Payroll and payroll-related expenditure are the largest cost of an HHA. Payroll is the vehicle used to pay employees for their time. Employees receive different rates of pay based on their job function, education, length of service, and role within the agency. Employees can be paid per visit or hour, or by shift, or salary, or a combination. Payroll processing is complicated by varying pay rates based upon activity, weekday versus weekend, and productivity bonuses.

In Table 2–1, the patient received a total of 12 nursing visits, 7 physical therapy visits, and 18 home health aide visits. The people who performed these visits want to be paid by the agency for their services. If the nurses, therapists, and aides are employees of the HHA, then they would be paid through the payroll system. If the nurses, therapists, and aides are employees of another organization that has sub-contracted with the HHA to provide temporary staff or an independent contractor that has contracted directly with the HHA, then they would be paid through the accounts payable system. The difference between employees and independent contractors is basically one of control and goes beyond the scope of this book, but the method of payment remains the same.

Additionally, all of the support staff who made those visits possible would like to be paid for their services. This is the function of the payroll system. The payroll system records all of the source information and converts it into paychecks for all of the employees. The conversion process takes into consideration employee pay rates, taxes, and employee benefits. System output does not stop at employee checks; there are internal and external reporting requirements associated with payroll and accounting requirements.

Payroll systems require a minimum amount of information to be functional. At a minimum, the payroll system requires the employee's name, address, social security number, W-4 elections, voluntary withholding elections, and pay rate. Payroll systems become more complex when human resource considerations come into play. Human resource considerations include vacation time, sick time, personal time, leave of absence considerations, health benefit elections, and so forth. The payroll and human resources functions complement each other.

The function of payroll calculation can be accomplished internally or externally. An agency may choose to outsource its payroll requirements to a third party, so it does not have to worry about producing checks, quarterly and annual reporting requirements, and all the other headaches generally associated with payroll. However, data collection requirements will still remain the same.

Source of Payroll Information

Payroll information can be gathered in numerous ways, and it is up to each individual agency to determine the methodology that works best for it. Some agencies may require that all employees punch in at a time clock as soon as they enter the agency and punch out before they leave. Another agency may choose to have its employees initial a time sheet. Once collected, someone should approve them prior to processing.

The complexity of an agency will also determine whether time studies or continuous time records will be the source of payroll information. A complex agency may need to keep track of its employees' time by the type of job tasks or functions that they are performing. Further clarification may require that the employee identify time spent by payor, by activity, by primary or secondary business process, or between companies.

Some agencies may choose to have field staff time calculated based on information required as part of the documentation process. Information can be attached to documentation entered directly from lap-top computers or scanned into the payroll system. Employees may keep start and stop times for patient visits, travel time, documentation time, and time spent on case conferences. Additionally, time will be differentiated between time spent in the direct provision of patient services and paid time off, such as vacation, sick, or personal time.

Employee Costs

The cost of an employee is far greater than the salary or hourly rate that the employee is paid. Employees receive fringe benefits such as paid time off (PTO); health benefits; and other agency-designed benefits, such as pension contributions, deferred benefit plans, and continuing education. The payroll system is often managed in conjunction with human resources. Human resources controls all employee information from interview through termination. The human resources function complements the payroll function by designing policies and procedures that help to make clear what the agency's expectations are of the employee. Additionally, the human resources function is to maintain compliance with external rules and regulations, such as the Americans with Disabilities Act and the Family Leave Act, and monitor state unemployment and workers' compensation claims.

The components of an employee's cost consist of gross wages, benefits, and employer's taxes. Gross wages are an employee's salary, the number of hours multiplied by the employee's rate, overtime, retroactive merit increases, or bonus monies paid by the agency. Bonuses might be paid to field staff as an incentive to take on difficult cases, to increase the number of visits, or for myriad reasons. Bonuses to administrative staff may be due to an incentive system designed by the chief executive officer (CEO).

Benefits are provided to employees as an incentive to retain qualified help and to keep employees healthy. The concept of PTO is to enable the employee to have a balance between family and work life. Employers recognize that people get sick or have personal tragedies throughout the course of the year and provide a PTO benefit instead of penalizing the employee. Employers can design PTO plans with increases in the number of days based on employment category or years of service. Additionally, some employers have a probationary period before a new employee becomes eligible for PTO and other benefits.

Employers will also design health benefit plans. Some employers will pay the entire cost of health insurance for the employee only. Others will pay for employees and their families. Health insurance is an expensive benefit to offer and has forced some agencies to set a cap that they will provide toward their employees' health insurance, thus leaving their employees to contribute the balance.

Employer taxes are a large portion of employee cost. Employers are responsible for matching the social security taxes that are withheld from every employee's paycheck. Employers are also responsible for state and federal unemployment taxes. In addition, employers are responsible for workers' compensation insurance for all of their employees. The workers' compensation insurance premium is calculated on gross wages.

PAYROLL TAXES

Once gross wages have been calculated, it is possible to determine the amount of taxes that will be withheld from each employee's paycheck. Employees complete a W-4 withholding form that determines the level of federal taxes that will be withheld from an employee's paycheck. The amount of the federal withholding will fluctuate based on gross pay earnings, the employee's filing status, and the number of exemptions claimed.

Social security is also withheld from every employee's pay. Social security tax is determined as a percentage of an employee's gross earnings up to a ceiling amount. State and local taxes are also withheld from employees' wages. These taxes are determined by the local taxing authority and can be determined by a flat percentage method, a graduated scale, or a flat amount. Payroll systems need to be able to determine where gross wages were earned to calculate proper withholdings of local and state tax. This presents a particular challenge to agencies that cover wide geographic areas.

It is the responsibility of the employer to withhold taxes from employees prior to issuing them a paycheck. Withheld payroll taxes are deposited on behalf of employees by their employer. The employer is responsible for completing monthly, quarterly, and annual statements that reconcile withholdings. An employer that does not make timely deposits of payroll taxes will be fined. Serious violations could lead to imprisonment.

Other Withholdings

Employers are also responsible for the garnishment of employees' wages. Garnishment of an employee's wages is usually due to a court order seeking payment from the employee. Typical examples are the repayment of school loans, alimony, and child support. Formulas can be rather complex and are determined by comparing gross and net pay amounts.

Employees can voluntarily withhold money from their paychecks. Voluntary withholdings could be for 401K contributions, sunshine or coffee funds, United Way contributions, or numerous other actions requiring employee contributions. Voluntary withholdings and garnishments become the employer's responsibility to make sure the funds wind up in the proper place.

Cash Flow

The payroll process represents a major cash flow consideration for an HHA. Employees are usually paid on weekly or biweekly cycles. An agency will need to have sufficient cash to cover the net pay of its employees and all tax deposits that need to be made on their behalf. This is normally the single largest cash flow item that an agency will encounter. Some agencies try to coordinate payment of their employees with receipt of PIP checks. Other agencies that are not on PIP have to have sufficient funds to cover payroll.

One of the cash flow difficulties is due to the timing of collections. Average collection cycles for an HHA can run anywhere from 30 to 120 days from the end of a billing period. If an agency provides services during the month, and it takes 15 days to get an invoice out to the payor from the end of the month, then another 90 days to receive payment, in theory, the agency has paid out eight or more payrolls before collection can take place. This requires significant working capital reserves; otherwise, there will be some very unhappy employees.

Reporting Requirements

The payroll system summarizes payroll for the entire year by employee, gross pay codes, payroll tax accounts, and other withholding accounts. The system identifies payroll costs on a pay period basis and will provide accounting with summaries of total payroll activity for reporting purposes.

Financial reporting is composed of several parts. The first part is the activity that took place to arrive at total gross wages. This is a combination of hours, overtime, salary, and bonuses. More importantly, it includes HHA payroll cost identified by person. Each person can be grouped into a department by function or organizational purpose for reporting in the financial statements. Personnel groupings can depend on whether employees provide patient services or perform administrative functions. However, this does not help the agency understand how much money it is spending for different functions within the agency. Understanding what functions or jobs were performed in arriving at gross wages is commonly referred to as a *labor distribution*. Labor distribution is a management tool as well as a source of information for financial statements.

Depending on the size and complexity of an agency, one person may perform multiple tasks. As an agency grows in size and complexity, management is interested in understanding how much money is being spent for different activities and departmental functions. At a minimum, a labor distribution should classify personnel by common groupings, such as clerical, supervisors, and management. More descriptive categories would include accounting, information systems, executives, billing department, schedulers, nursing management, home health aide supervisors, and so forth. Advanced reporting systems will identify all labor costs by the type of activity that is being performed.

When the labor distribution is known, it is possible to use this report for posting to the general ledger. Posting to the general ledger would recognize the expense associated with the payroll. Posting of payroll taxes and the net amount of the payroll checks will record the agency's obligations or liabilities.

As stated earlier, an employer has responsibility for submitting withheld payroll taxes. Withheld taxes are mailed by the employer to state and local taxing authorities. Federal withholding and social security are deposited in a local bank. Taxing authorities require employers to submit a monthly, quarterly, and annual reconciliation of withheld payroll taxes. Reconciliation of withheld payroll taxes requires the employer to complete a tax form that lists total number of employees for the reporting period, gross wages, payroll taxes withheld, deposits made by the employer, and any balance due. Different forms exist for local, state, and federal taxing authorities. The payroll system should be able to summarize this information for the HHA.

Additional reporting considerations include issuance of the employee's W-2 at year-end. The W-2 is a recap of all the employee's earnings, withheld taxes, and voluntary withholdings for the calendar year. The employer is responsible for distributing W-2s to its employees by January 31. Miscellaneous information that is often required from the payroll system is for unemployment claims, pension census, and union requirements.

PURCHASING AND ACCOUNTS PAYABLE

The purchasing function is used as a method of coordinating the purchasing activities of the HHA. This function is often the task of the office manager and is handled in an informal fashion, often by placing an order over the telephone. However, as agencies grow and become more formalized, the function of purchasing could be split out to a specific individual who has responsibility for gathering competitive bids, assuring that timely deliveries are made, and managing inventory. Formalization often requires a formal purchase order to accompany all purchase requests.

The coordination of the purchasing function helps to control an agency's expenditures. Expenditures can be controlled by requiring employees to forward purchase requisitions to their supervisors prior to submission to the individual who handles purchases. Often, supervisors are required to identify what general ledger account they want to charge the expense to, determine whether the expenditure had been budgeted, and determine what type of priority is required in receiving the requisitioned item.

The office manager may hold requisitions until he or she has an opportunity to satisfy minimum order requirements or until cash flow is adequate to place the order. When orders are delivered, someone in the agency will receive the order and sign for it. The delivery driver will leave the delivery receipt or receiver with the office manager. The office manager should forward this to accounts payable along with the original purchase order or request. This represents a confirmation of delivery, and the accounts payable clerk can match the supplier's invoice to the delivery ticket when the invoice is received.

Accounts payable is the process that summarizes and pays for all vendor and supplier obligations that the HHA may have incurred. Typical transactions that will be processed by accounts payable include rent checks to the landlord, loan payments to the bank, payments for leases, payments to suppliers, payments to independent contractors, and payments to repair people. The accounts payable function differs from payroll in that payroll is a vehicle to pay employees and keep track of their earnings. Accounts payable handles all nonemployee transactions.

An agency is required to send a statement of all monies paid to unincorporated vendors, suppliers, independent contractors, repair people, and so forth at calendar year-end. This statement is a 1099.

Source of Accounts Payable Information

The primary source for accounts payable transactions is the invoice. Invoices will be submitted to an agency for obligations that it has incurred. Sometimes the accounts payable clerk will have a signed delivery slip to match to an invoice; other times, the accounts payable clerk will have to have the invoice approved. Approval is a control feature that prevents the accounts payable clerk from increasing the agency's liabilities if someone is in dispute about the amount of or reason for the invoice.

Invoices can take many different forms. An invoice could list the items that were delivered, the patients who were seen by an independent contractor or subcontracting agency, or be a telephone bill. The accounts payable clerk will often place a face sheet on the invoice to identify the general ledger account number to which the invoice will be posted, the date the invoice was received, and special handling instructions. It is a good practice to attach an adding-machine tape to the cover sheet if multiple invoices are included.

The accounts payable clerk will enter invoices into the system. Invoices can be entered individually or in batch. Once the accounts payable clerk has entered all of the invoices into the system, it is a good practice to verify that they were entered correctly. Verification of data entry can be accomplished by running a tape of all invoices entered into the system and comparing it with the system edit total prior to posting. Additionally, the controller may want to review the general ledger classifications prior to posting.

Vendor Data

An accounts payable system has the ability to track information about the different vendors, suppliers, and professionals with which the agency does business. An accounts payable system will list unpaid or open invoices, payments, and balances due. The total balance due is the agency's accounts payable liability that is reflected in the financial statements.

Vendor data include information on the vendor or supplier: name, address, telephone and fax numbers, tax identification number, and payment terms. Charges for supplies will be dependent on the arrangement that an agency is able to work out with a vendor, delivery requirements, and volume of purchases. It is possible to negotiate with most vendors, although vendor alliances are often critical to the success of the agency. Low-cost vendors may not be willing to make an emergency delivery of supplies or be understanding when the agency is short on cash and cannot pay its vendors on a timely basis.

Cash Flow

Timely payments of accounts payable is another working capital requirement of an HHA. Vendors are no different from employees: they like to be paid on time. Often, an agency is able to negotiate payment terms of 30, 45, 60, or 90 days; however, when payments stretch beyond the negotiated terms, the vendor will be less likely to make an emergency delivery or extend additional credit.

Reporting Requirements

Data that have been entered into the accounts payable system are used for financial reporting. Each invoice that has been entered has a general ledger number assigned to it. The accounts payable process summarizes all invoices entered for the period and summarizes the activity by each general ledger account. This is frequently referred to as a *distribution report*. Unpaid invoices represent a liability or obligation to the agency, and paid invoices are considered a *cash disbursement*.

The accounts payable process produces an open payables report that identifies all unpaid invoices by vendor and the total amount due by vendor. The open payables report can be aged to show the approximate number of days that the obligation remains unpaid. Invoices that are not paid within normal payment cycles could indicate that the agency is having cash flow problems.

Another reporting requirement of the accounts payable system is to produce 1099s at calendar year-end. This document is reported to the Internal Revenue Service and summarizes the total amount of money that an HHA paid to its vendors.

FIXED ASSETS

A fixed asset system is used to keep track of all of the furniture, fixtures, vehicles, and equipment that an agency may purchase. Assets are recorded in the system at the cost of the asset plus all costs that were necessary to make the asset functional, unless the asset was donated; then the cost is the fair market value at the time the asset was gifted.

Assets within the system are identified by a description, invoice date, and other costs associated with it, and placed within a grouping that combines similar types of assets. For instance, a similar grouping may be all computer equipment. Every asset is estimated to have a useful life. Medicare determines useful life of assets by the American Hospital Association (AHA) guidelines. Financial reporting groups assets according to depreciation method selected.

Depreciation Methods

Depreciation methods vary by agency, but they must be applied consistently once adopted. Depreciation methods take the acquisition cost of an asset plus the cost associated with making it functional and subtract any estimated residual value the asset may have before calculating the periodic depreciation amounts. Agencies can use accelerated depreciation methods that weight an asset's useful life toward the first couple of years, when there is less likelihood of asset problems. Medicare requires the use of straight-line depreciation for purposes of cost reporting. This method spreads the cost of an asset evenly over the useful life of the asset. An example of an accelerated depreciation method that combines accelerated depreciation and the straight-line method of depreciation is the modified accelerated cost recovery system (MACRS).

Table 2–3 and Figure 2–2 demonstrate the concept of accelerated depreciation and the useful life of an asset. A computer was purchased for $2,000 and placed into service on July 1, 1995. For purposes of book depreciation, the MACRS depreciation method was utilized, and for cost reporting, straight-line depreciation is required. Table 2–3 and Figure 2–2 illustrate the concept of accelerated depreciation. Use of an accelerated depreciation method obviously makes sense for assets that have less value the older they become. This is usually due to advances in computer technology. Unfortunately, neither depreciation method accurately reflects the rate at which computer technology is becoming outdated.

Reporting

A fixed asset system records and tracks assets in a logical order. The system will calculate depreciation by any method the agency chooses and apply it to specific classes of assets. Monthly depreciation is automatically calculated by the system for ease of entry into the financial statements. An additional report that should be produced from the system includes the asset name, location, and tag or inventory number. This enables the controller, or his or her delegate, to verify that all assets listed on the financial statements are present and accounted for.

GENERAL LEDGER

The general ledger is the repository of all financial information. Information generated by the billing and accounts receivable processes, payroll, accounts payable, and fixed assets is maintained by the general ledger. Information that has

Table 2–3 Comparative Depreciation Calculation Using MACRS and Straight-line Depreciation (Cost of a Computer Purchased 7/1/95)

Depreciation	MACRS	Straight-line
Year 1	$ 400	$ 200
Year 2	640	400
Year 3	384	400
Year 4	230	400
Year 5	230	400
Year 6	115	200
Total	$2,000	$2,000

been generated by these systems can be entered into the general ledger manually or interfaced. Manual entry would require taking the summaries and reentering totals or all of the detail into the general ledger. If the systems were able to communicate with one another, they would be able to transfer data from one location to another. Each successive step refines the raw data until they are eventually produced in the form of financial statements. (See Figure 2–3.)

The general ledger collects information using a specific account numbering system. This system is referred to as a *chart of accounts*. The chart of accounts uses ranges of numbers to signify assets, liabilities, equity or fund balances, revenues, and expense classifications. Within each of these broad ranges are subgroups of accounts. For instance, assets can have subranges of account numbers identified for cash, accounts receivable, prepaid expenses, equipment, and accumulated depreciation.

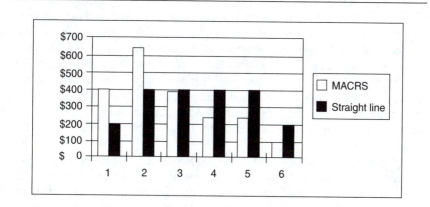

Figure 2–2 Graphical Comparison of Depreciation Methods

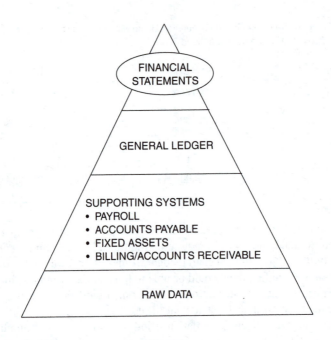

Figure 2–3 The Financial Reporting Hierarchy

The chart of account design is used consistently for all other financial applications. The reporting structure of the general ledger system should allow reports to be printed in detail or summarized depending on the users' requirements. Final output from the general ledger is the financial statements discussed in Chapter 1.

One of the primary reports produced by the general ledger system is the trial balance. The trial balance is a summary of account balances. The trial balance identifies changes in account balances for the reporting period. If the reporting period is the current month, then the trial balance will display last month's ending balances, current month's activity, and ending account balances. The ending balances from the trial balance are reflected on the balance sheet and year-to-date sections of the income statement for an HHA. Ending balances can be adjusted for reporting purposes.

Typical transactions that would be entered into the general ledger include billing, payroll, accounts payable activity, entries for depreciation, and adjustments to prepaid expenses. A prepaid expense could be a payment for an insurance policy or annual maintenance contract. The amount of the policy or maintenance contract will benefit future periods, so it is the accountant's job to reflect this as a prepaid expense and spread the benefit over the life of the insurance policy or maintenance contract. Often a monthly entry will be required to accomplish this.

Another typical entry is to accrue liabilities. An agency may have a liability for services performed but not yet paid. A common example is payroll. Payroll is paid on a weekly or biweekly basis. A payroll period may cover a specific two-week period but will not be paid for several days afterward. When payroll for the current month is paid in the following month, the accounting staff will be required to accrue the cost of the payroll. By accruing the cost of the payroll into the current month, the accountant is matching revenues of the current month with expenses of the current month even though the payroll is paid in the following month. Other accruals would include expenses that were part of the current month but not invoiced until the following month.

Entries are also required to reflect amortization of an agency's start-up costs, adjustments between current and long-term assets, calculation of bad-debt allowances, and any other transaction that has a financial bearing on the results of operation. It is important to note that accruals can be used to compensate for timing differences. For instance, an agency that has a pension program in place will probably make the pension payment in the following year. However, the pension expense is a cost of the current year. This cost can be reflected as one lump-sum entry to the agency or as monthly accruals to reflect pension liability over the course of the year. This is a preferred method, especially for PIP providers.

ACCOUNTING SYSTEMS

Manual Accounting Systems

Manual accounting systems are labor-intensive to operate and do not offer the reporting capabilities that managers require to make prudent and timely business decisions. Many start-up agencies are reluctant to invest in information systems to satisfy the clinical and financial requirements of running a home health operation. Unfortunately, this is an example of the old saying, "penny wise and pound foolish." The home health industry is labor-, regulatory-, and capital-intensive. An information system that can automate the repetitive tasks will enhance workers' productivity.

A typical manual accounting system would consist of three-by-five inch cards, a checkbook, and a ledger pad. During the month, visit activity would be recorded by patient on three-by-five inch cards. At month-end, activity would be summarized; totals would be written on the card; and an invoice or UB-92 would be completed by hand, a copy made, and the original mailed. This would be performed for the entire patient population month after month. The three-by-five inch cards would probably be stored by month, and as payments were received, cash would be recorded on a ledger sheet, and the payment listed on the patient's card. Every time a payment was received, the clerk would have to calculate the outstanding balance.

Concurrently, checks were issued to the employees who performed the visits. Payroll calculations were recorded on a ledger sheet by employee, and a check was handwritten. Invoices submitted by vendors and suppliers were filed in an expanding file folder alphabetically, and whenever there was spare cash in the checking account, someone would go through the expanding folder to determine who would be paid. This was probably accomplished by running a tape of open invoices by vendor to determine who and how much could be paid.

Often, the entire process was handled by the office manager, who had responsibility for ordering supplies, following up on receivables, responding to employee questions regarding withholding taxes and pay calculations, and negotiating with vendors and sales representatives. Reports that calculated visit activity by payor, referral source, or outcome were difficult to gather and probably not a high priority.

Year-end financial and cost reporting required assistance from either the local certified public accountant (CPA) or reimbursement consultant. Cost-reporting requirements called for accrual statements. This required the local CPA to summarize the ledgers for the entire year and then go through the boxes of three-by-five cards and determine how much money had been billed but not yet collected (accounts receivable) and determine what expenses had been incurred but not paid in the current year (accounts payable or accrued liabilities) to arrive at an accrual statement.

The cost reimbursement consultants required accrual statements to be able to complete the cost report. In addition, they needed statistics that reflected the total amount of visits that were performed by discipline, the pay source for those visits, the number of patients on service, and full-time equivalents. Furthermore, they were interested in determining the type of programs that were offered and wanted to understand some of the detail behind the financial statements that the local CPA prepared.

Automated Systems: Stand Alone

Automated systems reduced a great deal of the manual labor involved with billing, payroll, accounts payable, and general ledger functions. Repetitive tasks were automated, thereby increasing the volume of business that the office staff could manage. Automated systems also increased reporting capabilities and began to provide reports that could be used for the management of the HHA.

Automated systems require investment in a computer system. An agency will have several decisions related to automating the information-gathering processes.

Some decisions are dependent on the type of software applications that the agency requires, how much money it is willing to invest in software and hardware, and the applications that can be purchased "off the shelf."

Purchases of automated systems required an investment in computer hardware, software, training, and support. The benefits were increased flexibility with financial and management reporting and the ability to increase business volume without burning out the clerical staff.

Initial investments in computer systems were geared toward software that would satisfy the billing and accounts receivable requirements of the agency. Billing systems could be purchased for personal computers or minicomputers. Often, the accounting applications were on separate computers, and someone had to combine all the information to prepare financial statements.

Automated Systems: Integrated

The move to automated systems enhanced an agency's ability to produce invoices in a timely fashion, to manage cash more effectively, and to provide timely management reporting. However, the accounting department was still required to perform a great deal of repetitive tasks in order to produce monthly financial statements. The other phenomenon that occurred was that managers wanted more information, and they wanted it quicker. This presented a problem for the management staff because of the limitations imposed by transferring data from one system to another.

The development of integrated systems resolved this problem. An integrated system allows every component to speak to one another. This commonality allows information to be transferred from one component of the system to another by pressing a button. Integrated systems reduce processing time and increase reporting capabilities by allowing information to be merged from one section into another.

A major benefit to HHA managers is the increased analytical capabilities that an integrated system has to offer. Integrated systems will provide opportunities for combining clinical and financial data, what-if analysis, and very specific user-defined reports. These capabilities are becoming increasingly affordable and required for survival.

CONCLUSION

Chapter 2 identified several of the important supporting systems necessary to produce financial statements. These systems provide a tool for capturing enormous amounts of information about the patients who are served, the employees who provide services, and the vendors that provide services and supplies. When these data are accumulated into forms, they become information. Information is critical to the short- and long-term survival of the system, and its purpose exceeds financial reporting requirements. Information systems will become a necessary element of agency infrastructure, providing management with timely information regarding costs, quality, and outcomes.

Chapter 3

Accounting Functions

This chapter deals with some of the issues related to the compilation and review of an agency's financial statements and offers some practical suggestions for enhancing the internal reporting process. The chapter concludes with internal control concepts for protecting organizational resources.

Chapter 1 identified different types of financial statements. Financial statements are the end result or output of the accounting process. Chapter 2 reviewed some of the general processes that captured and collected information to produce financial statements. The process of compilation is the gathering of all data that pertain to the reporting period, review of processed material, and eventual presentation in a financial statement format.

Information is gathered manually or through automated processes. Once data have been gathered, they are entered into the general ledger. Some home health agencies (HHAs) will have accounting systems that interface with the general ledger; others will need to enter all transactions manually. Accounting systems that automatically interface data into the general ledger reduce the amount of time required to compile financial statements. Agencies that do not have automated systems will have to summarize transactions manually, then enter them into the general ledger. The degree of automation and the ability of the systems to interface with the general ledger package will determine the level of work required to produce financial statements.

TIMELY FINANCIAL REPORTING

A key point identified in Chapter 1 is the timeliness of financial statements. Timely financial statements assist management in making sound business decisions. Timely financial statements are the end result of the compilation and review process, which is dependent on many factors. One factor is whether accounting processes are manual or automated. Manual processes are slower and tend to be repetitious, whereas automated processes are quicker and more efficient.

Another factor that will determine compilation time is the operational issues that affect the gathering of organizational results for financial reporting. An agency that is unable to complete its monthly billing processes until 14 days after the month has ended will be unable to produce financial statements 7 days after the month has ended. Although this statement is rather obvious, it helps to underscore that there are multiple processes that affect timely financial reporting.

A third factor is accounting personnel and the prioritization of tasks. An agency that has an office manager whose responsibilities include many daily operational activities will experience greater difficulties in producing financial statements than an agency that has a dedicated accounting staff. Furthermore, accounting staff who have a multitude of activities may need to prioritize their activities to adhere to management's time schedule for the production of financial statements. One of the ways to accomplish the task of prioritization is to develop a closing schedule. A closing schedule indicates who is responsible for what activity and whether a completed activity will be an input to another activity or a completed process and directly entered into the general ledger.

THE CLOSING PROCESS

The closing process and subsequent publication of financial statements will be different for each agency. Variation will occur due to operational issues, systems limitations, and personnel issues. Utilization of a closing schedule helps to develop a timeline for anticipated completion of the financial statements. Of equal importance, it can be used as a continuous quality improvement (CQI) tool. When used as a CQI tool, one of the objectives is to increase the timeliness and, at the same time, the quality of the output. In this example, quality is the reduction of errors within the financial statements.

An example of a closing schedule could look like the following:

- Four working days after the month has ended, accounts receivable is to be closed, all bills printed, cash receipts entered, and month-end reports printed.
- Four working days after the month has ended, accounts payable is to be closed, month-end reports printed, and all invoices received for the current month accrued.
- Six working days after the month has ended, payroll reports are produced, and the month-end accrual is calculated.
- Eight working days after the month has ended, all journal entries must be entered into the general ledger and a trial balance printed.

- Ten working days after the month has ended, all balance sheet accounts have been analyzed, adjusting entries have been entered, supporting schedules have been completed, and financial statements have been produced and distributed.

A closing schedule that does not have the support of senior management will become a worthless piece of paper. In other words, the objective of the accounting department in producing financial statements within 10 working days after the month has closed must be the objective of all senior managers.

Closing Schedule Issues

In the above example, four working days had been allotted for closing of accounts receivable. This assumes that the agency has an automated billing system and that many activities are accomplished in a timeframe that allows for the completion of the billing cycle within four working days. Several of the assumptions inherent in a four-day timeline would require the agency to have an automated billing process; nursing documentation submitted within 24 hours after the visit was completed; and sufficient personnel for data entry, review, and printing of bills and reports.

If any one of the assumptions change, then the allotment of four working days will need to be expanded. For instance, if an agency subcontracts all of its therapy visits, and the provider only submits documentation every seven days, it would be impossible to adhere to the four-day closing schedule. It needs to be noted that the longer it takes to get bills out the door (i.e., completion of the billing cycle), the longer the agency will wait to be paid. Therefore, it is in the agency's best interest to require all documentation be submitted in a timely fashion and to expedite the billing process. This has caused some administrators to mandate that timely submission of paperwork become a job requirement and late submission be considered a career decision leading to the dismissal of the employee.

Closing of accounts payable in four days does not allot a great deal of time for most vendors to get their invoices submitted to the agency, approved, and recorded as a liability in the accounts payable system. Some invoices will arrive after accounts payable has been closed. These invoices can be manually accrued and therefore included in the current period. The closing process can be enhanced by identifying those vendors that are typically late and using that information to develop a month-end accrual composed of estimates. Additionally, a checklist can be developed to prevent missing estimates for the suppliers, professionals, and vendors that are typically late.

Once the accounts payable period has been closed, late invoices will be posted to the following accounting period. Adopting the practice of posting invoices to the first day of the subsequent month will enable the accounts payable person to reduce a step in the closing process, stay on top of entering data into the accounts payable system, and utilize the system to print out a summarized entry for purposes of the closing accrual.

Closing of payroll in six days after the month-end is dependent on several factors. Payroll is the largest expense that an agency will incur. An agency that is growing or utilizes independent or subcontracted field staff may experience substantial swings in weekly or biweekly payrolls. Therefore, a material misstatement of payroll expenses could occur. In this situation, an agency may choose not to estimate the last payroll expense but wait until the actual payroll expense is known.

Table 3–1 illustrates eight biweekly payroll cycles. Each payroll period begins on Friday and covers 14 days concluding on a Thursday. Payroll is paid eight days later, on the following Friday. Depending on an agency's closing schedule, payroll cost could be estimated (accrued) or recorded at actual cost. The above example illustrates several of the issues that an agency would encounter in processing its July financial statements.

Three payrolls were applicable to the month of July. One was paid in July, and two were paid in August. If an agency were to adhere to closing payroll within six working days, it would need to estimate three days' worth of payroll expense for purposes of July's financial statements. If the agency was concerned about estimating three days worth of activity, then it would need to wait until August 19 for the actual payroll results.

It is important to understand that July's payroll accrual would be for the payroll covering July 15 through 28 paid on August 5, and July 29 through 31 paid on August 19. Actual agency accounting policy dictates whether actual or estimates will be used for purposes of the financial statements.

Table 3–1 also illustrates a phenomenon with weekly and biweekly payrolls. When an agency pays employees on a biweekly period, there are two months every year that include three pay periods. The phenomenon delights employees but presents a cash flow challenge to the agency. The third payroll will not distort

Table 3–1 Schedule of Payroll Periods and Pay Dates

Payroll period	Pay date
June 17–30	Jul 8
Jul 1–14	Jul 22
Jul 15–28	Aug 5
Jul 29–Aug 11	Aug 19
Aug 12–25	Sept 2
Aug 26–Sept 8	Sept 16
Sept 9–22	Sept 30
Sept 23–Oct 6	Oct 14

accrual-based statements because the only additional expense that is reflected is payroll taxes.

Other issues related to closing schedules include the ability of staff to gather and reconcile information from external sources and write up the appropriate entries. Additionally, staff will need to perform analytical procedures, such as account reconciliation, and update supplementary schedules to support the financial statements. Some of the processes are redundant and can be automated, whereas others require manual preparation. Finally, a draft financial statement is prepared for review and closing entries.

Typical Entries

Entries will vary based on the size, complexity, and structure of the HHA. Additional variables include third-party arrangements, related party transactions, system automation, and interface of the accounting processes to the general ledger. As mentioned earlier, automated systems will reduce the amount of manual entries that will be required in the closing process. Further reduction of entries will be due to an integrated accounting system that automatically posts entries from accounts receivable, accounts payable, fixed assets, and inventory to the general ledger.

Typical month-end closing entries are listed below:

- posting of revenue and accounts receivable—gross,
- posting of contractual allowances,
- posting of cash receipts—accounts receivable,
- posting of cash receipts—miscellaneous,
- reversal of prior month payroll accrual,
- current month payroll entry (actually paid in the month),
- current month payroll accrual,
- current month payroll tax liability,
- amortization of prepaid expenses,
- amortization of intangible assets,
- depreciation,
- posting increases to accounts payable,
- posting of cash disbursements—accounts payable,
- posting of cash disbursements—manual or nonaccounts-payable, and
- posting of accrued expenses and liabilities.

The number of entries to the general ledger will be determined by an agency's accounting system, the complexity and structure of the agency. For the most part, the majority of entries are standard and will recur on a monthly basis. A way to streamline the closing process is to make up a master journal entry page for each major entry. The master page will be a completed journal entry except for the amounts. Every month, a copy will be made, and accounting personnel will enter actual amounts on the copy, thus reducing the repetitive task of writing out every account description and number each month.

Another approach is to develop the journal entry using spreadsheet software, such as LOTUS 1-2-3. This approach eliminates additional redundant tasks. Formulas can be entered to foot entries automatically to calculate cost allocation and reference date changes.

Many accounting packages have an option to handle recurring entries. This feature allows the user to enter the transaction once, then determine how many periods to which this entry will apply. The system will automatically post the entry to as many subsequent periods as the user has identified. An application for a recurring entry would include the amortization of start-up costs or any entry in which the amounts are known and consistent for multiple periods.

Reversing entries are used to reverse a prior month's accrual or estimate. Typically, reversing entries are marked with a large "R" or some other code to signify that the entry will reverse in the following month. Some agencies use different color paper to identify their reversing entries. An example of a reversing entry would be the July 15 to July 28 payroll paid on August 8. The entry would be posted to the month of July to reflect the matching of July revenue with July payroll expense. In the month of August, this entry would be reversed. The effect of reversing negates the fact that the payroll was actually paid in August. It is important to remember that the accounting staff will record the actual cash disbursement and related payroll cost in August; however, the reversing entry is an offsetting entry to the payroll cost, so none of the July payroll expense is reflected in the August financial statements.

The purpose of differentiating reversing entries from a standard entry is to signal preparers that they need to post the exact same entry to the following month in reverse format. This means that for July, the entry would debit the appropriate payroll expense accounts and credit accrued payroll. In August, the entry would debit accrued payroll and credit the appropriate payroll expense accounts. Often, accounting staff will make a copy of the original entry and place the copy in the following month's folder to remind themselves what entries need to be reversed. Most accounting software will reverse entries automatically if they are identified as reversing entries.

Appendix 3–1 has examples of several journal entries. Every agency will have different types of entries to include and exclude. For instance, a proprietary agency that is a C corporation will need to make provisions for taxes, whereas a nonprofit may need to track use of restricted funds; another agency will need to make a monthly estimate for pension liability.

Periodic Interim Payment Entries

Medicare-certified HHAs are paid by the Medicare program either on a claims-made basis or elect to be paid under the periodic interim payment (PIP) program. Accounting entries will vary dependent on whether the agency is reimbursed under claims made or PIP. The primary difference is that the PIP program accelerates cash flow to providers by issuing a flat amount every 2 weeks for 26 weeks. Checks are issued 14 days after the period ends. PIP payments will not correspond to remittance advice and, therefore, require the use of a clearing account.

The PIP clearing account is a method of reconciling payments made under the PIP program with remittance advice and outstanding receivables. When cash is received under the PIP program, cash is debited, and the PIP clearing account is credited. When remittance advice is received, the receivables are credited for their gross amount, the contractual allowance is debited for the amount corresponding to the claims processed, and the debit to the PIP clearing is debited for the net of the processed claims.

Chart of Accounts

The core of the general ledger system revolves around the chart of accounts. The chart of accounts is a listing of every general ledger account number that an agency uses. Every transaction that goes through the accounting process is assigned a general ledger number. A chart of accounts follows a fairly standard numbering practice. Ranges of numbers are assigned to assets, liabilities, fund or equity balances, revenues, patient care costs, and so forth. These numbers are then assigned to different transactions by the accounting personnel processing transactions.

A possible numbering sequence is listed below:

- 1000 to 1999, assets
- 2000 to 2999, liabilities
- 3000 to 3999, fund or equity balance
- 4000 to 4999, revenues and revenue offsets
- 5000 to 5999, direct expenses
- 6000 to 6999, indirect expenses
- 7000 to 7999, fixed expenses
- 8000 to 8999, interest and depreciation
- 9000 to 9999, nonoperating revenues

Balance sheet account numbers range from 1000 to 3999. Within the asset range, there are subcategories to differentiate current assets from long-term assets. Additionally, subranges would provide a sequence of numbers for cash, patient accounts receivables, allowances for doubtful accounts, prepaid expenses, furniture and equipment, depreciation, and so forth. The liability and equity sections would similarly use a sequence of subranges to identify various categories within their respective sections.

Numbering sequences depend on what information the agency is attempting to capture and what its internal and external reporting requirements are. The ultimate goal is to provide a mechanism to capture information in a fashion that facilitates reporting and provides the basis for a powerful analytical tool.

Profit and loss numbers range from 4000 to 9999, and determination of ranges to represent groups of numbers will depend on the ultimate use for the financial statements. One agency may be interested in using the account sequence from 6000 to 9999 to list all nondirect expenses in alphabetical order because it makes it easier to select numbers for coding accounting transactions. A second agency may choose to differentiate expenses by payor or department. A third agency may prefer to develop subranges that capture costs by cost center.

The power of the chart of accounts numbering system is enhanced by the use of prefixes and suffixes. (See Figure 3–1.) Use of prefixes and suffixes maximizes the account structure by adding extensions before and after the main number for additional classification combinations. A prefix is a numerical extension that goes in front of the main number and is used to differentiate accounts from a macro perspective. A typical prefix could be by company, location, or program. A suffix follows the main number and differentiates an account from a micro perspective. A typical prefix could be by department/discipline or payor. The ultimate power within the general ledger depends on the design of the chart of accounts and how easy it is for the agency's personnel to learn and use it. Some systems limit the users' ability to design a chart of accounts that will give the agency a mechanism to analyze its costs and make prudent business decisions. If this is the case, it would be wise for the agency to purchase a system that meets its current as well as future needs.

Additionally, agencies may need to consider additional prefixes and suffixes to capture more detail. (See Figure 3–2.) By adding prefixes and suffixes to the main account number, the organization does not limit the type of information that it can collect and increases reporting power. Agencies that have multiple locations and use a prefix classification for each location will be able to use the same general ledger structure for every location and every program that they offer.

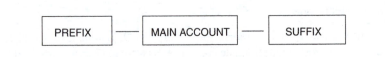

Figure 3–1 General Ledger Account Structure

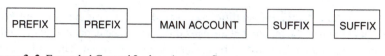

Figure 3–2 Expanded General Ledger Account Structure

THE REVIEW PROCESS

Once the initial entries have been entered into the general ledger, it is possible to begin the review process. The review process will generate several adjusting entries because of corrections, revision of estimates, missed entries, presentation purposes for generally accepted accounting principles (GAAP), or changes in the interim reimbursement rate.

Adjusting entries will also depend on the level of expertise of the accounting staff. Normally, adjusting entries are a part of the controller's or chief financial officer's (CFO's) review process, but there is no reason why a properly trained staff member cannot generate the adjusting entries prior to the review process. The review process is enhanced when accounting personnel generate supporting schedules, attach adding-machine tapes to the back of computational entries, and initial their work. Initialing of work indicates ownership and, hopefully, a sense of pride in output.

A sample of typical adjusting entries is listed below:

- entries resulting from the bank reconciliation,
- payor change,
- workers' compensation accrual,
- paid time off accrual,
- allowances for bad debt,
- reclassification of short-term versus long-term obligations, and
- reflection of current interim rate.

Bank Reconciliation

Bank reconciliations are a primary ingredient to the review of financial information prior to publication. Bank reconciliations help to determine whether all cash receipts and disbursements have been recorded on the financial statements and whether there are any miscellaneous bank charges that need to be reflected, and they keep track of all checks issued by the HHA that have not been cashed.

The process of reconciling looks at the bank's ending cash balance and compares it to the agency's cash book balance. Differences between bank and book balances are due to timing issues related to recording deposits, cashing of checks issued by the agency, and charges that have not been reflected on the agency's books. An example of a timing difference would be a deposit that was sent to the bank on the 31st of the month, but the bank did not post the deposit until the 2nd of the following month. This would represent a deposit in transit. Timing issues related to cash disbursements are referred to as *outstanding items*. Examples include checks that are written but not disbursed because of cash flow constraints, a payroll check that the recipient has not yet deposited, or a check issued and lost. The latter issue brings up the subject of void and manual checks. Void and manual checks must be handled properly; otherwise, they could distort an agency's financial statements.

It is recommended that bank reconciliations be done on a monthly basis and, if possible, prior to publishing financial statements. If the closing schedule does not allot enough time for completion of the bank reconciliation, then an adjusting entry will need to be made in the following period. Additionally, bank reconciliations need to be completed for all of an agency's bank accounts.

Table 3–2 is a bank reconciliation format. This format forces the individual who is reconciling the account to summarize cash receipts and cash disbursements. This format is useful for the reviewer to identify strange items that have cleared through the bank account. The format can also be used as a proof or review tool for the direct method of presenting the statement of cash flows. Furthermore, this format can be used as a tool for comparing forecasted cash receipts and disburse-

Table 3–2 Bank Account Reconciliation Format

	Prior month ($)	Receipts ($)	Disbursements ($)	Current month ($)
Bank balance (current month)	40,000	500,000	535,000	5,000
Deposits in transit (prior)				
Deposits in transit (current)				
Outstanding checks (prior)	(15,000)		(15,000)	
Outstanding checks (current)			20,000	20,000
Book balance (current month)	25,000	500,000	540,000	(15,000)

	Summary
Payroll paid on the 10th	$242,500
Payroll paid on the 24th	243,400
Accounts payable	54,100
	$540,000

	Summary
Transfer from depository	$500,000

ment reports to the actual ones. It is recommended that an outstanding-check list be attached to the bank reconciliation.

Payor Change

Payor changes are a fact of life in an HHA. Payor changes occur when a patient was admitted under one payor category, services have been provided and billed, then the claim is rejected because the patient is now covered under another plan. Proper review of a patient's insurance will correct this problem on the front end; however, there will always be an exception.

The exception will require removing charges from one payor and rebilling the proper payor. These changes need to be reflected on the financial statements. Good billing packages will provide a summary of all changes that have been entered into the system so that they do not become a reconciling problem for the billing and accounting staff. An example of the impact that a payor change has is shown in Table 3–3.

Table 3–3 illustrates several points. The first point is that improper verification of insurance costs the agency money. The cost is due to lost time collecting for services provided, time spent in researching the proper carrier to bill, and time spent revising and correcting entries to the billing system and accounting records. Furthermore, this is an example of a continuous quality improvement process that can be instituted by an agency. Tracking of the number of problems and the cost associated with improper front-end work will provide the initial benchmarks for an agency to surpass. A decrease in the amount of rebilling will have a positive bottom-line effect.

The second point that the illustration identifies is the decreased profit that the agency recognized for that patient. In this example, 20 nursing visits were billed to

Table 3–3 Journal Entry To Reflect Payor Change: 20 Nursing Visits Initially Billed to Commercial Carrier Now Billable to Medicaid

	Debit ($)	Credit ($)
The original entry		
Accounts receivable—commercial carrier (20 @ $95)	1,900	
Revenue—nursing		1,900
Reverse the original entry		
Revenue—nursing	1,900	
Accounts receivable—commercial carrier (20 @ $95)		1,900
The revised entry		
Accounts receivable—Medicaid (20 @ $55)	1,100	
Contractual allowance (20 @ $40)	800	
Revenue—nursing		1,900

a commercial carrier and then rebilled to Medicaid. This resulted in $800 less revenue to the agency because of a payor change.

Workers' Compensation Accrual

Workers' compensation is a cost of doing business. The annual premium for workers' compensation is estimated based on the most recent completed fiscal year payroll cost, and then when the year is completed, the workers' compensation rate is adjusted to reflect actual payroll cost. This process of retroactively billing can cause costs to be understated during a growth period and overstated during a period of decline.

One of the ways to reflect costs correctly is to develop a workers' compensation control schedule. The schedule calculates the actual liability and compares it to the annual premium, then accounting can either increase or decrease its accrual accordingly. Workers' compensation costs will vary by employee classification. Cost by employee classification will vary depending on the likelihood that an employee will be injured on the job.

Table 3–4 illustrates the concept of the workers' compensation accrual using three classes of employees. Workers' compensation rates are calculated based on $100 of payroll. The illustration assumes a rate of $1 per $100 of salaries for office workers, $5 per $100 of salaries for nurses, and $14 per $100 of salaries for aides.

In this example, the agency is enjoying significant growth over the prior year. The annual workers' compensation premium was estimated to be $30,000, or $2,500 monthly. Actual premiums for July would have been $3,450, or $950 greater than the estimate. This difference will be payable to the workers' compensation carrier after the year is ended and the audit completed.

Accruing actual workers' compensation costs and reconciling them against the estimate help an agency to reflect its proper cost of doing business, enhance reimbursement from cost-reimbursed payors, and identify the actual liability for workers' compensation expense. The illustration indicates that as of July, the agency had incurred a $3,300 workers' compensation liability.

Paid Time Off Accrual

Paid time off (PTO) is a term used for compensated time that employees can use if they are sick, are on vacation, or require personal time. PTO varies by agency, employee class, and length of service. Company policy dictates whether time can be accumulated and carried over periods.

Several issues arrive with PTO. The first issue is that PTO is a current period cost because the employee earns it in the current period even though he or she may not use the time. Another issue is that an employee's PTO may correspond to his or her anniversary year and not to the company's, thus requiring calculating the PTO accrual on an employee-specific basis.

Table 3–4 Estimation of Monthly Workers' Compensation Liability

	July salaries ($)	Rate	Liability ($)
Field nurses	30,000	0.05	1,500
Field home health aides	12,500	0.14	1,750
Office employees	20,000	0.01	200
Total	62,500		3,450

Annual premium	$30,000
Monthly premium	$2,500
Expense not recorded	$950 ($3,450 – $2,500)

	Actual	Estimate	Increase (Decrease)
January	$ 2,500	$ 2,500	$ 0
February	2,700	2,500	200
March	2,900	2,500	400
April	2,850	2,500	350
May	3,100	2,500	600
June	3,300	2,500	800
July	3,450	2,500	950
August		2,500	
September		2,500	
October		2,500	
November		2,500	
December		2,500	
Total	$20,800	$30,000	$3,300

The issue for financial reporting is recognizing PTO as an expense when earned, not when taken. This enables an organization to understand the proper cost of doing business and enhances reimbursement from cost-reimbursed payors.

Table 3–5 illustrates a simple example of the PTO liability calculation. Actual agency calculation would need to be customized to correspond to an agency's policies and procedures. Other considerations would include whether time is permitted to be carried into the next period and whether PTO follows the employee's fiscal year or the agency's fiscal year.

The cost per day calculation is derived by dividing the annual salary by the number of working days in the year. Working days was calculated by multiplying 52 weeks by 5 days per week. Liability is the result of multiplying cost per day by the number of days owed to the employee.

Allowances for Bad Debt

Bad debt is the result of services provided but never collected. Bad debt can occur for myriad reasons, including improper research of patient insurance on ac-

Table 3–5 Calculation of PTO Liability

Employee	Salary ($)	PTO days	Cost/day ($)	Earned	Used	Available	Liability ($)
Agaee, B.	17,500	15	67.31	15	6	9	605.77
Booth, W.	32,000	20	123.08	20	18	2	246.15
Fine, L.	12,000	15	46.15	15	10	5	230.77
Grimes, G.	23,000	15	88.46	15	15	0	0.00
Harrison, S.	18,900	15	72.69	15	12	3	218.08
Smith, T.	46,000	25	176.92	25	20	5	884.62
Veeche, R.	26,500	15	101.92	15	14	1	101.92
							2,287.31

ceptance of a referral, failure to determine secondary and tertiary insurance coverage, improper follow-up, improper documentation, denial of services provided, and so forth.

The allowance for bad debt is an estimate of the collectibility of an agency's receivables. The estimated allowance is directly correlated to the age of patient receivables. The older a receivable becomes, the more difficult it is to collect. One approach to estimating bad debt is the following, shown in Table 3–6. This method is arbitrary and does not take payment nuances into consideration. Additionally, depending on agency policies all receivables in excess of 150 days may get turned over to a collection agency. At that point, a reserve should be taken for the entire amount.

An approach that would have flavors of CQI in it is to develop a tickler file by payor. The tickler file would have a listing of contacts, their supervisors, telephone numbers, fax machine numbers, and all conversation with that particular carrier. Documentation should include specific nuances by carrier of what its billing requirements are, who the best person is to assist in researching a claim, and what its internal turnaround time is from receipt of a claim.

Table 3–6 Bad-debt Estimation Using Days Outstanding

Days	Amount to reserve (%)
0 to 90	0
91 to 150	25
151 to 210	50
211 to 270	75
271 and beyond	100

For instance, if a payor is holding claims for 60 days before releasing payment, initial follow-up should not be done until 60 days have passed. Additionally, by identifying carrier nuances, the reserve calculation can be structured based on carrier history and not arbitrarily assigned to the total of all outstanding claims.

Reclassification of Obligations from Short Term to Long Term

GAAP require that obligations be differentiated between short term and long term. Short term is the amount of the principal obligation that is expected to be paid within the next year. Often, an adjusting entry is required to adjust the short-term obligation balance. This is due to payments having disproportionate shares of interest and principal.

Table 3–7 illustrates an amortization schedule for the purchase of equipment. The equipment, which cost $15,000, will be leased for three years, and the interest rate is 8.5 percent. The principal amount would be summarized for the first 12 periods, June 1993 through May 1994, and this would represent the current obligation. The balance would be the long-term obligation.

Every time a payment was made, an adjusting entry would be required to transfer the next sequential principal payment out of long term and into short term. Interest would be recognized as payments are made.

Reflect Current Interim Rate

The rate Medicare pays for a visit is referred to as the *interim rate*. The interim rate is an average of total allowable costs divided by the total number of visits. There is no distinction between visit discipline and payment for medical supplies included in the interim rate.

The interim rate will change because of fluctuations in the volume of visits, changes in total cost, and changes in the discipline mix. The interim rate will also fall as volume increases. This concept will be explained in Chapter 4.

Increases or decreases to an agency's interim rate will have a financial impact to the agency. Therefore, it is prudent to calculate the changes in the interim rate to reflect properly the financial position of the agency. Calculation of changes in an agency's interim rate and analysis of cash receipts in relation to allowable costs will provide advance notification of potential overpayment problems or indicate that it may be time to request that the fiscal intermediary increase the interim payment to the agency rather than waiting until settlement of the cost report.

ACCOUNT ANALYSIS

Account analysis is a basic requirement of financial statement preparation. Account analysis helps to uncover potential problems, but of equal importance, it

Table 3–7 Equipment Lease Amortization Schedule

Date	Period	Principal ($)	Interest ($)	Extra principal	Balance ($)
	0				15,000.00
Jun 93	1	367.26	106.25		14,632.74
Jul 93	2	369.86	103.65		14,262.88
Aug 93	3	372.48	101.03		13,890.40
Sep 93	4	375.12	98.39		13,515.28
Oct 93	5	377.78	95.73		13,137.50
Nov 93	6	380.46	93.06		12,757.04
Dec 93	7	383.15	90.36		12,373.89
Jan 94	8	385.86	87.65		11,988.03
Feb 94	9	388.60	84.92		11,599.43
Mar 94	10	391.35	82.16		11,208.08
Apr 94	11	394.12	79.39		10,813.96
May 94	12	396.91	76.60		10,417.05
Jun 94	13	399.73	73.79		10,017.32
Jul 94	14	402.56	70.96		9,614.76
Aug 94	15	405.41	68.10		9,209.35
Sep 94	16	408.28	65.23		8,801.07
Oct 94	17	411.17	62.34		8,389.90
Nov 94	18	414.08	59.43		7,975.82
Dec 94	19	417.02	56.50		7,558.80
Jan 95	20	419.97	53.54		7,138.83
Feb 95	21	422.95	50.57		6,715.88
Mar 95	22	425.94	47.57		6,289.94
Apr 95	23	428.96	44.55		5,860.98
May 95	24	432.00	41.52		5,428.98
Jun 95	25	435.06	38.46		4,993.92
Jul 95	26	438.14	35.37		4,555.78
Aug 95	27	441.24	32.27		4,114.54
Sep 95	28	444.37	29.14		3,670.17
Oct 95	29	447.52	26.00		3,222.65
Nov 95	30	450.69	22.83		2,771.96
Dec 95	31	453.88	19.63		2,318.08
Jan 96	32	457.09	16.42		1,860.99
Feb 96	33	460.33	13.18		1,400.66
Mar 96	34	463.59	9.92		937.07
Apr 96	35	466.88	6.64		470.19
May 96	36	470.19	3.33		0.00
		15,000.00	2,046.48		

Note: Principal = $15,000; interest = 0.007083; term = 36; payment = $473.51.

supports the validity of the financial statements. Every balance sheet account should be supported by a subsidiary schedule, a control schedule, or some supplementary schedule supporting the account balance.

Wherever possible, account analysis should be supported with externally prepared documentation. Examples of externally prepared documentation include bank statements, copies of fixed asset invoices, contracts, lease or loan documentation, copies of interim rate changes, filed cost reports, and copies of submitted tax returns.

Often, account documentation is collected over the course of a fiscal year and stored in a three-ring binder by month. This method keeps all accounting documentation in one place and reduces the amount of work that external auditors may need to do. Hopefully, this will also reduce year-end audit fees.

Typical account analysis requirements and analytical support for the following account groups are shown below:

- Cash—bank reconciliation
- Patient accounts receivable—subsidiary schedule
- Other receivables—subsidiary or supplemental schedule, copies of notes, or contracts
- Prepaid expenses—supplemental schedule and copies of invoices
- Property, plant, and equipment—subsidiary or supplemental schedule, and copies of invoices
- Intangible assets—amortization schedule and supporting documentation
- Accounts payable—subsidiary schedule
- Accrued expenses—supplemental schedule showing estimate calculations
- Accrued payroll—payroll control schedule and filed tax returns
- Overpayments—supplementary schedule and copies of remittance advice
- Short-term obligations—amortization schedule and supporting documentation
- Long-term obligations—amortization schedule and supporting documentation

Cash

The main heading of cash can include many different accounts. Separate accounts would be identified for each operating, savings, and money market account that an agency owns. Every month, the agency will receive a bank statement from the bank or institution that is holding/investing its money. The process of reconciling bank balances to book balances will enable an agency to verify that it has properly accounted for all cash transactions that went through any of the checking, savings, or money market accounts for the month being reconciled. Copies of the bank statement and the internally prepared bank statement should be kept with the accounting records. The original bank statement should be kept with the canceled checks and filed in monthly sequence for future reference.

Patient Accounts Receivable

The main heading of patient accounts receivable includes many different payors, their respective outstanding balances, and their respective contractual allowances. A summary of the aged accounts receivable from the billing and accounts receivable system that reflects the outstanding balances by payor is an excellent subsidiary schedule for patient accounts receivable. The aged accounts receivable needs to be the same ending date as the specific balance sheet that it is supporting, and preferably the billing system will age receivables at gross and net. The gross aging will support the gross receivable balance and the net aging will confirm the contractual allowance balance by payor.

Table 3–8 is an example of an aged accounts receivable report. Differences in account balances indicate a problem between the billing and accounts receivable system and the general ledger. If the billing and accounts receivable system is manual or a stand-alone system the problem could be attributable to a change occurring and a correction being properly entered into the billing system but never entered into the general ledger. The problem could also represent a timing issue between entering transactions and running the report. These problems should be minimized with an integrated system.

The use of a subsidiary schedule allows the accounting staff to minimize the number of account numbers to set up for commercial carriers. Depending on the size of an agency, it may encounter hundreds of commercial payors. "The United States has 1,500 different third party payors, such as insurance companies and HMO's, with roughly 200 serving a given region."[1] To set up an individual account for each payor would be cumbersome. However, having one account labeled "commercial carriers" could be useful for many different small or one-time encounters with that particular payor.

Other Receivables

Other receivables is a general category for all money owed to the agency exclusive of patient receivables. If these receivables are tracked by an automated process, it is advisable to have a subsidiary schedule. If these receivables are tracked manually, the accounting staff should develop a supplemental schedule. Additionally, copies of promissory notes, contracts, or other documentation should be included as back-up.

Table 3–9 is an example of a supplemental schedule for an employee loan. The schedule identifies the loan recipient, the amount of the loan, the term of the loan, the interest rate, and when the loan is expected to be satisfied. In the example, the loan was made in March, and four payments have been made. Each payment consists of principal and interest. Interest is recognized in the month in which the payment is received.

Table 3–8 Accounts Receivable Aging

Payor	Total balance	Current	31 to 60 days	61 to 90 days	191 to 120 days	>121 days
AAA	17,082.50	11,126.50	5,826.00	130.00		
Aetna	750.00	750.00				
Alpha HMO	1,150.00		1,150.00			
BC of California	950.00				950.00	
BC of Indiana	4,250.00			4,250.00		
BC of Western	471.20	235.60				235.60
Delta	850.00			850.00		
Greater Atlantic	1,925.00		850.00	625.00	450.00	
HMO	32,985.00	20,365.00	10,520.00	1,500.00		600.00
Local 54	2,250.00		750.00	750.00	750.00	
Medicaid	20,703.00	5,826.75	6,025.75	3,450.50	3,650.00	1,750.00
Medicare	319,225.00	165,236.00	125,452.00	24,892.00	3,515.00	130.00
State Farm	8,870.00		5,620.00		3,250.00	
Prudential	1,000.00			235.00	765.00	
Wisconsin Life	15,000.00					15,000.00
Total	427,461.70	203,539.85	156,193.75	36,682.50	13,330.00	17,715.60
Percentage	(100)	(47.62)	(36.54)	(8.58)	(3.12)	(4.14)

Note: AAA = area agency on aging; HMO = health maintenance organization; BC = Blue Cross.

Table 3–9 Employee Note Receivable

Employee loan to: Jane Smith	3,000.00	Loan amount
Loan amount: $3,000	106.00%	Interest factor
Total for six-month term		
Interest: 6% simple interest	3,180.00	Total due
First payment due April	6	Number of payments
	530.00	Payment amount

	Loan ($)	Payments ($)	Balance ($)
January			
February			
March	3,000		3,000
April		500	2,500
May		500	2,000
June		500	1,500
July		500	1,000
August			
September			
October			
November			
December			

Prepaid Expenses

Prepaid expenses are the result of payments made in one month, but the payment has future benefit. Accrual accounting treats these benefits as assets and amortizes the expenditure over the life of the benefit period. Typical prepaid expenses include insurance policies, maintenance contracts, prepaid rent, and support arrangements.

Table 3–10 is an example of a prepaid expense control schedule. The schedule dedicates a column to each type of prepaid expense, and the rows identify current prepaid balances, increases to the prepaid account, and total amortization for the period. The illustration indicates that the fiscal year began with $20,100 in prepaid expenses. During January, a copier maintenance contract was added. The contract had an annual fee of $275, and its monthly amortization will be $22.92 monthly. Total expenses reflected on the income statement for the month of January are $2,572.92.

Use of a prepaid expense control schedule can be enhanced by instructing accounts payable personnel as to the differences between normal expenditures and prepaid expenses. Every time an expenditure is coded to the prepaid expense category, a copy of the invoice should be forwarded to the individual responsible for maintaining the prepaid control schedule. This not only provides back-up for the control schedule but also helps in determining the proper amortization. Addition-

Table 3–10 Prepaid Expense Schedule

	Workers' compensation ($)	Copier maintenance ($)	Quarterly rental ($)	Software maintenance ($)	Total ($)
January	20,000.00		100.00		20,100.00
Increase		275.00			275.00
Decrease	2,500.00	22.92	50.00		2,572.92
February	17,500.00	252.08	50.00		17,802.08
Increase				2,400.00	2,400.00
Decrease	2,500.00	22.92	50.00	200.00	2,772.92
March	15,000.00	229.16	0.00	2,200.00	17,429.16
Increase		150.00			150.00
Decrease	2,500.00	22.92	50.00	200.00	2,772.92
April	12,500.00	206.24	100.00	2,000.00	14,806.24
Increase					0.00
Decrease	2,500.00	22.92	50.00	200.00	2,772.92
May	10,000.00	183.32	50.00	1,800.00	12,033.32
Increase					0.00
Decrease	2,500.00	22.92	50.00	200.00	2,772.92
June	7,500.00	160.40	0.00	1,600.00	9,260.40

ally, inclusion of the coverage period in the column headings enhances the review process.

Property, Plant, and Equipment

Furniture, vehicles, improvements, and equipment are an agency's fixed assets. Fixed assets consist of furniture and equipment purchased for employees to conduct business. Fixed assets can include buildings and improvements to the buildings. When assets are purchased, they are capitalized and then depreciated over their useful lives. The useful life of an asset for purposes of Medicare follows American Hospital Association (AHA) guidelines. An agency's capitalization policy will determine the threshold for capitalization. Often, assets with a value of less than $500 will not be capitalized. These assets are normally classified as minor asset expenditures.

A fixed asset control schedule will list all assets purchased by an agency; the cost of the asset, including set-up expense; the acquisition date; the location of the asset; the asset's life; the asset's serial number, if available; and depreciation method. Assets are generally categorized by common grouping (e.g., all furniture in one section and all equipment in a subsequent section). Additionally, it is a good practice to identify each asset with an internal identification number for physical inventory purposes and for proper identification at the time of disposal.

Table 3–11 illustrates a fixed-asset control schedule. The control schedule identifies the amount of depreciation that has been taken since acquiring the asset. The schedule also identifies monthly depreciation on a monthly basis. The fixed asset control schedule is used to track assets, to provide the basis for the monthly depreciation entry by fixed-asset group, and to verify that the assets and accumulated depreciation on the books agree with the control schedule.

Intangible Assets

Intangible assets such as start-up cost, goodwill, and covenants not to compete are amortized over the life of the asset. Table 3–12 illustrates a simple amortization schedule for start-up costs. Start-up costs were $5,300 and are amortized over 5 years. On a monthly basis, the agency would recognize $88.33 in amortization expense. The amortization schedule enables the reviewer to verify that the accumulated amortization is correct on the financial statements.

Accounts Payable

Back-up for the accounts payable balance could be an open payables listing from the account payable system that has the same period end date as the account analysis period. Another alternative would be an aged accounts payable listing. Both reports should list, at a minimum, the vendor's name, the date of the liability, and the amount of the liability. Additional information would include a system-calculated age of the outstanding item, invoice numbers, description of invoice content, vendor terms, and discount availability.

If an agency utilizes a large number of independent contractors and subcontracted staff, the agency may want to consider separating fees from accounts payable items. Separation of fees provides the reader with a more realistic understanding of the organizational complexity involved with an agency.

Accrued Expenses

Accruing of expenses enables an agency to reflect correct period cost even though cash has not actually been disbursed. The review process tracks increases and decreases to the accrued expense classification. Accrued expenses can be an assortment of expenses all requiring separate account numbers or one category called accrued expense with a supplemental schedule that identifies the components that comprise the aggregate balance.

Table 3–13 is an example of a supplemental schedule used for analyzing the accrued expense account balance. In this example, pension was accrued during the previous year and will be remitted at the end of March of the following year. This

Table 3–11 Fixed Asset Control Schedule

Asset	Acquisition date	Cost ($)	Depreciation method	Life	Year-end accumulated depreciation	January expenses	January accumulated depreciation
Furniture							
Desk (24)	March 92	10,000.00	Straight line	20	1,416.67	41.67	1,458.34
Chairs (35)	March 92	5,000.00	Straight line	15	944.44	27.78	972.22
Printer stand	March 92	155.00	Straight line	15	29.28	0.86	30.14
Total		15,155.00			2,390.39	70.31	2,460.70
Equipment							
Copy machine	March 92	859.00	Straight line	5	486.77	14.32	501.09
Computers (5)	March 92	9,000.00	Straight line	5	5,100.00	150.00	5,250.00
Printers (3)	March 92	1063.00	Straight line	5	602.37	17.72	620.09
Laser printer	January 94	753.33	Straight line	5		12.56	12.56
Total		11,675.33			6,189.14	194.60	6,383.74
Grand total		26,830.33			8,579.53	264.91	8,844.44

Table 3–12 Start-up Cost: Amortization Schedule (Total Start-up Cost = $5,300)

	Start-up cost
Beginning balance	3,356.74
January expense	88.33
Balance	3,268.41
February expense	88.33
Balance	3,180.08
March expense	88.33
Balance	3,091.75
April expense	88.33
Balance	3,003.42

is also true for the annual audit costs. Notice that the current-year accrual estimates a monthly expense, thereby spreading the cost over the entire year instead of recognizing it in the period paid.

Table 3–13 Accrued Expense Schedule

	Pension ($)	Year-end audit ($)	Joint Commission on Accreditation of Healthcare Organizations ($)	Miscellaneous ($)	Total ($)
January	25,000.00	15,000.00	0.00	0.00	40,000.00
Increase	2,083.33	1,250.00			3,333.33
Decrease					0.00
February	27,083.33	16,250.00	0.00	0.00	43,333.33
Increase	2,083.33	1,250.00	1,000.00	500.00	4,833.33
Decrease		(15,000.00)			(15,000.00)
March	29,166.66	2,500.00	1,000.00	500.00	33,166.66
Increase	2,083.33	1,250.00	1,000.00		4,333.33
Decrease	(25,000.00)			(500.00)	−25,500.00
April	6,249.99	3,750.00	2,000.00	0.00	11,999.99
Increase	2,083.33	1,250.00	1,000.00		4,333.33
Decrease					0.00
May	8,333.32	5,000.00	3,000.00	0.00	16,333.32
Increase	2,083.33	1,250.00	1,000.00		4,333.33
Decrease					0.00
June	10,416.65	6,250.00	4,000.00	0.00	20,666.65

Often, expenses will be accrued because of an event that will happen at a later point in the year. In this example, the agency is anticipating a large bill from the Joint Commission on Accreditation of Healthcare Organizations for completing the certification process later in the year. When the bill is finally paid, the accrued balance would be zeroed out. Additionally, the accruing of expenses may be necessary on a monthly basis due to timing issues.

Accrued Payroll

Payroll is the largest expense of an agency. Payroll cost is the gross wages paid to employees, fringe benefits, employer's payroll taxes, unemployment taxes, and workers' compensation. Development of a payroll control schedule enhances the review process and provides a mechanism to identify potential problems. The schedule identifies payroll by pay period and pay date. Columns are set up for each type of payroll category that an agency has and for each withholding by type. Gross payroll and withholding taxes are entered into each respective column. The schedule summarizes gross pay and net pay. Totals should be compared to system reports, third-party payroll reports, or internally prepared totals.

A separate column is for the actual cash amount of the payroll. Cash can differ from net payroll because of manual or void checks entered through the payroll system. The difference would be the amount of the manual or void checks.

The columns representing gross payroll will be debits to the financial statement, and the withholdings will be credits to the balance sheet. When one reviews the payroll tax liability accounts, the payroll control schedule is helpful to determine whether entries have been posted to the proper account and tax payments made on a timely basis.

The payroll control schedule is summarized on a quarterly basis. This assists in reconciling total gross payroll for financial reporting purposes to gross payroll for quarterly tax reporting. Additionally, federal tax deposit amounts are identified by period, unemployment taxable wages, and unemployment liabilities. Copies of tax returns should be kept with the control schedule. Often, it is helpful to identify the check number of all remittances and the remittance date.

Furthermore, the payroll control schedule can be used for monitoring workers' compensation liability. Workers' compensation is calculated on gross payroll and is a natural addition to this schedule. Additionally, the control schedule can be increased to include as many gross pay columns, withholding columns, and other calculations that an agency may need.

Overpayments

Overpayments are monies incorrectly paid to an agency. A check will be received and deposited, but the overpayment will not be noticed until cash receipts are being applied. Overpayments represent a liability to the agency and should be returned. Medicare requires a quarterly statement be submitted that says that no overpayments have been received.

If overpayments are received and are not refunded to a subsequent period, it is helpful to track the payor, patient name, patient number, and amount of the over-payment as back-up for the liability. When money has been disbursed, it is helpful to keep track of the check date and number.

Short- and Long-Term Obligations

Support for short- and long-term obligations can be accomplished by develop-ing an amortization schedule for each obligation. Account back-up would include supporting documentation, an amortization schedule, and a summary schedule if multiple obligations are run through the same accounts. The amortization, or sum-mary, schedule is used to determine what portion of the obligation should be clas-sified as current versus long term. Additionally, the control schedule can be used to substantiate general ledger balances.

Profit and Loss Analysis and Supporting Documentation

Supporting schedules are a helpful way of explaining income statement results. Net income is the direct result of the mix of services provided, the payor mix, costs of providing services, and overhead. Any change in any of those variables will have an effect on the agency's bottom line. Often, displaying changes graphically enhances the reader's understanding of variable relationships.

Reports of this type include

* breakout of activity by visits and hours,
* visits and hours by payor, and
* visits and hours by referral source.

Additional considerations for profit and loss analysis and reporting is to make sure that expenses such as officers' life insurance, entertainment, meals, deprecia-tion, amortization, interest, and advertising are separated appropriately. These ac-counts have different reporting requirements for internal financial reporting, Medicare reporting, and tax reporting.

INTERNAL CONTROL

Internal control is a pervasive concept that requires the participation of all em-ployees within an organization and is no longer the domain of the accounting staff. The accounting staff may help to set up financial controls to protect assets. Inter-nal control considers all processes, both internal and external, that could positively or negatively affect an agency's mission and is the responsibility of multiple cross-functional levels of an agency. Internal control identifies critical success factors to monitor how well programs and product lines are doing and provides a foundation for CQI and risk management.

The concept of internal control has specific relevance to an agency's financial statements. Financial statements are the result of external situations, such as reimbursement mechanisms, and internal processes, procedures, and inputs that shape the final report card known as financial statements. Of equal importance, internal control is made of the internal procedures and processes that shape the organism or entity. Shaping occurs through the monitoring and management of change. Additionally, without clear and open communication channels and a sound operational and ethical base, the organism will never grow to its full potential.

> Internal control is not one event or circumstance, but a series of actions that permeate an entity's activities. These actions are pervasive, and are inherent in the way management runs the business. A business can be viewed as a system comprising two sets of processes:
> - The first, often termed the value chain, is directly related to an entity's fundamental purposes, consisting of activities such as inbound, operations, marketing and sales and services processes.
> - The second, support functions, includes activities such as administration, human resources, technology and procurement processes.
>
> Each of these business processes, which are conducted within or across organization units or functions, is managed through the basic management processes of planning, executing and monitoring. Internal control is integrated with these business processes and is a part of the management processes that causes them to function and monitors both their conduct and continued relevancy.
>
> This conceptualization of internal control is very different from the perspective of some observers who view internal control as something added on to an entity's operational activities and exists for fundamental business reasons. It is "built in," rather than "built on," and is part of an entity's infrastructure.
>
> This reality has important cost implications. Most enterprises are faced with a highly competitive marketplace and a need to contain costs. Adding new procedures separate from existing ones adds costs. By focusing on existing operations and their contribution to effective internal control, an enterprise can avoid unnecessary additional procedures and, perhaps, reduce costs.[2]

Figure 3–3 illustrates an internal control model consisting of nine components.

> Integrity, ethical values and competence, together with factors comprising the control environment, provide an atmosphere in which people

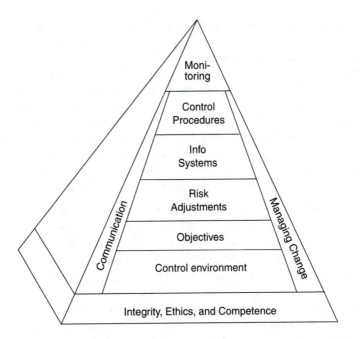

Figure 3–3 Internal Control Model. Reprinted with permission by Coopers & Lybrand.

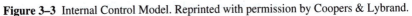

conduct their activities and carry out their responsibilities. These two components serve as the foundation for the other components. Within this environment, management establishes objectives and related strategies, assesses risks to their systems and control procedures to address those risks. Communication systems facilitate the flow of pertinent information throughout the organization and procedures exist for managing the changes the entity faces. The entirety of the process is monitored and modifications made as conditions warrant.[3]

Integrity, Ethical Values, and Competence

This is one of the base elements of the internal control model. This speaks about the agency's employees, especially senior management. "Certain organizational factors can influence integrity and ethical behavior. Ethical values and moral guidance should be communicated throughout the organization, by word and deed. A formal or informal code of corporate conduct—and the way that management lives with and enforces it—communicates an entity's expectations about duty and integrity to employees, suppliers and customers."[4]

The work environment is no different from an extension of the family. When a younger child observes the older child not paying attention to the rules, then it is alright for the younger child to disobey the rules. Truth telling, honesty, and consistency help to build a child's value system. This is no different in the workplace. Employees who observe managers bending the rules for themselves or others figure the same set of circumstances should apply to them. Managers who lie, ignore regulatory compliance, do not practice what they preach, or distort information send signals to their internal and external customers that there is an integrity problem within the system.

The concept of integrity and ethical values is set at the top with the board of directors. Each subsequent layer of staff should want and will be willing to do the right thing if examples are provided by senior management. Additionally, values will be affected by the type of people hired, incentive plans, the agency's mission, and how well management lives that mission.

Control Environment

"The control environment, together with integrity, ethical values and competence sets the 'tone at the top' of an organization. Control environment factors include the board of directors, management's philosophy and operating style, organizational structure, assignment of authority and responsibility, and human resource policy and procedures."[5]

Each agency will have a different type of control environment. One agency will have one office with a centralized management team, another agency will have multiple branch offices with decentralized support services, and a third agency will share resources with a sister organization. Assuming that the organizational design is appropriate to obtain the agency's organizational objectives, the next questions are at what level are decisions being made, are they consistent with policies and procedures, and are the individuals who are making the decisions authorized and accountable.

The control environment attempts to ensure that decisions are made within policy and procedure guidelines and that the individuals making those decisions are technically competent to make sound business decisions. Agencies that attempt to empower employees and push decision making down to their lowest level will have different internal control requirements from an agency that continues to require all decisions be made at the top. Success is dependent on employee competence and the agency's training programs. Additionally, if mistakes or problems do occur, they should be used as educational tools to prevent future problems.

Objectives

"By setting objectives and subobjectives, an entity can identify critical success factors, the key things that must go right if goals are to be attained. These critical success factors are for the entity, a business unit, a function, a department, or an individual. This framework enables management to identify measurement criteria for performance, with focus on critical success factors."[6]

Critical success factors could include

- maintenance of a specific payor mix;
- maintenance of a specific case mix;
- maintenance of a specific number of patients on service;
- the amount of time between acceptance of a referral and the first visit;
- the achievement of a specific outcome, within a certain amount of days, for a specific homogeneous group;
- the average age of accounts receivable not exceeding 75 days;
- financial statements distributed within six working days of the close of the month; and
- billing errors and denials less than 0.5 percent of total volume.

Development of critical success factors is a necessary ingredient to monitoring the strategic, operational, financial, and regulatory issues of an agency. Critical success factors can be developed at the entity level, the branch level, department level, or employee level. Deviations from the benchmarks may be due to positive or negative events and the passage of time. It is up to the management staff to determine if corrective action is required.

Risk Assessment

Every business has risk associated with it. Home health is no exception. Agency risk can be caused by external events, such as adverse weather conditions, decisions of union staff to strike, the ability to receive financing for business growth or working capital, loss of a referral source, loss of a major contract, and a changing reimbursement environment. Agencies also face internal risk, such as employee dishonesty, malpractice issues, information system failure, fire, employee turnover, and many other potential sources.

Agencies should do a comprehensive risk analysis.

> Risk analysis is not a theoretical exercise. It is often critical to the entity's success. It is most effective when it includes identification of all key business processes where potential exposures of some consequences exist. It might involve process analysis, such as identification of key dependencies and significant control nodes and establishing clear responsibility and accountability. Effective process analysis directs special attention to cross-organizational dependencies, identifying: where data originates, where it is stored, how it is converted to useful informa-

tion and who uses the information. Large organizations usually need to be particularly vigilant in addressing intracompany and intercompany transactions and key dependencies. These processes can be positively affected by quality programs with a "buy-in" by employees to achieve stated objectives. This can be an important element in risk containment.[7]

Risks should be reviewed on a regular basis to look at the current and future business environment. For instance, a decision to enter into a capitated contract will expose an agency to many different types of risk. If staff members are brought together to review potential areas of risk, then they will be able to understand what needs to be done, what critical success factors are necessary, and who is responsible for what areas. Additionally, these findings should be reviewed on a regular basis.

Information Systems

The original systems in home health were developed for data processing. These systems focused on getting bills out the door. This type of data processing system is being replaced by the information system. Information systems need to capture clinical and financial data. Relationships need to be developed between these data so the agency can use the data for the measurement of outcomes, assessment of intervention mix, and determination of pricing for negotiation purposes.

This shift will turn the information system into a competitive asset for an agency. Therefore, it is important that the asset is protected from harmful actions. Harmful actions can be deliberate or accidental, and appropriate safeguards need to be instituted to protect the asset from competitors, disgruntled employees, down-time, power surges, incorrect purging of data, and access to confidential records and information by unauthorized personnel. Safeguards need to include multilevel password protection and obsolescence.

Internal control assessments include determining whether the information system is being used to its maximum potential. Questions raised by this type of assessment would include the following:

- Are the staff properly trained in the retrieval of information?
- Can information be extracted when desired and in the format desired?
- Does retrieval require the use of a programmer?
- What is the processing speed?
- Can reports be customized for ad hoc reporting purposes?

Additionally, as informational needs change, can the system be adapted to handle the changing requirements of the agency, or will the agency be at a competitive disadvantage?

Control Procedures

"Control procedures include actions taken within an entity to ensure adherence to the policies and procedures established to address risks affecting achievement of the entities' objectives. Control procedures fall into one or more categories: operations, financial reporting, and compliance. They may include actions as diverse as checking or verifying that specific required actions took place properly over time, and securing facilities or segregating certain duties to prevent unauthorized or otherwise improper or erroneous actions from occurring."[8]

Control procedures are at many levels within the agency. The chief executive officer (CEO) and board of directors perform a top-level review of the results of the agency. They will look at the results of the agency in relationship to changes in the community, review results of strategic directions currently in process, and suggest alternative courses of direction.

The next lower level of review is the director level. This level may have responsibility for specific product lines; branch operations; programs; departments; or activities such as finance, operations, and information systems. The review requirements and controls implemented at this level prevent problems from being passed upstream. This level is concerned with contract compliance, regulatory compliance, and strategic and operational variances. Additionally, the players at this level need to be fully informed as to potential opportunities that can be exploited and determine what steps need to be taken to realize those opportunities. Conversely, problems can be corrected as well. Problem correction will occur by working with the respective staffs to understand whether problems are the result of external or internal situations. According to W. Edwards Deming, 85 percent of an organization's internal problems are due to the systems and processes developed by management; the other 15 percent are due to employees.

Both the CEO and director levels will utilize performance indicators or critical success factors to review the results of operation. Indicators can include ratios or relationships such as financial ratios, the number of patients assigned to a team or case manager, the number of visits per employee, gross profit by product line or payor, payor mix, visit mix, or myriad other indicators. The purpose of these indicators is to provide management with a tool that can give it quick notice of unusual trends or circumstances that warrant further research. Every indicator will have an indirect or direct relationship to the financial statements.

The next lower level is the transaction level. This level includes financial controls over assets, physical controls, information processing, and policies and procedures. Financial controls rely heavily on the processes of authorization, approval, and separation of duties. The purpose of authorization is to prevent incurring of obligations and disbursing of assets by personnel who do not have that specific responsibility. The process of approval is the acknowledgment that a disbursement or obligation is appropriate and, therefore, the agency's responsibility.

The concept behind separation of duties is to separate the function of custody of assets from the disposal of assets, from billing and posting cash, and from posting invoices and issuing checks. Separation of duties may not be 100 percent feasible in small agencies, but, wherever possible, it is advisable. If separation of duties is enforced, then the only way that fraud and embezzlement can occur is when two people work together. This is known as collusion.

Physical controls include a physical inventory count to match inventory items on hand to those in the books and records. Other physical controls include making sure an organization's cash and assets are kept in a safe place, reconciled, and protected from unauthorized access.

Information processing controls include system checks for required and accurate information, data or edit checks, and control totals to be included when entering information into the system. Other information system controls include multilevels of passwords to prevent unauthorized access, prevention of automatic data purging, back-up procedures, and internal system documentation that records who has accessed the system and what files were accessed. Additionally, information system controls are further defined to separate software, hardware, access controls, and electronic data interchange.

Policies and procedures provide the base guideline for an agency's control environment. Policies and procedures cover the functions of accounting, human resources, clinical operations, and financial operations. Policies and procedures should be reviewed on a regular basis, used as a training tool, and updated to reflect changes in organizational policies. Additionally, all employees should be well versed in the agency's policies and procedures, and supervisors should be asked to contribute so that the policies and procedures are owned by everyone.

Communication

"Effective communication must occur down, across, and up the organization. All personnel must receive a clear message from top management that control responsibilities must be taken seriously. Each individual must understand his or her role in the internal control system, as well as how individual activities relate to the work of others. They also need a means of communicating significant information upstream. Additionally, there needs to be effective communication with external parties—customers, suppliers, regulators, shareholders, and others."[9]

Communication is paramount in a dynamic environment. Managers must listen to employees when they bring their problems, concerns, or questions to their superiors. If managers do not listen and act on what employees are saying, then employees will not want to share their ideas. Additionally, management needs to move away from the concept of blame and judgment, to correction of the problem for the greater good of the organization.

Managing Change

> Conditions external to and within an entity will continue to change, and mechanisms need to be in place to identify and effectively deal with the changes. Circumstances that demand special attention include changes in regulatory or economic environments, new personnel in key positions, new or revamped information systems, rapid growth, new technology, new lines or products or activities, and restructurings. To the extent practical, control mechanisms should be forward looking, so that the impact of important changes can be anticipated and relevant actions taken.[10]

Home health managers need to consider how changes will affect their operations. What new risks will they encounter as a result of managed care and increased competition? Will their information systems meet their current and strategic needs? Are the financial and operational controls that are in place sufficient for the new environment? Are the staff apprised of the requirements necessary to succeed? Forgetting to address any of the above issues could have a negative impact on the financial viability of an agency, so, therefore, control mechanisms have to be forward-looking. Of equal importance, once trends or changes are identified, will the agency be willing to make the changes necessary, or will the agency ignore the problem, hoping that it goes away?

Monitoring

Monitoring of internal controls is ongoing. In reality, the controls get built into the system and enhanced as part of an agency's CQI processes. It is important to remember that controls are only as good as the personnel who have implemented them. Additionally, if the controls are ignored, then they are worthless.

Furthermore, controls are a mechanism to enhance the overall viability of an agency. Evaluation of internal benchmarks, critical success factors, and ratios against industry standards can help administrators determine how well they are doing in comparison to their competitors. However, by combining the internal control processes with system enhancement and CQI measures, there will always be room for improvement.

The goal of integrating internal controls into the agency's infrastructure is to build valuable processes that will help an agency accomplish its mission, remain financially viable, and be forward thinking in its processes. Hopefully, the end result will allow agencies to continue to provide high-quality services, remain fiscally responsible, and be operationally successful in a very dynamic marketplace.

CONCLUSION

Financial reporting must be based on a sound set of facts and figures. The examples outlined identified several integral tools necessary to support the financial reports of an agency. Typically, these tools are used in conjunction with management efforts to address internal control within the agency. The changing structure of today's organization requires that the responsibility for internal control be expanded beyond the domain of the finance department. Responsibility needs to be known and practiced by all members of management and the board. Otherwise, customers, both internal and external, will lose faith in management credibility. If this should happen, the organization's mission may be seriously threatened.

NOTES

1. E.O. Teisberg, et al. Making Competition in Health Care Work, *Harvard Business Review* (July–August 1994): 131–41.
2. Coopers & Lybrand, *Internal Control—Integrated Framework*, Exposure Draft. (New York, NY: March 12, 1991), 53.
3. Coopers & Lybrand, *Internal Control—Integrated Framework*, 58.
4. Coopers & Lybrand, *Internal Control—Integrated Framework*, 59.
5. Coopers & Lybrand, *Internal Control—Integrated Framework*, 69.
6. Coopers & Lybrand, *Internal Control—Integrated Framework*, 79.
7. Coopers & Lybrand, *Internal Control—Integrated Framework*, 95.
8. Coopers & Lybrand, *Internal Control—Integrated Framework*, 111.
9. Coopers & Lybrand, *Internal Control—Integrated Framework*, 123.
10. Coopers & Lybrand, *Internal Control—Integrated Framework*, 129.

Appendix 3–1

Sample Journal Entries

Journal Entry 1: Revenue Recognition
Any Home Health Agency
July 19XX

Description	Account #	Debit ($)	Credit ($)
A/R—Medicare		194,850.00	
A/R—HMO		40,750.00	
A/R—Medicaid		5,500.00	
A/R—Commercial		18,575.00	
Revenue—skilled nursing			133,000.00
Revenue—physical therapy			11,875.00
Revenue—occupational therapy			8,550.00
Revenue—speech therapy			5,250.00
Revenue—medical social services			7,000.00
Revenue—home health aide			94,000.00
Revenue—medical supplies			
		259,675.00	259,675.00

Prepared by:
Approved by:

Journal Entry 2: Record Contractual Allowances
Any Home Health Agency
July 19XX

Description	Account #	Debit ($)	Credit ($)
A/R—Medicare		1,150.00	
A/R—HMO			9,250.00
A/R—Medicaid			2,375.00
A/R—Commercial			
Contractual allowances		10,475.00	
		11,625.00	11,625.00

Prepared by:
Approved by:

Journal Entry 3: To Record Cash Receipts
Any Home Health Agency
July 19XX

Description	*Account #*	*Debit ($)*	*Credit ($)*
Cash—Operating account		240,865.00	
A/R—Medicare			190,000.00
A/R—HMO			33,000.00
A/R—Medicaid			770.00
A/R—Commercial			17,000.00
Overpayment liability			95.00
		240,865.00	240,865.00

Prepared by:
Approved by:

Journal Entry 4: To Record June 17 to 30 Payroll Paid July 8
Any Home Health Agency
July 19XX

Description	*Account #*	*Debit ($)*	*Credit ($)*
RN		16,650.00	
Home health aide		12,800.00	
RN managers		4,038.46	
Home health aide managers		1,153.85	
Quality assurance		1,269.23	
Intake		1,230.77	
Clerical—records		400.00	
Clerical—billing		600.00	
Clerical—accounting		961.54	
Clerical—payroll		846.15	
Clerical—scheduling		673.08	
Clerical—data entry		560.00	
Director of nursing		1,442.31	
Administrator		1,730.77	
Controller		1,384.62	
Federal withholding			4,200.00
FICA			3,499.17
State withholding			1,143.52
Local withholding			1,829.63
United Way			25.00
Garnishments			35.00
Cash—payroll			35,008.46
		45,740.78	45,740.78

Prepared by:
Approved by:

Journal Entry 5: To Record July 1 to 14 Payroll Paid July 22
Any Home Health Agency
July 19XX

Description	Account #	Debit ($)	Credit ($)
RN		15,984.00	
Home health aide		11,616.00	
RN managers		4,038.46	
Home health aide managers		1,153.85	
Quality assurance		1,269.23	
Intake		1,230.77	
Clerical—records		390.00	
Clerical—billing		645.00	
Clerical—accounting		961.54	
Clerical—payroll		846.15	
Clerical—scheduling		673.08	
Clerical—data entry		560.00	
Director of nursing		1,442.31	
Administrator		1,730.77	
Controller		1,384.62	
Federal withholding			4,105.28
FICA			3,360.32
State withholding			1,098.14
Local withholding			1,757.03
United Way			25.00
Garnishments			35.00
Cash—payroll			33,545.01
		43,925.78	43,925.78

Prepared by:
Approved by:

Journal Entry 6: To Record July Payroll Tax Liability
Any Home Health Agency
July 19XX

Description	Account #	Debit ($)	Credit ($)
Payroll taxes—RN		2,550.10	
Payroll taxes—home health aide		1,867.82	
Payroll taxes—RN manager		617.88	
Payroll taxes—HHA manager		176.54	
Payroll taxes—administrator		1,759.16	
FICA			6,859.49
FUTA			22.16
SUTA			89.85
		6,971.50	6,971.50

Calculation
FICA taxable wages—RN		32,634.00	
FICA taxable wages—home health aide		24,416.00	
FICA taxable wages—RN manager		8,076.92	

FICA taxable wages—home health aide manager	2,307.69	
FICA taxable wages—administrator	22,231.92	
FUTA taxable wages—RN	1,246.44	
FUTA taxable wages—administrator	1,523.45	
SUTA taxable wages—RN	1,246.44	
SUTA taxable wages—administrator	1,320.77	

Prepared by:
Approved by:

Journal Entry 7: To Reverse June Accrued Payroll

Any Home Health Agency
July 19XX

Description	Account #	Debit ($)	Credit ($)
RN			15,000.00
Home health aide			14,000.00
RN managers			2,692.31
Home health aide managers			1,153.85
Quality assurance			1,269.23
Intake			1,230.77
Clerical—records			400.00
Clerical—billing			600.00
Clerical—accounting			961.54
Clerical—payroll			846.15
Clerical—scheduling			673.08
Clerical—data entry			560.00
Director of nursing			1,442.31
Administrator			1,730.77
Controller			1,384.62
Accrued payroll		43,944.63	
		43,944.63	43,944.63

Prepared by:
Approved by:

Journal Entry 8: To Accrue July 15 to 28 Payroll Paid August 5

Any Home Health Agency
July 19XX

Description	Account #	Debit ($)	Credit ($)
RN		14,245.00	
Home health aide		11,700.00	
RN managers		4,038.46	
Home health aide managers		1,153.85	
Quality assurance		1,269.23	
Intake		1,230.77	
Clerical—records		375.00	
Clerical—billing		735.00	
Clerical—accounting		961.54	

Clerical—payroll	846.15
Clerical—scheduling	673.08
Clerical—data entry	350.00
Director of nursing	1,442.31
Administrator	1,730.77
Controller	1,384.62

Accrued payroll	42,135.78
	42,135.78 42,135.78

Prepared by:
Approved by:

Journal Entry 9: To Record Cash Disbursements

Any Home Health Agency
July 19XX

Description	Account #	Debit ($)	Credit ($)
Federal tax deposit—July 8 P/R		11,198.34	
Federal tax deposit—July 22 P/R		10,825.92	
2nd qtr state withholding		6,588.87	
2nd qtr local withholding		10,542.18	
2nd qtr FUTA		1,875.00	
2nd qtr SUTA		3,500.00	
United Way		50.00	
Garnishments		70.00	
Transfer to P/R account—July 8		35,008.45	
Transfer to P/R account—July 22		33,544.99	
Postage meter		250.00	
Cash—operating account			113,453.75
		113,453.75	113,453.75

Prepared by:
Approved by:

Part II

Reimbursement Issues

Chapter 4

Retrospective Reimbursement

Home health agencies (HHAs) are paid for services provided in either a prospective or retrospective manner. An agency that is paid prospectively knows exactly what it will be paid for services that have been provided. An agency that is paid retrospectively will not know what its final payment will be until all of its costs and records have been reconciled and audited.

Agencies that choose to participate in the federally funded Medicare program are currently retrospectively reimbursed. Participation in the Medicare program requires satisfaction of the conditions of participation and annual filing of an agency cost report. The purpose of the cost report is to gather direct and indirect costs into a format that was devised by the Health Care Financing Administration (HCFA) to apportion overhead costs to reimbursable and nonreimbursable cost centers.

Retrospective reimbursement requires the filing of a cost report that follows the Medicare principles for reimbursement and is subject to review by the agency's fiscal intermediary (FI). Actual reimbursement for Medicare services is not known until the audit process has been completed, and the agency receives a notice of program reimbursement from its FI.

COST RELATED TO PATIENT CARE

Additionally, retrospective reimbursement is cost based. This means that a provider is reimbursed for reasonable cost incurred in the delivery of patient care and maintaining the facility that supports the provision of patient care. The Code of Federal Regulations (CFR) §413.9 identifies costs related to patient care:

> Principle: All payments to providers of services must be based on the reasonable cost of services covered under Medicare and related to the care of beneficiaries. Reasonable cost includes all necessary and proper

costs incurred in furnishing the services, subject to principles relating to specific items of revenue and cost. However, for cost reporting periods beginning after December 31, 1973, payments to providers of services are based on the lesser of the reasonable cost of services covered under Medicare and furnished to program beneficiaries or the customary charges to the general public for services, as provided for in §413.13.

Definitions:

1. Reasonable Cost—Reasonable cost of any services must be determined in accordance with regulations establishing the method or methods to be used and the items to be included. The regulations in this part take into account both direct and indirect costs of providers of services. The objective is that under the methods of determining costs, the costs with respect to individuals covered by the program will not be borne by individuals not so covered, and the costs with respect to individuals not so covered will not be borne by the program. These regulations also provide for the making of suitable retroactive adjustments after the provider has submitted fiscal and statistical reports. The retroactive adjustment will represent the difference between the amount received by the provider during the year for covered services from both Medicare and the beneficiaries and the amount determined in accordance with an accepted method of cost apportionment to be the actual costs of services furnished to beneficiaries during the year.
2. Necessary and Proper Cost—Necessary and proper costs are costs that are appropriate and helpful in developing and maintaining the operation of patient care facilities and activities. They are usually costs that are common and accepted occurrences in the field of the provider's activity.

Applications:

1. It is the intent of Medicare that payments to providers of services should be fair to the providers, to the contributors of the Medicare trust funds, and to other patients.
2. The costs of providers' services vary from one provider to another and the variations generally reflect differences in scope of services and intensity of care. The provision in Medicare for payment of reasonable cost of services is intended to meet the actual costs, however widely they may vary from one institution to another. This is subject

to a limitation if a particular institution's costs are found to be substantially out of line with other institutions in the same area that are similar in size, scope of services, utilization, and other relevant factors.

3. The determination of reasonable cost of services must be based on cost related to the care of Medicare beneficiaries. Reasonable cost includes all necessary and proper expenses incurred in furnishing services, such as administrative costs, maintenance costs, and premium payments for employee health and pension plans. It includes both direct and indirect costs and normal standby costs. However, if the provider's operating costs include amounts not related to patient care, specifically not reimbursable under the program, or flowing from the provision of luxury items or services (that is, those items or services substantially in excess of or more expensive than those generally considered necessary for the provision of needed health services), such amounts will not be allowable. The reasonable cost basis of reimbursement contemplates that the providers of services would be reimbursed the actual costs of providing quality care however widely the actual costs may vary from provider to provider and from time to time for the same provider.

CFR §413.9 offers providers a great deal of latitude in determining the cost structure of their HHAs. The FIs recognize that services will vary depending on the type of patients that is being serviced by the agency. An agency's client base can affect utilization patterns, time of service, and the amount of medical supplies consumed. Additionally, administrative costs will depend on the work force required to support the provision of patient care and satisfy the myriad business activities required to operate an HHA.

This section also identifies the concept that costs should not be borne by individuals not covered by the Medicare program. This statement is slightly contrary. When costs are disallowed by the FI or visits shifted from Title XVIII to other, this increases the cost of service for non-Medicare patients. However, this point is quickly forgotten.

LESSER OF COST OR CHARGE PRINCIPLE

Costs not only have to be reasonable, but also an agency is reimbursed at the lower of cost or charges. If the HHA's costs are lower than its charges, the FI will base reimbursement on the HHA's actual cost. If charges are lower than actual cost, then reimbursement is based on charges. CFR §413.13 states "in comparing costs and charges under the lesser of costs or charges principle . . . the reasonable cost for items and services and the customary charges for those same items and services are to be aggregated. Total reasonable cost of covered items and services is compared with total customary charges for those items and services, separately for Part A and for Part B."

An exception to this principle would be for a nominal charge provider. A nominal charge provider is a provider whose charges are 60 percent or less of its reasonable aggregate cost. Charges are less than cost because the provider's customary practice is to charge patients based on their ability to pay. A nominal charge provider is reimbursed for actual cost.

The Limits

Providers are faced with another limitation when considering reasonable costs. Reasonable costs cannot exceed per-visit limitations developed by the Health Care Finance Administration (HCFA). CFR §413.30, limitations on reimbursable costs, states that reimbursable provider costs may not exceed the costs estimated by HCFA to be necessary for the efficient delivery of needed health services. HCFA may establish estimated cost limits for direct or indirect overall costs or for costs of specific items or services or groups of items or services. These limits will be imposed prospectively and may be calculated on a per admission, per discharge, per diem, per visit, or other basis.

Procedure for Establishing Limits

In establishing limits under this section, HCFA may classify providers by type of provider (for example, hospitals, skilled nursing facilities, and home health agencies) and by other factors HCFA finds appropriate and practical, including

- type of services furnished;
- geographical area where services are furnished, allowing for grouping of noncontiguous areas having similar demographic and economic characteristics;
- size of institution;
- nature and mix of services furnished; or
- type and mix of patients treated.

Estimates of the costs necessary for efficient delivery of health services may be based on cost reports or other data providing indicators of current costs. Current and past period data will be adjusted to arrive at estimated costs for the prospective periods to which limits are being applied.

Prior to the beginning of a cost period to which revised limits will be applied, HCFA will publish a notice in the *Federal Register* establishing cost limits and explaining the basis on which they were calculated.

Exceptions

Limits established under this section may be adjusted upward for a provider under the circumstances specified in Paragraphs (f)(1) through (f)(8) of this section. An adjustment is made only to the extent the costs are reasonable, attributable to the circumstances specified, separately identified by the provider, and verified by the intermediary.

> (f)(2) Extraordinary circumstances states that if the provider can show that it incurred higher costs due to extraordinary circumstances beyond its control. These circumstances include, but are not limited to, strikes, fire, earthquake, flood, or similar unusual occurrences with substantial cost effects . . . there may be an opportunity to seek relief from the limits.
>
> Any provider that applies for an exception to the limits established under paragraph (f) of this section must agree to an operational review at the discretion of HCFA. The findings from any such review may be the basis for recommendations for improvements in the efficiency and economy of the provider's operations. If such recommendations are made, any future exceptions shall be contingent on the provider's implementation of these recommendations.

The limits were devised as a method of controlling HHA expenditures. In 1987, a lawsuit brought against HCFA by Representatives Harley Staggers (D-WV) and Claude Pepper (D-FL) caused Medicare utilization policies to be rewritten, increasing services that beneficiaries could receive. This increase in utilization has caused Medicare Part A costs to increase substantially since 1988. The increase in Part A, visit utilization, is illustrated by Table 4–1.

COST APPORTIONMENT

The reimbursement formula is the lower of cost, charges, or limits. This formula can then be applied to the cost apportionment methodology to arrive at total program costs. CFR §413.53, determination of cost of services to beneficiaries, explains the cost per visit calculation methodology. For cost reporting periods beginning on or after October 1, 1980, all HHAs must use the cost-per-visit by type-of-service method of apportioning costs between Medicare and non-Medicare beneficiaries. Under this method, the total allowable cost of all visits for each

Table 4–1 Total Medicare Home Health [Services] Benefit Payments

Federal fiscal year	Part A	Part B	Total	Change from prior year	Visits per 1,000 enrollees	Average charge per visit* ($)
1985	1,908	40	1,948	11.7	1,329	55
1986	1,939	32	1,971	1.2	1,256	58
1987	1,815	35	1,850	–6.1	1,153	61
1988	2,010	46	2,056	11.1	1,144	64
1989	2,251	56	2,307	12.2	1,313	64
1990	3,352	75	3,427	48.5	1,889	64
1991	4,995	62	5,057	47.6	2,219	69
1992	6,986	75	7,061	39.6	3,717	59
1993	9,529	101	9,630	36.4	4,660	61
1994	12,533	121	12,654	31.4	5,702	63
1995	15,074	140	15,214	20.2	6,446	65
1996	17,217	162	17,379	14.2	6,898	68
1997	19,127	188	19,315	11.1	7,045	72
1998	20,518	217	20,735	7.4	7,108	76
1999	21,932	250	22,182	7.0	7,166	79

Note: Based on FY95 president's budget assumptions. HCFA revises historical estimates slightly with the data available each year.
*Based on Part A alone.
Source: HCFA, Division of Budget. Adapted from Table 5–10, Green Book, Overview of Entitlement Programs, House Ways & Means Committee, July 15, 1994.

type of service is divided by the total number of visits for that type of service. Next, for each type of service, the number of Medicare-covered visits is multiplied by the average cost per visit just computed. This represents the cost Medicare will recognize as the cost for that service, subject to cost limits published by HCFA (see §413.30).

Table 4–2 illustrates the calculation of the lower of cost, charges, or the limits. In this example, the aggregate cost is lower than the aggregate amount of the limits, or charges; therefore, reimbursement would be based on costs. Often, providers will set their charges slightly higher than the existing limits. This assures them that they will not have a lower of cost or charge problem.

Additionally, limit problems are normally a function of volume. Table 4–3 assumes that an HHA has $850,000 of overhead expenses, such as administrative salaries, rent, utilities, and all of the support functions that make patient care possible, and the variable cost of service is $30.95. Table 4–3 demonstrates how the cost per visit declines as volume increases. This is because overhead expenditures do not increase proportionately with volume.

Table 4–3 also illustrates that the average limits remain fixed given a consistent discipline mix; therefore, providers that have large amounts of overhead will need

Table 4–2 Illustration of Lower of Cost, Charges, or Limit Calculations

	Cost ($)	Total visits	Medicare visits	Cost/ visit ($)	Program cost ($)
Reimbursable cost					
Skilled nursing	1,350,000	18,000	14,000	75.00	1,050,000
Physical therapy	235,000	4,000	3,400	58.75	199,750
Speech therapy	240,000	4,000	360	60.00	21,600
Occupational therapy	32,200	600	280	53.67	15,028
Medical social services	50,450	500	400	100.90	40,360
Home health aide	440,000	11,000	10,400	40.00	416,000
Total	2,347,650	38,100	28,840		1,742,738

			Limits		
Program limits					
Skilled nursing			14,000	82.65	1,157,100
Physical therapy			3,400	81.20	276,080
Speech therapy			360	83.65	30,114
Occupational therapy			280	87.90	24,612
Medical social services			400	120.30	48,120
Home health aide			10,400	48.25	501,800
Total			28,840		2,037,826

			Charges ($)		
Program charges					
Skilled nursing			14,000	100.00	1,400,000
Physical therapy			3,400	90.00	306,000
Speech therapy			360	90.00	32,400
Occupational therapy			280	90.00	25,200
Medical social services			400	90.00	36,000
Home health aide			10,400	60.00	624,000
Total			28,840		2,423,600

to do a higher volume of visits to prevent a limit problem. Additionally, Table 4–3 also illustrates the concept of break even. The break-even formula is as follows:

$$\text{Break even} = \frac{\text{Fixed cost}}{\text{Contribution margin}}$$

Break even implies that a business will not lose money on the services provided, thus it covers its variable and fixed expenses. Table 4–3 illustrates that an HHA

Table 4–3 Analysis of Cost per Visit versus Average Medicare Cost Limits per Visit

Visits	Program cost ($)	Cost/ visit ($)	Average limit ($)
5,000	1,004,774	200.95	70.66
10,000	1,159,548	115.95	70.66
15,000	1,314,322	87.62	70.66
20,000	1,469,096	73.45	70.66
25,000	1,623,871	64.95	70.66
28,840	1,742,737	60.43	70.66
30,000	1,778,645	59.29	70.66
40,000	2,088,193	52.20	70.66
45,000	2,242,967	49.84	70.66
50,000	2,397,741	47.95	70.66

Note. Assumptions: overhead = $850,000; variable cost per unit = $30.95.

with $850,000 in fixed overhead and a variable cost of service of $30.95 would not have a limit problem at approximately 21,400 visits. This illustrative computation ignores the fact that the average limit figure of $70.66 is dependent on discipline mix.

The concept of break even is misapplied in the Medicare context. The analysis illustrates when an HHA could lose money due to limit problems; however, there is no opportunity to make a profit for visits performed in excess of the break-even amount. This is because the Medicare program only reimburses for reasonable costs and does not offer providers an opportunity to make profits. When Medicare transitions to prospective payment, and there is an opportunity to make a profit, there will be a substantial increase in competition.

Accounting Records and Reports

HHAs are required to keep their books on the accrual method of accounting. Accrual accounting recognizes expenses when incurred and revenues when earned. Furthermore, CFR §413.20 states that the principles of cost reimbursement require that providers maintain sufficient financial records and statistical data for proper determination of costs payable under the program. Standardized definitions, accounting, statistics, and reporting practices that are widely accepted in the hospital and related fields are followed. Changes in these practices and systems will not be required in order to determine costs payable under the principles of reimbursement. Essentially, the methods of determining costs payable under Medicare involve making use of data available from the institution's basic accounts, as usually maintained, to arrive at equitable and proper payment for services to beneficiaries.

At a minimum, providers must be able to identify visits by discipline and payor, direct costs by general service, and reimbursable and nonreimbursable cost centers. Within each cost center, costs should be identified by the major columns, such as administrator, supervisor, nurse, therapists, aides, and others to facilitate cost reporting. Additionally, direct costs are differentiated between employee salaries, employee benefits, transportation costs, and purchases of contracted services. Administrative expenses should be maintained by cost center.

Ideally, an HHA will set up its chart of accounts to separate employee benefit cost by cost center (i.e., the payroll taxes, workers' compensation, health insurance, life insurance, etc., that apply to skilled nursing, physical therapists, home health aides, and administrative employees). In the event that the agency's payroll and accounts payable systems are not set up to accommodate this type of classification, benefit costs can be prorated.

Table 4–4 demonstrates how employee benefit cost could be prorated to different cost centers. This method is better than leaving employee benefit cost to be distributed through the administrative step down; however, the objective of cost reimbursement is to maximize reimbursement. Wherever possible, it makes sense to capture accounting data in a fashion that enhances the reimbursement process. Ideally, any cost that is related to a specific cost center should be directly costed to that cost center instead of allocated through the administrative step down.

Stepping down of administrative cost is nothing more than prorating administrative cost to reimbursable and nonreimbursable cost centers. This methodology attaches the largest amount of administrative cost to the cost center that has the largest amount of direct expense. Often, direct cost is no more than a function of

Table 4–4 Prorated Employee Benefit Cost

	Wages ($)	Prorated benefits ($)
Administrative	75,000	10,786
Skilled nursing	125,000	17,976
Physical therapy	50,000	7,190
Home health aide	60,000	8,628
Total	310,000	44,580

	Benefits
Payroll taxes	30,380
Workers' compensation	2,450
Health insurance	10,000
Life insurance	1,750
Total	44,580

volume and rate; therefore, of the six disciplines, skilled nursing will receive the largest portion of the overhead.

Additionally, the step-down methodology indiscriminately prorates costs to reimbursable and nonreimbursable cost centers. The problem from a reimbursement perspective is that providers lose money when administrative costs are prorated to nonreimbursable cost centers. Furthermore, this method ignores the activities that were responsible for these costs and how the costs relate back to the services that were provided. Provider Reimbursement Manual (PRM) PRM §2328 offers an exception to the allocation of overhead to home-health-based hospices. The cost of inpatient care provided under contract for an HHA-based hospice may be excluded from the statistical basis used to allocate administrative and general cost. The amount of cost excluded must be based on auditable records of the actual cost to the HHA for care provided to hospice patients under an arms-length contract with a nonrelated provider of inpatient care. All other hospice costs will receive overhead from the parent HHA through the required step-down process.

There are two additional cost-finding options available to HHAs. Both of these options require approval from the FI, and the provider must have a relatively sophisticated accounting system in place to take advantage of the following options. The first option is the use of direct assignment of general service costs. Administrative expenses are captured and classified by cost centers. The allocation process first assigns directly identified administrative expense and then steps down administrative expense that is common to both reimbursable and nonreimbursable cost centers. The second option is the use of unique cost centers. Unique cost centers are similar to the process used for cost centers one through four. The allocation statistics for these cost centers could be square footage or dollar value in the case of capital-related building, fixtures, and movable equipment. Transportation could use actual cost or miles as an allocation base. The allocation statistic would first assign costs based on the statistic, and the residual would be stepped down.

Direct Assignment

Direct assignment of general and administrative expenses requires the prior approval of the FI. Requests for approval must be made in writing 90 days prior to the beginning of the cost reporting period. The intermediary must respond in writing, and once approved, the cost report must be submitted in the approved format until a request is made to change it back to the previous cost-finding method. Additionally, it needs to be noted that if the provider fails to keep its accounting records in a proper fashion, the FI will not allow direct assignment and require the agency to use the traditional cost-finding process.

Requests submitted to the FI should identify how the general and administrative category will be subdivided. For instance, if the request is to separate home health administrative expenses from hospice administrative expenses, then the requesting provider would identify three cost centers to capture general and administrative expenses. The first cost center would be the HHA, the second cost center would be the hospice, and the third cost center would be other general and administrative expenses that apply to both the HHA and the hospice.

These cost centers would be established on the provider's chart of accounts, and during the normal accounting processes, direct assignment of administrative support staff time would be assigned to the appropriate cost center. Assignment of time is based on the activity that was performed by the employee and the operation the activity supported. If the activity was for the sole purpose of one cost center, then that is where it should be charged. If the activity supported more than one cost center, then it should be charged to the general support cost center. Assignment of personnel needs to be supported by continuous time records. Time studies are estimates and therefore are unacceptable for direct assignment of costs.

Continuous time records are recorded every day by the agency's personnel. The time records should include the employee's name, how his or her time was spent during the course of the day, and a description of the activities that were performed during the day. Time should be kept in 15-minute increments. Time records are then submitted to payroll and summarized, and then payroll cost is charged to the respective cost centers based on actual duties performed within the agency. Employer costs, such as payroll taxes, health insurance, workers' compensation, and pension cost, should follow the distribution on a pay period basis.

In this example, payroll and payroll-related expenses would be charged to either HHA, hospice, or the other cost center. General and administrative expenses not related to patient care but directly assignable to either the HHA or hospice would be charged to the appropriate cost center. Cost charged to specific cost centers (HHA or hospice) must be factual and auditable. Any cost that supports both cost centers would be chargeable to other. The cost-finding process would first assign the general and administrative expense that belonged to the HHA to the home health cost centers, then assign the general and administrative expenses that belong to the hospice to the hospice cost center on the cost report. The other costs would follow the traditional cost-finding process of stepping down expenses to each cost center.

Furthermore, PRM §2307 states that to accommodate additional general service cost centers, the provider must add additional columns to the allocation worksheets or attach a supporting worksheet with similar information to document the step-down of costs to those cost centers benefiting from the general service cost centers. Any modifications necessary to worksheets after the cost allocation must also be approved by the intermediary as part of the request for direct assignment of costs.

Unique Cost Centers

Use of unique cost centers requires prior approval of the FI, which is required to respond in writing. Request for approval should be done prior to the beginning of the cost-reporting year and, although not explicitly stated, should be submitted 90 days prior to the beginning of the cost-reporting year.

Providers requesting the ability to change the order of allocation of general and administrative expenses must be able to convince the FI that costs will be accumulated in the proposed cost centers on an ongoing basis and that the statistics used as part of the allocation process will accurately measure the amount of services charged to each cost center, be auditable, and result in a better cost-finding methodology. An example of a unique cost center would be billing. Billing cost would be accumulated within the general ledger chart of accounts during the year. As part of the cost-reporting process, an additional column would be added on the B-1 schedule identifying the statistical basis to allocate the costs accumulated in the general ledger.

Unique cost centers are prohibited for the six home health disciplines. This is unfortunate because there are different costs involved with services offered in each of the six disciplines. For instance, the nursing discipline includes routine nursing and high-technology nursing. By combining these types of services, the agency cannot use the cost report as a reliable tool to determine its average cost per visit. Other factors include the length of the visit, travel time, contact time, and documentation cost.

Periodic Time Studies

The provider reimbursement manual differentiates between continuous time records and periodic time studies. Periodic time studies are in lieu of ongoing time reports and represent estimates of time spent. Periodic time studies can be used for unique cost centers if the following conditions are met.

- The time records to be maintained must be specified in a written plan submitted to the intermediary no later than 90 days prior to the beginning of the cost-reporting period to which the plan is to apply. The intermediary must respond in writing to the plan, whether approving, modifying, or denying the plan, prior to the beginning of the cost-reporting period for which the plan is to apply.
- A minimally acceptable time study must encompass at least one full week per month of the cost-reporting period.
- Each week selected must be a full week (Monday to Friday, Monday to Saturday, or Sunday to Saturday).

- The weeks selected must be equally distributed among the months in the cost-reporting period (e.g., for a 12-month period, 3 months of the 12-month period and 3 of the 12 weeks in the study must be the first week beginning in the month, 3 weeks the 2nd week beginning in the month, 3 weeks the 3rd, and 3 weeks the fourth).
- No two consecutive months may use the same week for the study; for example, if the second week beginning in April is the study week for April, the weeks selected for March and May may not be the second week beginning in those months.
- The time study must be contemporaneous with the costs to be allocated. Thus, a time study conducted in the current cost-reporting year may not be used to allocate the costs of prior or subsequent cost-reporting years.
- The time study must be provider-specific. Thus, chain organizations may not use a time study from one provider to allocate the costs of another provider or a time study of a sample group of providers to allocate the costs of all providers within the chain.

The intermediary may require the use of different or additional weeks in the study in its response to the provider's request for approval and may prospectively require the changes in the provider's request as applied to subsequent cost-reporting schedules.

Written Requests

Written requests to the FI should be very clear as to what is being requested. The request should state whether the cost-finding method requested is for direct assignment or unique cost centers. The request should identify how the change will lead to a more accurate measurement of cost in consideration of the different activities that take place at the respective agencies. Requests are most likely to be approved if the HHA can convince the FI that it has the financial systems in place to accomplish this type of reporting, the personnel that will be charged to different categories, the type of expense classifications that will be charged to different categories, and a sample of the continuous time records or studies that will be used to support assignment of personnel cost.

The intent is to receive approval in writing from the FI, then capture costs according to the plan that was outlined for the FI. There is a cost attached to increased documentation, and once approved, it will be the responsibility of all employees to record their time in relationship to the activities that were performed. Adherence to the approved plan will hopefully prevent problems on the back end with the FI.

ACCRUED EXPENSES

Accrual accounting requires recognizing liabilities when incurred. Liabilities are the result of normal business transactions. Liabilities are differentiated as short and long term. The unpaid portion of a mortgage, bank loan, or note payable represents a liability to the agency. This group of liabilities would have a short-term and a long-term component. The short-term component is expected to be paid within one year. Money owed to employees for salary, vacation, sick time, or other fringe benefits that was not paid to the employee during the accounting period represents liabilities. These are short-term liabilities.

PRM §2305 states that short-term liabilities must be liquidated within one year after the end of the cost-reporting period in which the liability is incurred. Generally, liabilities are liquidated by disbursing cash, although liabilities can be liquidated through the transfer of assets such as stock or the reversal of the original accrual. Accrual reversal could present a problem for the agency if the expense is significant. If the accrued expense is disallowed for the cost-reporting year because it was reversed in the following year, it is important to remember that that expense needs to be added into the year that booked the accounting reversal.

There are several exceptions to this rule. The first exception would be if the agency is unable to pay the liability within one year. The agency must notify the FI in writing that it is unable to pay the liability within the one-year time limit. The agency must explain why it is unable to pay the liability and when and how it intends to liquidate the liability. The FI can extend the agency up to two additional years to pay the liability.

Other exceptions apply to interest paid to The Mother House or other governing body (PRM §220), members of organizations having arrangements with the provider (PRM §704.5), reimbursement of vacation costs (PRM §2146.2), and sections that mandate liquidation with 75 days after the end of the cost-reporting period.

One area that the 75-day rule applies to is the compensation of owners and stockholder employees. PRM §906.4 states that payment to owners for salaries and bonuses must be made within 75 days after the close of the cost-reporting period. If payment is not made within the cost reporting period, or within 75 days thereafter, the unpaid compensation is not includable in allowable costs either in the period earned or in the period when actually paid.

Money owed to stockholder employees and owners must be supported by a note payable. The note payable must be negotiable, be in writing, contain an unconditional promise to pay a specified amount on demand, and include a specified future time for payment of the liability. Additionally, the note must be payable to the bearer of the note or to the order of a specific individual.

Accrued expenses can also include fringe benefits. Expenses that are incurred by employers on behalf of their employees that are in excess of their salary are referred to as fringe benefits. Fringe benefits can include pension, educational, and paid time off expenses incurred by an employer to attract and retain qualified employees, improve morale, and enhance organizational efficiency. Fringe benefits are allowable if the costs are reasonable and related to patient care (PRM §2102.1, PRM §2102.2).

Paid time off is generally recognized when an employee is compensated even though he or she is not working. This may be because the employee is sick, is home taking care of a sick child, is on vacation, or is attending to a personal matter. Depending on the agency's personnel policy, there may be an opportunity to increase an agency's Medicare reimbursement by converting from a cash method of recognizing paid time-off expenses to an accrual method.

An agency can keep its books and records on the accrual basis for accounting purposes but only reflect its paid time off liabilities when paid. An agency may have a liability to pay employees even though the fiscal year has ended. This may be due to benefit cycles that do not correspond to the agency's fiscal year. In this example, the employee has earned the right to vacation or sick time but has not taken it by the end of the fiscal year. Employees have until the end of the calendar year to take their vacation time; otherwise, they will lose it. The agency can accrue for purposes of cost reporting all unpaid but owed vacation, sick, and personal time. It is important to remember that once this practice is started, it must be continued and that the accrual must be supported by the agency's personnel policy. Additionally, employer payroll taxes applicable to vacation, such as Federal Insurance Contributions Act (FICA), must not be accrued in the period when the vacation costs are accrued but treated as a cost in the period when the vacation costs are paid.

Vacation costs are reimbursable when costs associated with vacation pay are earned in the cost-reporting period. Earned vacation costs must be supported by payroll records kept by employees. Records should be consistent with the employer's vacation policy for the entire organization. Vacation pay must be reasonable in consideration of compensation levels and other determining criteria.

If the vacation pay policy is consistent among employees, vacation pay can be carried forward consistent with the organizational policy. In the event that vacation policy is inconsistent, then vacation pay can only be carried forward for two years. Furthermore, PRM §2146.2 states that the time limitation for owners is consistent with organizational policy and supersedes the 75-day compensation rule.

Fringe benefits can also include pension cost. Pension is a deferred compensation benefit that is earned while employees are working but is not available to the employees until they retire. Employees can choose how they want to receive their pension benefits. The pension benefit is a wonderful opportunity in a cost-reimbursed world. As long as the pension plan meets the conditions for a formal plan, and is funded by the agency, this becomes a great benefit to the employees.

PRM §2142 offers the following definition of a pension plan.

A pension plan is a type of deferred compensation plan which is established and maintained by the employer primarily to provide systematically for the payment of definitely determinable benefits to its employees, usually over a period of years, or for life, after retirement. Such a plan may include disability, withdrawal, option for lump-sum payment, or insurance or survivorship benefits incidental and directly related to the pension benefits. Such benefits are generally measured by, and based on, such factors as age of employees, years of service, and compensation received by the employees. A plan designed to provide benefits for employees or their beneficiaries to be paid upon retirement or over a period of years after retirement shall be considered a pension plan, if under the plan either the benefits payable to the employee or the required contributions by the provider can be determined actuarially.

In order for a plan to be considered funded for purposes of Medicare cost reimbursement, the liability to be funded must have been determined, and the provider must be obligated to make payments into the fund. Funds existing at the discretion of the provider are not considered valid; such plans will be treated as direct pension plans, and payments will be allowed only when paid to the beneficiary.

OPERATING EXPENSES

Medicare has developed guidelines in determining whether cost is reasonable and necessary for patient care. Costs that are incurred to generate new business or increase utilization are nonallowable expenditures. Providers may choose to incur costs that are not allowable under the Medicare program. It is recommended that these costs be handled as an A-5 adjustment to lower program cost. Some providers adopt the approach that they will "bury" the cost, and let their FI find nonprogram cost. This approach can cause the FI to dig deeper to find other costs that should be disallowed. More importantly, this approach could negatively affect an agency's cash flow if it is reimbursed under the Periodic Interim Payment (PIP). Current-period cash flow will be reduced based on prior cost report settlements to reflect the difference between reported and settled costs. This factor is then applied to reduce the current period's payment stream.

Costs are also evaluated from the perspective of a prudent buyer. The concept of a prudent buyer is one who refuses to pay more than the going price for any item or service; therefore, providers should take advantage of purchase discounts and volume purchases and attempt to seek the best deal available. This concept is especially important in evaluating purchased service agreements.

Advertising Costs

Advertising costs are allowable if they relate to the provision of covered services to Medicare beneficiaries or to maintaining the facility. These costs include telephone directory advertising to list the agency's telephone number and services, classified advertising to recruit personnel, and costs related to a positive public image. Costs that are incurred to increase utilization of services, promotions, publicity, or fundraising activities are nonallowable.

Contracted Services

Contracts that are in excess of five years or have an automatic renewal are considered unallowable cost. This does not include contracts with a duration in excess of five years due to a specific election to continue by the HHA. Additionally, contracts with fees contingent on the HHA's reimbursement, profit, or billed charges are considered nonallowable.

Depreciation

Depreciation expense must be based on an asset's historical value as supported by the original invoice when acquired or the fair market value at the time of donation. Depreciation expense must be clearly identifiable in the HHA's trial balance, supported by a depreciation control schedule that identifies total depreciation expense by asset and includes the agency's capitalization policy. The depreciation schedule would identify the depreciation methodology employed, useful life, current and accumulated depreciation, and book value for every asset within a particular classification. The capitalization policy defines the level that purchases are capitalized versus treated as minor equipment and expensed. Often a threshold of $500 is established for small equipment purchases.

Depreciation expense methodology includes straight-line depreciation, sum of the years method, or the declining balance method. Additionally, Medicare recognizes the half-year and actual time depreciation methods for determining first- and last-year cost.

Educational Activities and Seminars

Educational cost is allowable for part-time education at properly accredited institutions for undergraduate and graduate work. Allowable expenses include tuition, textbooks, and materials. Seminar and related travel expenses are permitted in that they further the quality of patient care or enhance organizational efficiency. The intermediary may have a problem with seminars in "exotic locations" and try to deem them luxury expenses. This is a potential subjective judgment area and is best supported by identifying travel research that indicates that the seminar in the exotic location was cheaper than a "traditional location."

Home Health Coordination

This type of cost has received a great deal of attention over the past several years. The provider reimbursement manual segregates this type of service into four areas: (1) home health coordination activities, (2) patient solicitation activities, (3) discharge planning activities, and (4) education and liaison activities.

1. *Coordination Activities*—This is the cost of explaining the agency's policies and procedures to the patients and their families once the referral has been made to the agency. Coordination activities include assisting in establishing a definitive home care plan prior to discharge that includes assessment and coordination of the appropriateness of requested services, medical supplies, and appliances. Coordination also includes ensuring that the HHA is ready to meet the patient's needs at the time of discharge. This entails making arrangements for any special medical supplies or appliances, making arrangements for training agency personnel regarding unfamiliar procedures or problems pertaining to the patient's care, and communicating information regarding the patient to the agency. These costs are allowable.

2. *Patient Solicitation Activities*—This type of cost is not allowable. Activities related to patient solicitation include, but are not limited to, visiting patients or reviewing patient charts before they have been referred to the HHA and attempting to persuade patients, physicians, or hospital personnel to refer to the HHA.

3. *Discharge Planning Activities*—This is a cost that is part of the hospital function and, therefore, not an allowable cost of the HHA. Any cost related to predischarge activities will be disallowed because it is felt to be a duplication of services. Additionally, this can be construed as payment for referrals, which creates much larger problems.

4. *Education and Liaison Activities*—Cost to educate other members of the health care system such as physicians and hospital administrators concerning the benefits of home health care is an allowable costs. Liaison activities can also include the development of home care policies and procedures.

Some HHAs may choose to provide nonallowable services to the hospital, physicians, and others in the health care community. This choice may be an exceptional, prudent decision from a business perspective, albeit a nonreimbursable one from Medicare's perspective. It is recommended to keep continuous time records of the personnel who perform these types of functions and to deduct the nonallowable portion from the cost report voluntarily at the time of filing.

Interest

Interest is a cost incurred by an agency when it finances its operations externally. Interest expense could be due to loans for buildings, credit line borrowings for working capital, or lease arrangements to purchase computers and office furniture. Interest is an allowable expense that requires supporting documentation such as amortization schedules, invoices from banks, or other externally prepared documentation. Interest expense must be clearly identified in the agency's general ledger, related to the reporting period, and supported by some form of loan documentation. The loan documentation is a means of supporting short- and long-term liability balances.

Interest income is to be offset against interest expense, unless the interest income is the result of income earned from grants, gifts and endowments, funded depreciation, qualified pension funds, deferred compensation funds, and interest earned as a result of judicial review by a federal court. Interest paid to related parties is generally nonallowable.

Medical Supply Cost

The HHA's trial balance should separate medical supply cost into two components. Routine supplies are a cost of providing patient care. The cost of these supplies is included in the visit cost and is nonbillable. Examples include cotton balls, adhesive tape, and tongue blades. Nonroutine supply cost represents the agency cost for supplies that are billed to the patient. Examples of nonroutine supply cost include catheters, enemas, and dressings. Nonroutine medical supplies are marked up over cost anywhere from two to three times cost. Additionally, the HHA should have a consistent policy for charging Medicare and non-Medicare patients.

Noncompetition Agreement Cost

A fee paid to a seller not to compete with the purchaser for a stated number of years is amortized over the life of the agreement. This cost is not related to patient care and, therefore, is nonallowable.

Organizational Cost

Organizational cost is the cost of incorporating. Allowable cost includes legal and accounting fees required for the establishment of the corporate charter. Unallowable costs are costs related to the sale and issuance of stock. Organizational cost is amortized over a 60-month period.

Owners' Compensation

Compensation of owners, executives, and other senior personnel could cause a potential reasonable cost issue from the FI's perspective. Compensation is a potential problem because of the requirement that it be reasonable. In order to evaluate the reasonableness of compensation, the FI will evaluate the total compensation package against comparable compensation levels within the same geographic area. Additionally, compensation is determined by the type of services that the agency provides, the size of the agency, the number of personnel who are employed by the agency, the owners' qualifications, their educational background, and the actual duties and services that are provided by the owners. Total compensation is considered to include salaries, benefits, deferred compensation packages, and other services and assets that are provided for the personal benefit of the owners.

Compensation issues have become rather complicated. The changing industry requires HHAs to attract skilled individuals to guide their respective agencies. The intent of this regulation is to prevent undue enrichment on the part of owners; however, expanding this rule to include key personnel hampers the agency's ability to attract qualified personnel. Additionally, the mechanism of compensation evaluation is very subjective. Providers that have had cost disallowed do have the option of appealing and requesting that their case be reviewed by the Provider Reimbursement Review Board (PRRB). Unfortunately, even if the decision is decided in favor of the provider, the agency still suffers because of the disallowed costs negatively affecting cash flow until they are actually paid.

Additionally, it is important for owners to document their time and activities, especially if they are involved in multiple companies. More documentation supporting the owners' involvement in day-to-day activities will help prevent arbitrary decisions on the FI's part.

Purchased Management and Administrative Support Services

HHAs receive management and support service proposals on a regular basis from individuals and management companies that claim to be able to provide services in a more efficient manner than the agency's staff can. The FI is concerned that, if the agency chooses to purchase these services, the services are needed, do not represent a duplication of existing services, the costs are reasonable, and the agency is adhering to the prudent buyer clause when negotiating and evaluating the benefits received from a management service agreement.

PRM §2135 has outlined four areas that the FI considers when evaluating management contracts to determine whether the costs are reasonable:

1. whether the contract results from competitive bids that are reasonable and within industry norms for similar services;
2. whether the contract is between unrelated parties;
3. whether the contract provides for services that are designed to accomplish within a prescribed timeframe clearly stated goals and objectives based on the needs of the provider; and
4. whether the provider maintains adequate documentation of the services rendered and the status of the stated goals and objectives.

In addition to the cost of the management contract being reasonable, the HHA needs to keep records and documentation to support the cost of the purchased services. It is suggested that documentation that supports the fees charged for management services include a copy of the contract(s) and any amendments. Periodic progress reports must be submitted by the management organization. An analysis should show the efforts of the provider to comply with the prudent buyer principle guidelines in assessing its needs, establishing the goals to be attained, evaluating the available alternatives, and choosing the terms of the contract. Board minutes or other documentation must show continued reassessment of the effectiveness of the services and detailed identification of the services actually received during the period. Any other documentation available, such as visit or contact reports, minutes of committee meetings, cost/benefit analyses, and so forth, that would support the receipt of services and substantiate the attainment of the goals and objectives desired and the reasonableness of the fees paid, is needed.

Additionally, any contract that the HHA enters into that has a value of greater than $10,000 over a 12-month period must have a clause in the contract that allows the Secretary of Health and Human Services and the U.S. Comptroller General (or their representatives) access to the subcontractor's books, documents, and records to verify the extent of costs and services provided under the contract. This clause must be included in the contract for services to be covered for Medicare reimbursement. Furthermore, the clause needs to allow access to the related parties that may be dealing with the subcontractor.

Related Parties

A related party is one who has the ability to influence decisions. Decisions can be influenced either through direct or indirect control, common ownership, or affiliation. For purposes of common ownership, this includes anyone who is related to the owner either through blood, marriage, or adoption. The concept of related parties is to prevent a related organization from generating a profit from the Medicare program; therefore, all transactions are reduced to cost. Cost must follow the same guidelines for allowable cost as if it was originally incurred by the agency. Related party cost is allowable as long as it is reasonable and was incurred to furnish services to patients or facilities and services to the provider.

An agency that has related party cost included in its allowable costs must make available sufficient documentation to support the costs. Additionally, the FI may request access to the books and records of the related organization to determine whether the allocation methodology was appropriate.

PRM §1010 identifies an exception to the related party principle. The exception identifies four criteria that must be met to enable the HHA to be granted an exception from the related party principle. The first section states that the supplying organization must be a bona fide, separate organization and legal entity and not an operating division of the agency. The second requirement is that the HHA represents a small portion of the services that are provided by the related party, these services are offered to other nonrelated purchasers within the competitive market, and the price for these services is easily ascertained. The third requirement is that the services, facilities, and supplies are not a basic element of patient care and that these services are not normally performed by the HHA staff. The final requirement is that the charge to the HHA must be the same as charged to other customers within the open market.

Start-up Costs

Cost incurred by an HHA prior to licensure should be capitalized and amortized over 60 months. Amortization is treated as a general and administrative expense and spread across all payor groups. Expenses that are typically treated as start-up expenses include administrative and nursing salaries, rent, utilities, insurance, interest, employee training costs, repairs and maintenance, housekeeping services, and any other allowable cost attributable to the start-up period.

Taxes

In general, taxes levied against an HHA are allowable costs except for federal, state, and local income taxes. Fines and penalties are not allowable costs.

COST REPORTING

All HHAs participating in the Medicare program are required to file an annual cost report. New providers can choose a cost-reporting period of at least 1 month but not more than 13 months, and providers that have no Medicare activity can file an abbreviated cost report. The cost report is due by the last day of the third month following the close of the period covered by the cost report. For cost reporting periods ending on or after June 27, 1995, cost reports are due no later than 5 months following the close of the cost-reporting period. An additional 30-day extension is available if the agency can demonstrate to the FI that there is a good reason for the extension, and it submits a written request and receives approval. If the cost report is not received after the grace period, interim payments will be suspended, and the FI has the ability to deem all interim payments from the beginning of the cost-reporting period an overpayment.

Providers that voluntarily or involuntarily terminate participation in the Medicare program or experience a change in ownership must file a final cost report 45 days from the date of termination from the Medicare program. Payment for plan of treatments submitted prior to cessation from the Medicare program will continue to be paid. Additionally, if an agency can reasonably demonstrate a need to the FI and convince the FI in writing, it is possible to change the cost-reporting year. The agency must submit a written request to the FI 120 days prior to the proposed year-end, and if the FI is convinced that the change has merit, then the FI will notify HCFA of the change 30 days prior to the proposed period-end.

The cost report is a series of sequential forms that allows the agency to record its costs and statistics that relate to the cost-reporting year. The cost report is submitted with a check in the event that the agency has been overpaid, a copy of the agency's financial statements, and HCFA Form 339. The HCFA Form 339 is a questionnaire that the FI uses to expedite the settlement process. The form consists of 14 sections that include questions about financial data and reports, the provider organization and operation, capital-related costs, interest expense, insurance, deferred compensation and pension plans, educational activities, nonpaid workers, cost to related organizations, purchased services, provider-based physicians, intensive-care-type inpatient hospital unit, home office costs, and bad debts. The agency completes this form by responding yes, no, or not applicable to the questions in each section. Affirmative responses will require the submission of additional information. Furthermore, the entire form package includes additional questionnaires related to the provider-based physician section.

The cost report is HCFA Form 1728-86. The cost report is broken into six primary sections: (1) certification and statistics, (2) reclassification and adjustment of trial balance expenses, (3) cost allocation and cost allocation statistics, (4) apportionment of patient service costs, (5) reconciliation of costs and payments, and (6) financial statements. Form 1728-86 includes additional forms for HHAs that qualify as certified outpatient rehabilitation facilities.

The cost report is set up to identify agency cost by cost centers. Cost centers are defined as general service cost centers, reimbursable cost centers, or nonreimbursable cost centers. Cost apportionment spreads the general service costs such as general and administrative expenses between reimbursable and nonreimbursable cost centers.

The goal of the cost report is to provide a standardized format for reporting expenses incurred in the provision of home health care. The cost report provides separate pages and specific columns to identify employee salaries, related benefits, contracted services, and general and administrative costs. Providers then have an opportunity to reflect adjustments that may increase or decrease allowable costs.

From the provider's perspective, the goal of the cost report is to maximize reimbursement. The accounting system should capture costs in a fashion that enhances agency reimbursement. Specifically, an agency should strive to reduce the amount of agency expense that is allocated using the cost apportionment process. General and administrative expenses that are prorated to reimbursable and nonreimbursable cost centers based on the relationship of total expenses for that cost center to the total of all cost centers have very little bearing on how and why the cost was actually incurred. Therefore, the goal is to assign as much of an agency's operating expenses directly to the cost centers that benefited from incurring the expense.

This can be accomplished by identifying expenses by department and/or discipline. For example, expenses that would relate to the discipline of nursing would include the salaries and wages of nurses who performed nursing visits, the cost of benefits and taxes that are attributable to the wages that were paid, and other costs related to the provision of nursing visits. This can include specifically identifiable transportation costs, contracted nursing services, medical supplies related to the nursing visits, and possibly nursing supervision. This costing methodology should be followed for each discipline and/or department.

Furthermore, if the agency is providing multiple services, programs, or product lines, the accounting system should identify direct, indirect, and overhead-related expenses as they relate to the specific service, program, or product line being offered. This is a good practice from a management perspective and helps to enhance the reimbursement process providing the agency has requested and received approval from its FI. Ultimately, the agency should strive to identify as much cost as possible directly before the cost apportionment process takes place.

If an agency only offers skilled, intermittent services from its Medicare-certified agency, and it is providing a large volume of visits, then it may question what value the enhanced accounting system may offer since it is sufficiently under the limits. The extra effort required to capture expenses by discipline and department will provide the agency with a head start in a prospective payment environment. An agency that does not have a sophisticated accounting system in place will never know whether it is losing or making money on a per visit basis.

Furthermore, identification of per visit cost from the cost report is perhaps one of the most misleading pricing/costing mistakes an agency could make. The cost report identifies a cost per visit for purposes of reimbursement only. The cost report ignores length of service, skill level for particular services, service requirements, and support activities. This process gives an equal value to all visits. Additionally, indirect and general and administrative costs are allocated based on the relationship of direct cost per discipline to the total cost of all disciplines. This process ignores the activities and processes that would make the cost per visit higher or lower for a specific payor, type of service, program, or product line.

Many agencies have chosen to create separate entities to enhance the reimbursement process. This strategy is often used to segregate product lines, such as skilled intermittent visits from private duty programs. The cost apportionment process is based on total direct expense, so if a skilled, intermittent visit had a direct cost of $30, and a private duty shift had a direct cost of $200, then 1 private duty shift would receive almost 87 percent of overhead dollars allocated during the cost apportionment process. In reality, the amount of effort to schedule or oversee the visit versus the shift might be 50/50. Additionally, if a time study were performed, the amount of effort that may be required could indicate that 70 percent of the effort is related to billing the skilled, intermittent visit versus 30 percent for the private duty shift. Often, these companies would be managed by shared personnel and have common costs. The home office cost report is a mechanism to identify common costs and charge the costs back to the company that benefited by the services that were performed.

Home Office Cost Report

The home office cost report, HCFA Form 287-92, was devised by HCFA to report efficiencies in the health care delivery process. Efficiencies are gained through not replicating staff and taking advantage of consolidated operations. The home office cost report is required for providers that operate, own, or control multiple businesses of which a Medicare-certified home health agency is one of the businesses. The home office cost report identifies shared or common services and seeks to identify costs back to the individual components that received benefit from the common services.

Home offices can vary greatly based on the number of related organizations within the related organizational structure. The home office structure can be relatively simple such as is shown in Figure 4–1. In the example below, home office personnel could reside in either entity. The cost-reporting methodology would remove home office cost from any of the components and then redistribute the cost back to the specific entities that benefited from the home office cost. Cost that is charged to the HHA must follow the guidelines of reasonableness and be necessary for the provision of patient care; otherwise, the cost will be nonallowable. Additionally, it is helpful to employ the use of cost centers in the accounting system. Cost centers would identify costs that support the home office operation and the entity operation. When completing the home office cost report, specific ac-

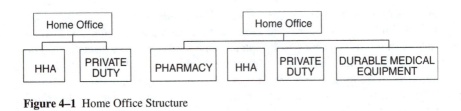

Figure 4–1 Home Office Structure

counts could be referenced for inclusion in the cost report. The total cost could then be adjusted to exclude nonallowable program cost. Total remaining cost would then be distributed to the entities by three possible methods.

The first methodology is direct costing. Direct costing can take place during the year and as part of the cost-reporting process. For example, if one of the entities performs the majority of administrative activities, such as the purchasing of services, normally it will place purchases for all of the companies at one time to take advantage of quantity discounts or vendors will itemize invoices by specific company but issue only one invoice instead of invoicing all companies. If this happens, it is important to trace how the goods and services are consumed by each company and to have a sophisticated accounting system track and support the cost, source of the transaction, and distribution of expenses for purposes of intercompany accounting. If the intercompany approach is utilized, it is important to have sufficient detail of all transactions that went through the intercompany accounts, support beginning and ending balances with subsidiary schedules and analysis, and have copies of actual invoices on file.

Direct costing can occur for specific individuals who share their time and efforts between multiple companies. Identification of time, effort, and projects should be made as part of a continuous time study. Identification of how an employee spends his or her time will enhance the cost-finding process so that the appropriate portion of the employee's salary, benefits, and payroll taxes is charged to the proper entity, thereby not distorting patient costs.

Another costing methodology is the functional allocation. The functional allocation determines a specific statistic to serve as a base for allocating services. For instance, if payroll is a centralized function that supports all entities, then a functional allocation could be determined based on the number of checks issued to the respective entities. A centralized purchasing function could allocate costs functionally based on the number of purchases made or requisitions handled.

Home office costs that are not allocated directly, or functionally, would be treated as residual cost and allocated in a pooled cost methodology. The pooled cost methodology is identical to the cost apportionment methodology utilized for allocating general cost centers on HCFA Form 1728-86. The allocation process assigns the largest amount of overhead to the entity that has the greatest accumulated cost in relation to total cost. Therefore, the direct or functional allocation methodology provides a better allocation mechanism than pooled cost. Attempts should be made to utilize these approaches before resorting to the pooled cost approach.

The home office structure is available for providers that control multiple entities. The allocation process remains the same; however, there may be a need to create multiple home offices.

In Figure 4–2, there would be three home offices. A home office would be set up for common personnel for Region A and Region B. A corporate home office would charge support cost to both Region A and Region B.

Interim Rate

Upon entry into the Medicare program, an interim rate is set for each provider. The interim rate can be established based on the organization's financial statement, budgeted program costs, or rates of comparable providers in the area. Providers submit bills manually and electronically to their local FI, which pays them based on the interim rate established for the agency. The interim rate is the same for every type of visit and includes the cost of medical supplies. Additionally, agencies that have experienced an increase or decrease in costs subsequent to establishing the interim rate can request that the FI change its interim rate to reflect program costs accurately.

The interim rate is the result of dividing total allowable costs by the total number of visits actually performed or anticipated. Total visits include all payors within the HHA and, therefore, attach an equal cost weighting to every type of visit and every payor, regardless of the amount of services required by a specific payor.

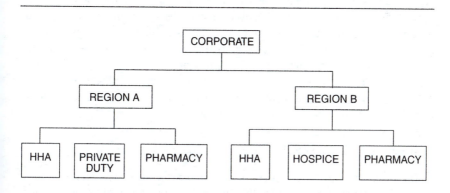

Figure 4–2 Home Office Structure for Providers that Control Multiple Entities

Within the program, there is an opportunity for retroactive adjustments. Interim payments are made based on estimated cost. A retroactive payment cannot be made until the end of the cost-reporting period. An initial retroactive adjustment is possible on receipt of the cost report. The initial settlement will consider whether there have been problems with the particular provider in previously submitted cost reports, whether the submitted cost report indicates any potential cost disallowances, and total interim payments made to the agency.

Periodic Interim Payment

Providers can choose to participate in the PIP program if they meet the initial and ongoing requirements of the program. The PIP program was established to help providers with cash flow problems by providing a steady stream of payments based on estimated program costs. PIP payments are made biweekly and cover a two-week period.

Entrance into the PIP program requires that providers must have patient service cost for Medicare beneficiaries in excess of $25,000 annually. Medicare must represent in excess of 50 percent of an agency's payor mix. The agency must have filed a completed cost report and have the ongoing ability to report cost, charges, and visit statistics on a regular basis.

Acceptance to the program is based on the FI's judgment of whether there is the potential for overpayment to the provider. The concept of overpayment comes into play with termination from the PIP program. Providers can be terminated from the PIP program if the provider feels that the likelihood of an overpayment exists because of declining utilization, improper filing of PIP reports, submission of invoices, or impending bankruptcy.

PIP reports are due 30 days after the close of each quarter. If an agency's volume is increasing, then it will probably file for a lump-sum adjustment. A lump-sum adjustment is the difference between actual cost for the quarter and the estimated payments that the agency received. If visit volume decreases, then the agency will need to submit a check for any overpayments it may have received.

Additionally, entrance into the PIP program provides the agency with a huge cash inflow. The agency will begin to receive its biweekly PIP checks and still receive payments for claims submitted under the claims-made basis. This should help the agency to reduce any outstanding loans.

Provider Statistical and Reimbursement Report

The FI provides every provider with a summary of the claims that have been paid and the charges associated with those claims. It is imperative that providers track and summarize payments that they have received from the Medicare program. Providers should create a log of visits that have been paid and compare it to the monthly provider statistical and reimbursement (PS&R) report that is provided by the FI. The purpose for this reconciliation is to make sure that the visits reported on the PS&R are exactly what has been reflected within the records of the agency. The PS&R statistics are the same statistics that the FI uses for settlement of the cost report. Therefore, if the PS&R is incorrect, the agency could be significantly penalized by the incorrect data. By keeping an internally prepared log that is auditable, an agency can contest incorrect statistics that the FI may attempt to use in the settlement of the agency's cost report.

Chapter 5

Prospective Payment

The previous chapter dealt with retrospective reimbursement from the perspective of the Medicare program. Retrospective reimbursement is a payment methodology that reimburses Medicare-certified home health providers for costs of providing patient care. Actual costs are never known until the cost report is filed and the fiscal intermediary (FI) approves the filed cost report. Under a prospective payment methodology, the fee for providing services is known in advance.

The primary concern under a retrospective reimbursement methodology is to follow the program rules and regulations. Rules and regulations were designed to keep costs at a reasonable level. Specifically, providers were required to keep costs at the lower of costs, charges, or limits. This type of structure placed a ceiling on total reimbursement for low-volume providers, while large-volume providers were less affected by the lower of cost, charges, or limits formula. This type of payment system does not provide the opportunity to make a profit; consequently, there is little or no incentive for providers to control their operating costs.

In a prospective payment environment, there is an opportunity to make a profit. Payment for services is known in advance, and home health agencies (HHAs) will have an incentive to control their costs. This transition may be a little difficult for some providers due to the cost-reimbursed payment system being relatively risk-free. As payment vehicles transition from cost-reimbursement mechanisms to prospective payment models, the amount of provider risk will begin to grow. This chapter will contrast cost reimbursement to different types of prospective payment systems, such as fee-for-service, discounted fee-for-service, episodic payments, per diem, and per capita.

ACCESS TO CARE

The basic premise is that a reimbursement system influences provider decisions on admissions, services provided, cost control, staffing, and related items. Of course, non-financial considerations are critical in a provider's decision process, including the patient's medical condition, availability and capability of caregiver support, other resources in the community, quality of care objectives, professional standards, and ethical considerations. Although such factors can mitigate and even override financial incentives, our assumption is that financial incentives must be carefully considered by agencies in order to maintain their financial viability.[1]

Under a cost-reimbursed payment system, providers are very rarely discouraged from admitting patients onto service. In fact, the cost-reimbursed system encouraged providers to increase the amount of services that were being provided. This worked as long as the agency had signed physician's orders that supported a plan of treatment, and services were consistently provided in relationship to the plan of treatment; otherwise, there was the risk of having visits denied. Denial of services was the only risk that providers encountered from an operational perspective.

In 1987, a lawsuit was brought against the Health Care Financing Administration (HCFA) because of "increasing Medicare paperwork and unreliable payment policies."[2] The successful outcome of this lawsuit increased the amount of home health services that could be provided to Medicare beneficiaries. Providers adopted a new philosophy. The new philosophy was to maximize visits. Visits were maximized by increasing home health aide services and breaking visits that held multiple skilled components into separate visits. Table 5–1 shows the increase in Part A expenditures as a result of the lawsuit. It also needs to be noted that the increase in the volume of visits is attributable to several factors other than increased utilization. These forces include the graying of America, increased acceptance of home health care services, increased technological advances, and increased emphasis on decreasing hospital length of stay.

The concept of visit maximization is purely driven by administrative decisions. Visit maximization was a strategy adopted to make sure that all fixed and variable costs were reimbursed within the program formula of the lower of cost, charges, or limits. From an access of care perspective, this strategy provided more services and possibly helped to cause a dependence on the part of the patient for continuing services.

Cost reimbursement has been utilized by Medicare and some of the state Medicaid programs. Some of the state Medicaid programs follow the Medicare guidelines and offer cost-reimbursed payment structures to program providers. Other states have adopted a prospective payment methodology in an attempt to control health care expenditures. Beyond defining payment for services prospectively, state Medicaid programs attempt to control utilization by requiring precertification prior to providing services.

Table 5–1 Total Medicare Home Health Services Benefit Payments*

Federal fiscal year	Part A	Part B	Total	Charge from prior year	Visits per 1,000 enrollees	Average charge per visit**
1985	1,908	40	1,948	11.7	1,329	55
1986	1,939	32	1,971	1.2	1,256	58
1987	1,815	35	1,850	−6.1	1,153	61
1988	2,010	46	2,056	11.1	1,144	64
1989	2,251	56	2,307	12.2	1,313	64
1990	3,352	75	3,427	48.5	1,889	64
1991	4,995	62	5,057	47.6	2,219	69
1992	6,986	75	7,061	39.6	3,717	59
1993	9,529	101	9,630	36.4	4,660	61
1994	12,533	121	12,654	31.4	5,702	63
1995	15,074	140	15,214	20.2	6,446	65
1996	17,217	162	17,379	14.2	6,898	68
1997	19,127	188	19,315	11.1	7,045	72
1998	20,518	217	20,735	7.4	7,108	76
1999	21,932	250	22,182	7.0	7,166	79

*Based on FY95 president's budget assumptions. HCFA [Health Care Financing Administration] revises historical estimates slightly with the data available each year.
**Based on Part A alone.

When a provider elects to participate in a program that pays for services prospectively, there is the potential to limit patient access to services. Providers will be unwilling to provide patient care if the fee they receive is less than the total cost of providing care unless they have the ability to offset losses against funds generated because of their nonprofit status or profits from other payors.

Therefore, if the payment for services is less than the cost of providing services, providers will lose money in a prospective payment environment. Providers that lose money when providing services will not remain in business very long. Profits are essential to the long-run financial viability of an organization, and this does not differentiate between proprietary HHAs and nonprofit HHAs. Profits are used for investment in the future; purchase of furniture, equipment, information systems, research, and development; and repayment of loans. Without profits, the HHA will not be able to provide services, and access to care will be threatened.

Once the transition has been made away from cost-reimbursed payors, HHAs will need to begin to consider the relationships between revenue, variable costs, fixed costs, and volume. Additionally, this is the first introduction into the concept of provider risk. The elements of risk include rewards, losses, and uncertainty. In a prospective payment environment, provider risk is the relationship between revenue on a per visit, hourly, episodic, or capitated basis; total agency costs; and the volume of services.

One of the tools that is available to help understand the relationship between rates and volume is the break-even analysis formula (Figure 5–1). Break-even analysis identifies what price is necessary to break even in relationship to volume estimates or what volume is necessary to break even given a specific pricing methodology. Integral to this computation is determining what an agency's total costs will be to provide services. Total cost is composed of a fixed component and a variable component. The fixed component consists of truly fixed costs that will not fluctuate with volume and costs that are semifixed. Semifixed costs will remain fixed for certain levels of volume and then fluctuate incrementally with large volume increases. The variable component will fluctuate directly with every unit of service provided. The difference between the payment amount for each unit of service and the variable cost to provide a unit of service is known as the *contribution margin*.

$$\text{Break even} = \frac{\text{Fixed cost}}{\text{Contribution margin}}$$

In a simplified example, if an agency has $1 million of fixed cost, has a variable cost of $50 per unit of service, and will receive $100 for each unit of service, then break even would occur at 20,000 visits. This is the point where the revenue line and the total-cost line intersect. If the agency only generates 15,000 visits, it will report a loss of $250,000. Visits in excess of the break-even amount will generate a profit of $50 for every visit that is performed in excess of 20,000 visits.

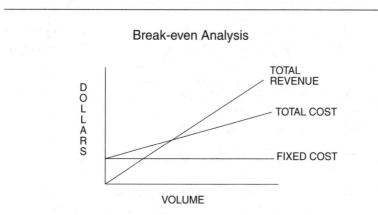

Break-even Analysis

Figure 5–1 Graphical Representation of Break-even Analysis

Changes in the contribution margin will alter the break-even point. Changes will occur because of negotiation of a lower payment rate for each unit of service or fluctuations in the variable cost. For example, if the actual variable cost was $45 for each visit, then break even would occur at 18,182 visits.

Beyond Medicaid prospective payment is a prospective payment system that is no longer mandated but is dependent on the patients' insurance coverage, or contractually negotiated between the payor and the provider. In the case of commercial insurance, an HHA has an opportunity to establish a specific charge structure for the services that it provides. Commercial carriers are then billed for services that are provided to their policy holders. Private pay, or commercial insurance, has been a very lucrative payor source for HHAs.

Commercial carriers limit access to home health services through definition of benefit clauses within individual policies. Each policy could have different home health benefits. Benefits would have been predetermined by the type of coverage that the policy holder purchased. Access to home health services depends on the amount of services included in the policy, type and amount of home health services, and total dollar limitation for home health services. Beyond actual policy limitation, commercial carriers began to employ case managers to determine appropriate levels of care to control their expenditures and to review charges in relationship to rates that have been predetermined as being usual and customary charges for specific types of services.

In general, access to care was only limited because of specific policy limitations or the patient not having the financial resources to pay for services. This unfortunately caused traditional indemnity policy rates to increase on a regular basis, and in an attempt to control rising health care costs, health maintenance organizations (HMOs) were created. HMOs were able to offer employers lower rates to cover their employees because they were able to control the cost of providing health care services.

One of the ways that HMOs were able to obtain lower rates is that they offered providers the promise of a large volume of visit activity in return for a discounted per visit rate. The discounted per visit rate could be for each discipline or type of service. The discounted per visit rate would be prospectively determined for each discipline, and then it was up to the provider or the HMO to determine utilization. It is important to note that access to care could be limited because a patient was not actively enrolled within the HMO program or because of the utilization practices of the HMO. From a financial perspective, if the discounted per visit fee exceeds the agency cost per visit, then the payment structure was not a source of access to care restriction.

Using the cost structure from the above simplified break-even analysis, if the HHA negotiated with the HMO to accept $75 for every unit of service that it provided, then the HHA would need to receive 40,000 visits from the HMO before the HHA would cover its costs. It is important to understand several items related to the revenue, cost, and volume decisions. First, total costs will increase from $2 million to break even at $100 per visit to $3 million to break even at $75 per visit. This may require an infusion of cash to meet the increased working capital requirements. Second, the provider should question whether the HMO will be able to provide 40,000 visits to the agency or whether this is solely a ploy to get the agency to reduce costs to a level that the HMO is interested in paying. The other consideration is, what happens to the agency when it goes from a contract that provides 20,000 visits to one that provides 40,000 visits? What effect will the increased volume have on fixed costs? There is a good possibility that fixed costs will increase by some amount. It may be necessary to add personnel, recruit additional staff, train new hires, buy new furniture and computer equipment, or expand the size of the office. If fixed costs increased by $50,000, the break-even volume would now be 42,000 units. From a visual perspective, a discounted per visit arrangement has the effect of causing the aggregate total revenue line to shift downward toward the total cost line as the contribution margin narrows, causing the point where the revenue and total cost lines cross to shift to the right (Figure 5–2).

HHAs that exist in a fee-for-service environment can approach the offering of services from the perspective of a profit center mentality. A profit center approach is volume-dependent and will become more profitable as volume increases and costs remain fixed. Inherent in this paradigm is the concept that HHAs are paid for production, whereby more services are better, services are illness-based, and service provision follows a fee-for-service orientation. This mindset will transition to a cost center approach as payment mechanisms shift utilization responsibility to the provider and eliminate volume payment methodologies.

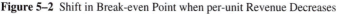

Break-even Cost

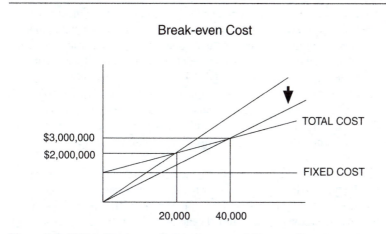

Figure 5–2 Shift in Break-even Point when per-unit Revenue Decreases

As risk increases, HHAs will need to adopt a much different paradigm when providing services. The new paradigm will force providers to provide more services for less money, transition from quality assurance to quality improvement, and adopt a systems orientation that focuses on outcomes, processes, and process improvement. Success will be a measure of low-cost, high-quality services instead of how far the "rules and regulations" can be stretched. Agencies will quickly learn that the strategies of success in a cost-reimbursed world potentially will cause failure in a prospective payment system that is driven by managed care organizations (MCOs). This is because MCOs will say, "This is what we want," and it is up to the HHA to provide the services within the payment structure, or the MCO will find an agency that will.

SHIFTING OF RISK

Payors quickly realized if they were going to control rising home health expenditures, they needed to develop payment methodologies that transferred the responsibility for controlling utilization to the HHA. The use of case managers and preauthorizations created an adversarial relationship between patients, home health providers, and the payor. HHAs found themselves in the role of patient advocates attempting to persuade case managers via telephone that a particular patient required more services because of his or her unique situation. By changing the payment structure, payors quickly realized that they could shift utilization responsibility to the HHA. This type of prospective payment is accomplished by paying a fixed amount based on an episode of care, a day's worth of care, or a life of coverage.

Access to care will be limited under an episodic or per diem payment structure if anticipated service levels and related costs exceed the fixed payment amount. Providers will be unwilling to accept patients onto service if specific service requirements will exceed the payment structure, unless this is a one-time event, and all other cases are profitable. Even with the HHA sharing responsibility for appropriate utilization levels, there will be cases in which providers will not accept a patient onto service unless provisions are made for specific outliers. An example of an outlier would be a chronic case that would remain on service for months, and the episodic payment structure was for cases with a normal duration of several visits or a limited timeframe.

In Figure 5–3, an episodic or per diem payment is demonstrated as a fixed payment. A per diem rate will cover one day, whereas an episodic rate could be for a fixed time period or for an entire illness episode. When an HHA provides services that cost less than the fixed payment, it will generate a profit. If the cost of services provided exceeds the fixed payment, then the HHA will lose money. Inherent in

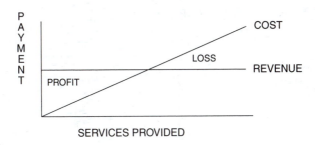

Figure 5–3 Episodic Payment Structure

the illustration is the concept of time. Patients may require more intense services on admission into the home health program. Initially, the agency will provide services with costs that exceeds the per diem reimbursement. The longer the patient remains on service and if service intensity decreases, the aggregate payment should exceed the aggregate cost of patient care; otherwise, it will have a problem.

From a financial perspective, HHAs must determine whether they will be able to provide services for less than the fixed payment amount. Also, they will begin to explore how to become more efficient in the provision of services. Increases in service efficiency will positively affect the HHA's bottom line. Efficiency may be the result of providing fewer visits. This could be accomplished by combining multiple skilled interventions into one visit instead of three. The savings that would accrue from reducing total visits would be slightly offset by the increased cost of the longer visit. Actual costs would also depend on specific agency payment policies.

Table 5–2 could reflect the cost of postsurgical wound care. Here, the patient was on service for approximately 15 days, received nursing care, and was charged for medical supplies. The cost reflected in Table 5–2 represents the direct and indirect costs of providing care. The episodic payment will need to exceed direct and indirect costs for providing care and generate a residual. The residual is used to satisfy loan repayments and fixed-asset expenditures and to contribute to agency profit.

In this situation, if the episodic payment is less than $435.34, the agency will lose money on this specific case. The agency will need to evaluate the mix of all possible cases to determine the appropriate levels of indirect and fixed expenses to assign to each case. Beyond break even, agencies need to understand how much profit each case will generate. It is the mix of cases that will determine overall agency profitability.

Table 5–2 Evaluation of the Episodic Payment Structure

Expenses	Units	Cost ($)	Total ($)
Direct expenses			
Nursing visits	7	42.00	294.00
4 × 4s (box)	1	8.76	8.76
Gauze (box)	1	2.15	2.15
Tape (package)	1	1.95	1.95
Subtotal direct			306.86
Indirect expenses			95.62
Fixed expenses			32.86
Total			435.34

The break-even formula can be expanded to include the concept of profitability.

$$\text{Break even} = \frac{\text{Fixed cost} + \text{profit}}{\text{Contribution margin}}$$

A simple break-even formula could be calculated on the above case using the following agency characteristics. The agency had fixed cost of $1 million, and the agency wanted a $150,000 operating profit. In this example, fixed cost included all indirect costs of patient care. The episodic payment is $750 per case, and the agency's variable cost is $306.86. The agency would need 2,595 cases to generate a $150,000 profit.

Reality is much more complex than this example because each case will have different service requirements. The episodic payment may fluctuate based on specific patient requirements. Understanding break even would require calculating the contribution margin for each possible case and then extending the result by the frequency with which the case may occur. Other considerations include different contribution margins based on discipline, medical supply category, and payor. The sum of this result can then be compared against anticipated fixed cost and profit levels.

Additional analysis may require reviewing service levels within the episodic payment structure. Service levels could fluctuate because of patient demographics, the presence of a caregiver in the home, or the employee or team providing care. Service levels could also fluctuate because they encompass several different patient groups. Each patient group could have different frequencies and contribution margins attached to it.

An agency that has a financial objective of a 10 percent bottom line will need to make sure that on average the episodic payment structure is generating enough residual after direct, indirect, and fixed expenses to satisfy this objective. If the 10 percent bottom line goal will not be met, then it will require evaluating whether the goal is realistic. The evaluation may determine that only specific cases can be accepted in order to have an annual operating profit of 10 percent. If this is unrealistic, then only three choices remain. First, the agency can attempt to negotiate better pricing on the front end. If this is not possible, then the agency needs to reduce the cost of providing care. Reduction of the cost of care is achieved through building efficiencies into the delivery process and reducing waste and overhead costs. The last choice is to revise the financial objective downward from 10 percent, to seek alternative services to offer, or to look for other business opportunities.

A per capita payment methodology is similar to an episodic payment system in that the payment stream is fixed. The difference, however, is how the payment works. In an episodic payment system, the payment stream may be based on a patient, a specific patient problem, or a combination of factors. In the hospital environment, payment is structured based on diagnosis-related groups (DRGs) that correspond to specific medical diagnosis. In the home health setting, the episodic payments could be dependent on a classification based on nursing diagnosis. Nursing diagnosis would encompass many patient characteristics, such as primary problem, complicating problems, activities of daily living, and presence of a caregiver.

Under a per capita payment methodology, providers will be paid a flat rate based on the number of covered lives that they negotiate to provide home health services for if needed. Per capita rates are determined based on units of 1,000 lives, anticipated types of services, and service levels. Rates are determined based on the number of covered lives on a monthly basis and the services that are to be provided. This is normally referred to as *per member per month* (Table 5–3).

Table 5–3 Computation of a per Member per Month Rate in a Capitated Payment Structure

Services	Visits	Total cost ($)
Skilled nursing	55,000	2,175,250
Physical therapy	31,000	1,302,000
Occupational therapy	6,000	240,000
Speech therapy	4,500	171,000
Medical social services	2,500	125,000
Home health aide	70,000	1,750,000
Supplies		58,627
		5,821,877
Covered lives	(500,000)	
Annual covered lives	(500,000 × 12)	6,000,000
Per member per month		.97

In Table 5–3, home health usage for a population consisting of 500,000 managed care beneficiaries totaled $5,821,877. To arrive at monthly cost on a per member basis, multiply the number of managed care beneficiaries by 12 to arrive at the total annual number of covered lives. This result is then divided into cost to arrive at the monthly cost per member. Per member per month rates may result in differentials due to the population being covered, such as Medicare, Medicaid, or commercial beneficiaries. Factors such as age and sex could affect per member cost.

Per member per month rates could be actuarially determined.

> No longer can the actuary use conventional actuarial approaches to estimate the anticipated use rate and cost of services. The actuary must consider when, where, and why the services will be pursued. This requires that the population be segmented into those who are willing to use the managed care system all of the time, most of the time, and never. Only when this distribution of enrollees is known can the actuary have any hope of accurately projecting or anticipating the healthcare cost. The actuary can help predict likely patterns of enrollee choices and also conduct retrospective analyses summarizing prior enrollee choice patterns.
>
> Widely differing demographic distributions (that is, age and sex, health status, family size mix) are anticipated in each of these categories. Since demographic characteristics are key determinations of actual utilization and cost characteristics, the projected assumptions will vary by each type of projected population. In addition, the local competitive situation will determine the actual mix of enrollees.[3]

HHAs that do not have a sufficient understanding of a population's utilization and service requirements should either use an actuary to estimate resource consumption or negotiate a fee-for-service arrangement until they can develop sufficient data to assume risk.

In the capitated payment system, access to care is potentially limited because the HHA has an incentive to provide the minimum amount of services possible. The less services that are provided, the more profits the agency will be able to retain. Providers will need to evaluate their entire cost structure and clinical protocols to determine where efficiencies can be built into the system. Applying costs and clinical protocols that have been developed for the Medicare patient population could create a major disadvantage to the HHA. Depending on the type of capitated contract that is entered, there may be an entirely different demographic requirement to consider when providing care. Additionally, beyond controllable provider cost is the cost of the unknown. This is the cost associated with providing services to a specific population that requires more services than originally forecasted. This is also known as an increase in utilization.

Capitation payments put home care providers at greatest financial risk. When capitation is used by the HMO or Preferred Provider Organization (PPO) it shifts the cost risks of the entire covered population onto the provider organization. Under the capitation approach home care providers will have to render services to all referred cases. The risk is greater under this form of payment because of the many variables that need to be controlled in order for it to work to the provider's advantage. The home care provider must first be able to control the costs of the services rendered, the amounts of labor, supply and equipment to be used and the length of the treatment/service period. What makes this difficult is that the home care provider can be affected greatly by unexpected and increased numbers of complex cases, catastrophic cases, and referrals from the HMO and PPO physicians. While capitation payments place the provider organization at greater risk many of the risks can be reduced by limiting the types of cases included in the capitation plan and the costs that the provider must absorb when a capitated plan is negotiated.[4]

RISK

Risk can take many different forms as HHAs begin to transition away from cost-based reimbursement (Figure 5–4). The simplest definition of risk is the degree of probability that loss may occur. In this example, an agency will either generate a profit or a loss from providing a particular service. The concept of risk becomes more complex when volume uncertainty is added into the profit equation. To expand on the previous example, now an agency will generate a profit or loss depending on the volume of referrals that it receives or services that it provides in relationship to its revenue and cost.

$$\text{Profit} = ((\text{revenue} \times \text{volume}) - (\text{cost} \times \text{volume})) - \text{fixed expenses}$$

$$\text{Where volume} = (\text{patients} \times \text{service requirements})$$

Uncertainty will have different effects on the equation depending on how controllable the unknown elements are. In the above equation, volume represented an unknown, and depending on the volume of patient services, an agency could either generate a profit or lose money. The unknown element is minimized in a fee-for-service environment. As the payment structure changes, risk is increased because the revenue stream is flat; however, the volume of services remains uncertain. Uncertainty will increase because utilization is semicontrollable.

In a cost-reimbursed environment, risk is minimal. HHAs that are exclusively composed of Medicare activity will have 100 percent of their cost reimbursed by

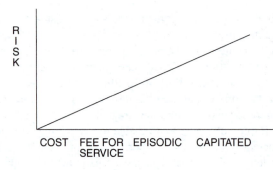

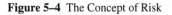

Figure 5–4 The Concept of Risk

---

the Medicare program. This includes owner compensation, pension plans, benefits, continuing education, and auto allowances. As long as providers can substantiate that all costs are reasonable and necessary to provide patient care, and their aggregate costs follow the lower of the cost, charges, or limits formula, then 100 percent of their costs will be reimbursed.

This situation is similar to depositing savings in a passbook account. Annual interest will be nominal, but there is a high confidence level that all deposits in a federally insured savings account will remain intact and that there is no possibility that the principal will erode.

When an agency's payor mix changes from 100 percent cost reimbursed to include patients with other types of insurance, it begins to increase its risk. Risk is very controllable in a fee-for-service environment, and the analysis is straightforward. Risk is simply understanding whether the fee that would be paid to the agency exceeded the cost of providing care and whether the compensation is sufficient to cover any dilution in the agency's Medicare reimbursement.

The controllable element in the fee-for-service situation is the relationship between the prospectively determined rate of compensation for a unit of service and the agency's costs. Direct cost and indirect cost of providing care are controllable at the agency level. Other controllable elements would be determining what services had been approved and whether there were limits in the amount of care or the frequency of care. All elements of the volume equation are controllable.

When providers enter into discounted fee-for-service arrangements with HMOs, Medicaid programs, or other payors, they increase their risk. The elements of controllability from the HHA's perspective remained the same except for anticipated volume. Volume was not in the agency's control, and depending on the specific circumstances, an agency could have its financial viability threatened.

Financial viability could be threatened if actual volume multiplied by the contribution margin for each unit of service provided did not exceed the proportionate amount of overhead associated with this particular visit volume.

From a provider's perspective, risk is minimal with a per visit payment structure in relationship to the risk that is borne by the payor. Payor risk is due to the payor's inability to control the expenditure for home health services because of an inability to control the volume of services provided. Attempts at controlling the cost were implemented, such as precertification and benefit limitations. These attempts caused payors to realize that they needed the providers to control utilization; therefore, they began to transition into payment methodologies that transferred risk to the provider.

Episodic, per diem, and per capita payment systems accomplished this goal. From the provider's perspective, an episodic or per diem payment structure increases risk dramatically. The increase in risk will necessitate a more proactive stance to understanding the relationship between costs and service levels. The relationship between costs and service levels must be known at a patient problem level for episode and per capita payment systems. In addition, capitated payment systems require providers to understand the global service requirements of the population they will serve, monitor utilization levels, and proactively investigate any fluctuations from contractual parameters.

The shift to an episodic or per diem payment system will prospectively establish a flat rate for specific services. It will be up to the provider to determine whether it can deliver high-quality home health care services to ensure that a specific outcome is achieved within the constraints of the payment. Providers will be able to minimize risk by controlling utilization and understanding the relationship of direct and indirect costs to specific patient characteristics.

Success in an episodic payment system will depend on the agency's ability to negotiate with payors prior to accepting patients onto service. Providers will need to be able to quantify the amount of services that will be required for a specific patient when the referral comes in the door. Success will depend on the agency's ability to negotiate with a payor regarding specific patient characteristics and then control the delivery of care within defined parameters.

If an intake nurse or care coordinator is responsible for negotiating rates with payors prior to admission, then he or she will need to determine service requirements and costs based on information provided by the payor. If the only information that a payor has available is the anticipated medical diagnosis at discharge, then the intake nurse will need to review all the different patient problems that could be attached to a specific medical diagnosis. If the intake nurse can obtain additional information from the payor source, then pricing may become a little less generalized. The key is to begin to develop an agency database that is based on different patient characteristics, medical diagnoses, physician characteristics, and payor demographics. By developing specific groupings of patients, an intake nurse will feel relatively confident in determining service and cost requirements prior to admission to obtain the best possible pricing for his or her agency.

Reliance solely on the medical diagnosis is not a good indicator of resource requirements. The Georgetown study confirmed that "medical diagnosis does not have a high predictive power for resource consumption. A better indicator of resource consumption is the nursing diagnosis."[5] Nursing diagnosis will take into consideration all of the patient problems, including physiological, psychological, and environmental components; comorbidities; activities of daily living; and presence of a caregiver to assist the patient.

Therefore, to understand the total units of service by discipline and the related costs, a better indicator of resource consumption will be nursing diagnosis. If potential referrals can be identified in relationship to an agency's prior experience with a similar type of patient problem, then the intake nurse will have a sound starting point for negotiating with the payor. There will always be variation due to the human condition; however, the more data that can be accumulated by the agency, the better it will become in forecasting resource consumption, thus reducing one of the unknown variables in the volume equation. Furthermore, risk can be minimized further by understanding the approximate range of services within a patient classification and what constitutes normal variation from outliers.

As HHAs begin to evaluate previous cases by patient characteristics, they will begin to identify fluctuation in service levels. These fluctuations could be due to an improper classification of a patient within a specific group or normal random variation in service requirements. Normal variation will begin to identify low and high levels of service by discipline. It will be important for the agenvy to understand why these variations are taking place and to develop a pricing strategy that considers potential fluctuations. Pricing strategies will also need to consider a sufficient contribution margin to provide for those cases that miss the mark.

The positive side of risk is the opportunity to make a profit. Profits can be generated on an episodic or per diem setting if providers are willing to be innovative and build efficiencies into their processes. Efficiencies can occur as a result of combining multiple visits into one, changing the frequency of visits to enhance outcomes, or lowering indirect costs through advances in information systems. By understanding the relationships between patient requirements, service, costs, and patient outcomes, agencies can manage a large portion of the unknown components within this type of payment structure. It will be possible to negotiate changes in the fixed payment for outliers or potentially difficult patients if service levels are known and can be evaluated against the proposed payment. Providers that cannot negotiate a favorable return can decline to accept the referral. Declining a referral will need to be evaluated in light of organizational strategies as they relate to a specific referral source.

A fully capitated payment system potentially offers the most risk to a home health provider. Risk is highest because of an equation element that is totally uncontrollable by the HHA. The missing equation element is understanding the two components of volume: (1) the number of patients and (2) the service requirements of those patients that will determine actual utilization. This element is related to the population that the HHA has agreed to serve and the referring practices of the providers within the network. HHAs negotiate with an HMO or an MCO to provide home health services for a specific population. An MCO could be a PPO, insurance companies, self-insurance employers, unions, third-party administrators (TPAs), or the government. The population is based on the number of people participating in the HMO or MCO's health plan. If the population is typically a healthy, working-age population, then service requirements are going to be substantially less than if the population is a Medicare or Medicaid population.

HMOs or MCOs employ actuaries to forecast potential service requirements based on plan benefits, geographic area, age, and previous experience. The HHA is at a distinct disadvantage when negotiating with an MCO because it does not have the same information that the MCO has. It is imperative to get as much information as possible from the MCO to help in forecasting possible service requirements. Understanding service requirements and expectations will help providers determine whether they want to participate in a fully capitated or partially capitated capacity. Specific suggestions will be made in the managed care section for negotiating and forecasting service levels.

In a capitated payment system, the revenue is fixed. Managers must adopt a cost center mentality to survive. A cost center mentality looks at the management of costs and how efficiencies can be built into the system. This is because profitability is a direct result of cost containment, innovation, and efforts to build efficiency. Cost containment, innovation, and efficiency span both clinical and administrative disciplines.

Capitated contracts can place the HHA at full risk or at partial risk. "A home care provider can take on a full risk contract when it has assurance that the organization has utilization and cost management control systems in place and it has negotiated a contract that protects it from higher than usual referrals, catastrophic cases, complex cases, and, case mix changes."[6]

Other alternatives to fully capitated contracts can include shared risk or partially capitated contracts.

> Under a shared risk payment arrangement, the HMO (and PPO) share the losses and profits with the home care provider. If over the course of the contract period (or other specified time period) the home care provider's costs exceed the capitation, per diem or per case payments the home care provider and the HMO will share in the loss. The sharing

can be on an equal basis (50/50) or some other basis (e.g., 25% HMO/ 75% home care provider). With a shared risk arrangement the two parties also agree to split profits when the home care provider's costs are less than the payments received. Here again the sharing can be 50/50, 25/75 or some other agreed upon sharing ratio.[7]

Furthermore, a partial risk payment approach allows the HMO (and PPO) and the home care provider to change a full risk or shared risk arrangement whenever a specified loss or profit limit is reached by the home care provider. Whenever this aggregate profit (loss) limit is reached the two parties agree to either adjust the agreed upon payment amount or to revert to a discounted fee-for-service payment plan. The partial risk payment approach is used as a braking mechanism to end a full risk or shared risk payment plan that results in a financial problem to either party because of referral, utilization, cost and pricing problems.[8]

QUALITY

High-quality home health care can potentially be affected by changes in the payment system. Changes in the payment system could positively or negatively influence quality in home health care. "Because home health care is intended to enhance or at least maintain health, outcome measures can and should be used to assess the adequacy of care in areas of significant and measurable impact. Home care can affect many facets of an individual's health for which quality measures can be constructed, such as physiologic status, functional status, health-related knowledge, compliance, and satisfaction."[9]

Outcome measures determine changes between admission and discharge. Outcome measures can be as simple as assessing if defined goals were met or not met. Or, outcomes can look to identify results for continuous quality improvement purposes. If this is the intent, then an expansion of outcome measures may include met early, met late, and changed. Additionally, attaching reasons to each of the outcome measures that deviate from the original goal will enhance the analysis and learning processes. Goals will change based on specific patient characteristics. For instance, a postsurgical patient may have a goal established that his or her wound will heal, another patient may need to administer his or her own medications, while a third patient's goal may be a pain-free death.

A study conducted by the Center for Health Policy Research published a report entitled *A Study of Home Health Care Quality and Cost under Capitated and Fee-for-Service Payment Systems* that was funded by HCFA. The study was based on a random sample of 1,632 Medicare patients. The patients were from 38 different Medicare-certified agencies. Nine of the agencies were owned by HMOs, 14 had contractual relationships with HMOs as well as providing fee for service to other providers, and the remaining 15 were "pure" fee-for-service providers.

The study found very different utilization patterns between the different providers:

> HMO patients averaged 12.7 total visits and 3.1 visits per week, compared with 18.8 total visits and 4.4 visits per week for FFS [fee for service] patients during the 60-day period after admission. These utilization differences translated into substantial cost differences, with patient-level, longitudinal cost (resource consumption) of Medicare home health care considerably lower for HMO patients than FFS patients, even after adjusting for the less intense case mix of HMO patients. The average cost of home health care per Medicare HMO patient between admission and discharge or 12 weeks (whichever occurred first), unadjusted for case mix was about two-thirds the cost per FFS patient ($877 vs. $1,305). It appears that a volume-outcome relationship exists that points to a positive association between utilization/cost per episode and patient status outcomes in the home health field.[10]

This conclusion has many interesting implications for prospective payment mechanisms. First, different utilization patterns exist based on a provider's orientation. An HHA that is owned by an HMO will follow a similar pattern of health maintenance for all of its clients. Conceptually, health maintenance seeks to get patients in and out as quickly as possible. This is consistent with a cost center mentality versus a free-standing HHA that is practicing a profit center mentality and seeks to maximize visits.

A second notable finding is the relationship between more visits and better outcomes. This would suggest that to succeed in a managed care environment, providers must forsake quality patient care in exchange for financial viability. Therefore, it is important to be in agreement when contracting with an MCO as to the types of outcomes that are expected and the appropriate cost of achieving those outcomes.

QUALITY, SERVICE, AND PRICE

Competition in the managed care arena will be based on the factors of quality, service, and price. Managed care beneficiaries will not be happy with anything less than high-quality health care and, if not pleased, will enroll in other plans. Therefore, MCOs will want to enroll providers who can deliver quality outcomes and high service levels for the lowest price.

HHAs will need to determine what types of services they are willing to offer and how to price services accordingly. For instance, they will need to know what the cost is of visiting all patients 24 hours after acceptance of a referral or providing physical therapy services within 48 hours after acceptance of a referral. Additionally, agencies will need to know what type of patients they will receive from their referral sources.

If an agency contracts to provide services to a rehabilitation hospital, it had better know what types of patients it will receive and what the service requirements will be. Understanding current referral source patterns is certainly one component of developing service standards. However, HHAs need to work with the referral sources to understand what impact a change in referral source policy will have upon the HHA. What happens if the referral source decides to develop a program that will specialize in cancer patients? What impact will that have on the HHA's service requirements?

Along with the concept of service is the measurement of quality for services provided. Are the patients, payor, referral source, and HHA employees satisfied with the arrangement? Is there a plan to measure the satisfaction and quality outcomes and report the results to the payor, referral source, and employees? Evaluating standards of care and other agency-critical success factors can be used as a continuous quality improvement tool and as a marketing vehicle for other managed care contracts.

The combination of quality, service, and price will certainly dictate which agencies will receive managed care contracts. An analysis of provider cost was included in the results from the *Study of Home Health Care Quality and Cost under Capitated and Fee-for-Service Payment Systems*. The following schedule identifies the cost of the study participants in relationship to the limits for freestanding HHAs.

The costs displayed in Table 5–4 were taken from the cost reports for the freestanding and facility-based HHAs. The HMO HHAs were not required to submit a cost report but reported costs for purposes of this study. The costs reflected in the above schedule reflect the direct cost of providing care plus administrative expenses and hospital overhead (facility-based HHAs).

It is important to note that there is a significant difference between the cost of services for HMO HHAs and free-standing HHAs. This variance is attributable to the difference in mindsets. The HMO HHAs are part of a capitated MCO that functions with a cost center mentality. "Medicare-risk HMOs are paid a fixed capitation rate by Medicare, and they must provide all care within the constraint imposed by the resulting total revenue by beneficiary. This approach creates strong incentives for HMOs to constrain the use and cost of care."[11] The free-standing HHAs are functioning in a profit center mentality, in which the more visits they perform, the larger their return. Furthermore, this table does not speak to the differences in utilization but the total resources that are consumed for a unit of service. Therefore, as managed care begins to ratchet revenue streams downward, agency cost must decrease at a faster pace.

Table 5–4 Average Cost per Visit by Discipline

| | Agency cost (average values)* | | | |
| | | | FFS study HHAs | |
Discipline	National cost** ($)	HMO owned ($)	Free-standing ($)	Facility-based ($)
Skilled nursing	74.06	59.26	72.15	88.96
Physical therapy	71.19	54.85	69.86	92.72
Occupational therapy	70.80	56.43	69.30	81.22
Speech therapy	73.98	62.18	83.58	102.20
Medical social services	102.67	70.57	105.10	132.30
Home health aide	39.86	36.03	41.79	50.48

*Cost per visit from participating agencies' cost reports.
**Federal limits adjusted to January 1, 1991, for free-standing metropolitan statistical area (MSA), HHAs.

Source: *A Study of Home Health Care Quality and Cost under Capitated and Fee-for-Service Payment Systems* by P.W. Shaughnessy, R.E. Schlenker, and D.F. Hittle, p. D.4, Center for Health Policy Research, 1994.

MANAGED CARE

Management's Paradigm Shift

There will be many different levels of managed care. HHAs have been contracting with managed care providers for years. Most of the transactions have been via a fee-for-service payment system. As managed care pushes to eliminate the fragmentation in the health care delivery process, the primary vehicle to accomplish this change will be the payment system. Payment systems will eventually transition to a fully capitated system that focuses on global capitation. Until this happens, providers will work within a fragmented delivery system whose slow metamorphosis is attempting to eliminate fragmentation by focusing on the continuum of care.

The transition from a cost-reimbursed payment system to one that is prospectively reimbursed will require management to change its approaches to the management of clinical and financial operations. This transition becomes compounded by managed care. The focus in the managed care environment will emphasize the delivery of high-quality health care at the lowest possible price. MCOs will say this is what they want, and it is up to the HHA to deliver. This will require beginning to adopt a systems orientation. A systems orientation will look at inputs, the process, and outputs across the entire organization. This orientation will move away from a follow-the-rules approach to one of finding creative ways to provide value to the patient, the MCO, and the agency's employees. Inherent in this transition are building systems that are proactive instead of reactive; using data for organizational learning instead of "I got you"; and adopting a collaborative approach to the provision of services, both clinical and financial.

PROVISION OF CARE

Management of the care delivery process in a prospective payment environment will be much different from that in a cost-reimbursed environment. One of the primary differences will be transitioning from a mentality of providing care to one of managing care. In a cost-based environment, HHAs had the ability to provide care to the patient population they served. The provision of care was determined by the physician and the primary nurse assigned to a patient. Services were provided that assisted patients in their healing process but sometimes went beyond what was medically necessary. For instance, home health aide visits could be ordered to help with household chores, light meal preparation, laundry, or shopping. Additional nursing may be provided because of a bond that has formed between the nurse and the patient.

Managed care will require looking at why services are provided and eliminating the ones that are not medically necessary. This is the concept behind managing care. Managing care is providing services that are appropriate and necessary. It is the elimination of services that "feel good" or were ordered because of an inability to "let go" and discharge a patient. One of the challenges will be to identify how different interventions have a greater impact on the overall well-being of a patient. It will be necessary to track the cost of different types of services in relationship to immediate and long-term outcomes. Understanding of the relationship between interventions, costs, and outcomes will enable providers to negotiate with MCOs to find the balance between the holistic approach of the community health nurse and the financial requirements of the MCO.

Managed care is the provision of more services for less cost. Managed care requires changing maximization of reimbursement strategies into operational efforts to build economies and efficiencies into the service delivery process. A required component is the transition from hand-holding to maintenance programs where patients and their caregivers accept accountability for achieving specific outcomes that measure their healing processes. Another element of the transition will be forgetting about Medicare rules and regulations. For visits to be reimbursable by Medicare, the patient had to be homebound. Under managed care, it may make sense to take the patient to a rehabilitation facility if it will enhance patient outcomes.

Measurement of patient outcomes will be critical in managed care. Patient outcomes will measure how successful clinical interventions were in the provision of care. This information will become part of the reporting regimen that will be expected by MCOs. The delivery of care will be evaluated on two levels. The first level will be the patient's outcome in relationship to the agency's assessment and choice of care plans. The second will be a patient satisfaction survey of the agency. The patient satisfaction survey may consider how knowledgeable the home health professional was, whether he or she was courteous, and how well he or she explained the patient's problems or exercises to the patient.

Patient outcomes will depend on the HHA's clinical expertise, how well its multidisciplinary teams interact with one another, and clinical pathway development. Clinical pathway use can serve the agency in determining appropriate clinical expertise for each step along the pathway. Utilization of teams in relationship to a clinical pathway will hopefully develop a common goal of a patient outcome instead of individual discipline goals taking precedence. Furthermore, the use of a clinical pathway system can be tied into the HHA's overall quality management program. Care can be evaluated prospectively instead of retrospectively, thus enabling agencies to develop outcome management systems.

ORGANIZATIONAL READINESS

Management of the home health delivery process will be essential for survival in a managed care setting. This will require the development of a strong management team. Managers must understand the financial implications of entering into risk-based payment structures. Each payment mechanism will have different levels of risk associated with it, and agency viability will be determined by how well management works together in transitioning into these different vehicles. "Providers should be familiar with the market for managed care services and the strengths of their own organization."[12] Transition ability will be determined by how willing management is to accept risk and to what degree it chooses to be at risk. This choice will also depend on the financial stability of the organization and the organization's ability to respond quickly.

As the level of risk increases, more will be required of management. Managers will need to determine what services add value and what services add cost. This is true for patient care and administrative activities. From a patient-care perspective, agencies will need the ability to forecast service requirements by groups of patients with similar problems and environmental characteristics and by managed care populations; to understand how contractual obligations from a patient-care and reporting perspective will differ by contract and population; and to determine what processes management must institute to manage proactively specific contracts, referral sources, and coordination of services.

Coordination of services will require developing communication protocols between team members. Team members could be representatives from each discipline who have case management responsibilities for groups of patients, or teams could be functional departments within the agency. Communication between teams will need to be consistent, to be timely, and to strive toward the codevelopment of specific outcomes that enhance the provision of care and administrative processes. Inherent in the concept of coordination and communication is the need for accountability in the provision of services. Services must be provided in a timely and consistent fashion to enhance the entire delivery process.

From an administrative perspective, managers will need to be accountable for all costs incurred by the agency. Beyond accountability for costs is the willingness to examine costs at all levels and then take corrective action. Examination of costs will look at specific program or product-line costs to determine whether they add value or represent nonvalue-added cost. Part of this process needs to include determining which costs are controllable and which costs are not controllable. This becomes one of the first steps toward the management of fixed, semifixed, and variable costs within the agency. Once everyone understands the composition of agency costs, and whether they move directly or indirectly with the provision of patient care, then informed strategies can begin to be implemented to reduce overhead and streamline processes.

True costs will not be found in the Medicare Cost Report. True costs will be found through the development of cost accounting systems designed to measure and monitor an agency's compliance with contractual obligations and actual costs in relationship to forecasts, budgets, and prospective payments. Examination of costs may include development and enforcement of productivity standards for all employees, determination of how much nonvalue-added time could be eliminated through process improvement efforts, or advances in information technology. The concept of efficient human resource management will become a critical element in the development of successful organizational strategies to compete in the managed care environment. Productivity standards will help to control costs and provide a base for determining appropriate staffing levels when forecasting potential changes in volume or type of services due to adding or deleting programs.

INFORMATION MANAGEMENT

Central to a successful organizational strategy is an information system that will collect data regarding key patient elements. Data collection will capture patient demographics at the time of referral, update the patient record for information gained during the patient assessment, and enable every subsequent action related to the patient to be added to the patient record. Subsequent actions could be visits or phone contacts from a case manager or any team member. Data collection would document interventions at each point along the clinical pathway and identify why variances were occurring at any point. For instance, maybe the clinical pathway was extended for an additional day because medical supplies were not delivered in a timely fashion, and the nurse was not able to teach the patient about wound management, thus requiring an additional visit.

Furthermore, the data collection process is enhanced by allowing the home health professional to access the patient record while in the patient's home. Review of the patient record will provide insights into what interventions have been performed, by whom, and whether they were effective. The information system should also provide on-line help if the professional has a question about changes in patient condition or about performance of a specific intervention. Real-time access to agency protocols and patient records will enhance the outcome management processes.

Once collected, data will need to be extracted in a fashion that enables management to make informed decisions. Informed decisions could include monitoring the progress of a particular patient or updating a physician or case manager who is inquiring about a patient's status. Systems that collect data at the point of patient contact and update immediately or overnight will enhance the HHA's ability to communicate with all of its clients.

Data collected will provide information about physician practice patterns, referral sources, payor characteristics, and patient problems. Patient problems need to be identified by geographic area, age, sex, team or employee, and specific patient characteristics. Costs need to be attached to patient problems to measure the cost of providing care. Costs will identify specific discipline cost, medical equipment and supply cost, and cost fluctuation by eventual outcome. Information systems will need to link the results of providing care with the costs of providing care and quality of care. Quality of care will be evaluated from a clinical and financial perspective.

Information systems will also provide data for ongoing analysis of operational results in comparison to plan, contractual requirements, and organizational objectives. Contractual requirements may require changing from a submission of invoice mentality to providing in-depth management reports about the population that received services. From an organizational perspective, the information system should have a modeling capacity to use data within the system for "what if" analysis regarding changes in operating protocols or staffing requirements or understanding how costs would change if low-cost services were substituted for more expensive services.

STRATEGIES FOR NEGOTIATING WITH MCOs

From a macro perspective, the transition to managed care is a balancing act. The balancing act requires understanding agency costs as they relate to the provision of services; understanding contractual requirements; and providing high-quality, cost-efficient care. Organizational strategies will differ between providers, but one common element exists for all providers. The key is to understand managed care requirements before entering into the managed care arena, carefully choose how to compete, and negotiate a managed care contract that includes operational safeguards. Inclusion of operational safeguards is a requirement if there is any uncertainty about how well the agency will be able to manage risk.

Structuring the managed care contract properly on the front end can be the difference between financial viability and insolvency. The goal is to have a win–win relationship between the MCO and the agency for the purpose of providing high-quality home health services to the plan's beneficiaries. Therefore, it is important to take the time on the front end to develop a relationship that works for both parties. From the perspective of the HHA, this means that the contract provides a sufficient return for services provided and a safeguard against many unknown variables. Otherwise, quality of services and access to care could be threatened.

Due Diligence

Before entering into an agreement with an MCO, it is important to understand as much as possible about the MCO. At a minimum, it is important to understand how the MCO is regulated, the MCO's organizational structure, and whether or not the MCO will have the ability to pay its bills.

> Among the most important facts is who is the payor in a managed care contract. If it is an HMO or insurer, it will be subject to state laws which regulate its fiscal solvency. It may also be subject to state laws which govern unfair claims practices as well as laws which require prompt payment. If it is an employer or third party administrator, there will be less state regulation since the plan is self insured and governed by a federal statute called the Employee Retirement Income Security Act (ERISA). In either case, providers should determine if the payor has the financial resources to support itself and its payments.[13]

Understanding the organizational structure will also help to determine whether plans utilize risk-based contracts or use primary gatekeepers to control utilization, or whether utilization is controlled through preauthorization mechanisms.

Financial considerations when contracting with an MCO include understanding the financial condition of the MCO. This may require reviewing the MCO's balance sheet and profit and loss statement, if available. It may also require reviewing specifics about individual programs or plans such as what kind of reserves does each plan have, what is the plan's medical loss ratio, and what are the plan's profit margins. Inherent in the financial results are indicators of overall plan success, quality, and acceptance. These indicators would include member retention, number of employers who dropped the plan for another plan, member satisfaction, and the results of a comparison of turnover rates in relationship to other plans.

A potential source of external information is the National Committee for Quality Assurance (NCQA) located in Washington, DC. NCQA's purpose is to accredit health plans for purposes of public disclosure. "NCQA accreditation is a nationally recognized evaluation that purchasers, regulators, and consumers can use to assess managed care plans. NCQA accreditation evaluates how well a health plan manages all parts of its delivery system—physicians, hospitals, other providers, and administrative services—in order to continuously improve health care for its members."[14]

Other issues to consider include what type of population is covered by the MCO, who is in the provider network, how are the physicians compensated, and what hospitals participate. Does the population consist of healthy working adults, or does it include beneficiaries who receive Medicaid and Medicare benefits? If the MCO offers different types of benefit plans, it is important to understand what services are included and excluded by plan, how the benefits relate to the referring and discharging practices of the provider network, and whether the plans have deductibles or copayment responsibilities. Understanding benefit plans by specific populations helps to forecast service requirements. "Check the benefits carefully; in certain plans, only a third of members are entitled to durable medical equipment (DME) or home infusion therapy (HIT)."[15]

Identifying plans that have deductible or copayment responsibilities forewarns the HHA not to have this become its responsibility for tracking and collecting. Collection of premiums is the MCO's responsibility, not the HHA's. HHAs that accept the responsibility for collecting copayments will increase their operational costs of providing services to the managed care population. The HHA will also run the risk of increasing its cost due to bad debt for uncollectible copayments. Additionally, attempting to collect the copayment at visit time could confuse the patient and muddle the purpose of the visit. This action may potentially cause dissatisfaction with the home health encounter.

If entering into a fee-for-service managed care contract, it is important to understand how utilization will be monitored. If utilization will be determined by the MCO, is it done prospectively or retrospectively? What is its utilization denial rate, and what recourse does the agency have for appealing denials? Utilization is dependent on patient eligibility. Patients who are not eligible for service present a potential cost to the HHA. It is important to determine how patient eligibility will be confirmed. Confirmation could be as a result of examining the patient's plan card. This does not ensure that the patient currently is covered; therefore, verification of eligibility should be done with someone in the MCO. In either case, "try to build in protection in the contract so that your reliance on the patient's card and telephone verification from the plan are sufficient to get paid."[16]

It is important to understand what a specific payor's practices and policies are prior to entering into a contractual relationship. "Payors often require that providers adhere to certain policies and procedures, often set forth in a Provider Handbook or Manual. The procedures can relate to quality assurance, utilization review, enrollee (or provider) grievances, appeals of claims, etc."[17] It is also important to understand whether service substitution is permitted, for example, having a licensed practical nurse (LPN) provide services that are within the scope of his or her technical ability that traditionally have been performed by a registered nurse (RN).

SCOPE OF SERVICES

While an agency is reviewing the policies and procedures of the MCO, the HHA should consider what services it wants to offer to the MCO. An agency can elect to provide all types of home health services or to provide limited services. In either situation, it is important to quantify for purposes of inclusion into contractual obligations the services that will be included or excluded. Service inclusion could be based on specific programs such as the following:

- Pediatrics
- Homemaker
- IV therapies
- Cardiac
- Respiratory therapy
- Geriatrics
- Hospice
- Medical equipment
- Rehabilitation
- Orthopedics
- Meals on wheels
- Supplies
- Obstetrics
- Psychiatric
- Home modifications
- Nutrition
- Wound care

Services can have limits attached to them. Limits can be based on the number of units provided to a specific patient. Units can include the number of hours, visits, medication doses, or supplies that would be furnished to a particular patient. Limits can be quantified in terms of total dollars, time on service, rental time before purchasing, number of patients on service at any one time, or diagnosis/disease. Diagnosis/disease limits can be spelled out by DRG; patient problem; or types of chronic cases, such as patients who have AIDS or cancer. Limits can also include specific patient treatment requirements, such as ventilators.

It is important to consider exclusion of specific cases and types of patients from capitated or episodic payments. Exclusion may simply require defining an alternative formula for compensating the HHA to provide services. Negotiating that all chronic cases be paid on a fee-for-service basis would help to reduce HHA risk. This represents a "carve out" or population refinement. HHAs may want to consider a provision for catastrophic losses. Stop-loss insurance is expensive and may be available through the MCO or commercially. Purchase of stop-loss insurance is a necessary cost in a capitated environment and should be figured into the cost of providing care when negotiating with MCOs. Stop-loss insurance can be purchased for individual occurrences or in the aggregate.

Programs can also be defined by the type of services that will be provided within each program. Program specifics may include intermittent visits, hourly services, shift care, personal care services, day care, or live-in services. Services would include or exclude disciplines, types of medical equipment, and IV therapies, such as the following:

- Nursing
- Speech therapists
- Home health aides
- Orthotics
- Preventive medicine
- Home dialysis
- Nursing aides
- Occupational therapists
- Social services
- Prosthetics
- Support groups
- Oxygen
- Physical therapists
- Nutritionists
- Pain therapies
- Braces
- Community education

- Therapy aides
- Pastoral services
- Enteral/total parenteral nutrition
- Wheelchairs
- Blood products

ACCESSIBILITY OF SERVICES

The scope of service would also need to be defined according to the geographic area that the agency is willing to cover, determination of what happens if a patient is seen for home health services outside of the network, and determination of what happens if the patient is hospitalized or requires emergency care while on service at the HHA. Agencies will need to review contractual requirements in light of the services that they propose to offer. For instance, it may be infeasible to provide around-the-clock nursing services or have every hospital discharge seen for home health evaluation 12 hours after discharge. All types of service delivery will need to be negotiated into the contract prior to signing. Anything that is not clarified could potentially increase the HHA's risk.

Accessibility will also be determined by how the HHA chooses to compete. For instance, if the HHA enters into a local managed care contract, the geographic area will be limited versus entering into a regional or national contract. Service accessibility will influence an agency's staffing policies, recruitment and retention efforts, and the need to form subcontract relationships with other providers to provide coverage.

Accessibility from the MCO's perspective can be expanded to include the concept of one-stop shopping. How easy it is for the MCO to make a referral will be an issue. Is the HHA a one-stop provider, or will the MCO be forced to make multiple referrals? From the perspective of the MCO, the one-stop shopper is preferred because of administrative ease, monitoring of compliance with the MCO's policies and procedures, and evaluation of patient satisfaction.

FORECASTING SERVICE LEVELS

In preparing to bid on these services, agencies need to obtain some information from the managed care organization, such as hospital utilization reports, summaries of outpatient utilization (therapies, home care, medical supplies, equipment, infusion therapies), total number of enrollees by payor source, and episodes of care reports. An extensive amount of information may be available from these reports, which include a beneficiary analysis of all services rendered to the client for a defined event. This allows extraction of average number of visits per diagnosis data, along with length of stay averages to be determined. These factors assist agency administrators in understanding the organization's utilization patterns and coverage items, allowing bids for services that are acceptable to both parties.[18]

Information obtained from the MCO can be combined with data within the HHA's information system. The HHA's bid preparation team can forecast levels of care using actual agency care guidelines. Care requirements can be determined by sorting actual results in the agency's database and then extrapolating against information obtained from the MCO. The results of this type of analysis may forewarn the HHA of potential problems from entering into contractual relationships with the MCO. For instance, if the MCO's utilization levels are below the HHA's, this is a good indication that the HHA may need to work on its utilization protocols prior to entering into a relationship with the MCO. Another possibility would be that the HHA used data from its cost-reimbursed Medicare population. These data will not offer a one-to-one correlation unless the MCO is covering a similar patient base. Therefore, it is best to try to match data obtained from the MCO by age, sex, geographic area, and type of service requirements.

If possible, attempt to get trend information by month, type of service, and discipline. Trend information by hospital discharge, physician groups, clinics, and other potential referral sources will help determine whether home care utilization is increasing.

> Utilization projections must be realistic. Experienced medical groups will not use services at the same rate as a newly formed independent practice association (IPA). Projections should address the likelihood of significant, uncontrolled utilization and the IPA doctor's unfamiliarity with ordering services. Trending should factor in the effect of educating doctors inexperienced in managed care over the term of the contract. Also, projections should be differentiated by product line, such as commercial, Medicare and Medicaid enrollees. Utilization of services within each plan will differ.[19]

Utilization needs to include catastrophic cases.

It is also important to remember that the agency's relationship with the MCO will change depending on the type of payment structure that is selected. "Under capitation payment to the HHA, the HMO has an incentive to maximize home health use (since its payments to the HHA are the same regardless of home health use), while the HHA has the opposite incentive to minimize such use. The incentives are reversed under the FFS payment arrangements between HMOs and

HHAs, in which case the HMO will have an incentive to minimize home health use, while the HHA's incentive will be to maximize use."[20]

DEVELOPMENT OF A BUDGET

Once services have been identified and potential service utilization forecasted, it is time to develop a budget. The development of a budget will serve many purposes. The primary purpose is to determine fluctuation from service requirements that could present a financial hardship for the agency or provide a source of renegotiation with the MCO. Changes in utilization may be due to changes in the MCO practice guidelines, additions or changes in the network, changes in benefits offered by the MCO, seasonality, or geographic expansion of the plan. These changes should be analyzed immediately by management and, if they could threaten the HHA negatively, communicated immediately to the MCO with the hope of enabling the HHA to renegotiate its payment rates. Additionally,

> differentiating between eligible and non-eligible members is critical for budgeting and assessing utilization.
>
> If a provider group is capitated to provide a single service, budgeting may be straightforward. But if multiple services are provided, budgeting issues increase exponentially. There is a tendency to overlook questions such as how eligible members who go outside your service area are to be treated. That can be an expensive situation if a member must have non-contracted providers render the treatment. Usually, the contracted provider group cannot obtain discounts from outside providers in keeping with the discounts demanded by the managed care contract.
>
> When capitating multiple services, assign each a reasonable allocation of the capitation and clearly define how each will be identified and tracked. A computer tracking system should be developed prior to the implementation of services.[21]

The information system can have all forecast assumption entered to facilitate monitoring contract utilization and compliance. Budget data can be identified by month, referral source, physician, team, medical diagnosis, or even nursing diagnosis to enhance monthly analysis.

ACTUAL UTILIZATION

> Newly capitated providers often underestimate the amount of preparation, planning and management necessary in the administration of a capitated contract. This is particularly true of providers who must reimburse other providers to perform some of the services covered under

capitation. In essence, some of the capitated providers find themselves owing large sums that they have failed to accrue. In several instances, the providers have already spent their capitation payment. To make matters worse, the more members that are enrolled, the further into debt the provider becomes. To justify to the HMO that the risk pool was inadequately funded, data is crucial. Conversely, if the HMO does not receive significant encounter data to substantiate the level of funding for the risk pool, it will be inclined to renegotiate the funding at a lesser amount for any subsequent contracts.[22]

OTHER FINANCIAL ISSUES

Assessment of organizational abilities and how they relate to the different prospective payment possibilities is key to the long-run viability of an HHA. Providers may want to consider partial capitation as a way to increase their business base, enhance their bottom line, improve the payor mix, eliminate collection problems, or simply increase their visibility to the managed care community. It is important to know which MCOs are in the community, whether they are moving toward capitated payment systems, and whether there is an opportunity to bid on a capitated contract.

Entering into a partially capitated contract enables HHAs to offer services that can control utilization. Services that may be uncontrollable will require HHAs to negotiate fee-for-service arrangements. The long-term element of this strategy is to transition into full capitation as organizational abilities warrant. This requires becoming extremely knowledgeable about the relationships between utilization and costs.

Whether in a partially capitated or fully capitated contract, it is important to try to minimize risk. Risk can be decreased by negotiating risk payment corridors, payment floors, and ceilings. Risk payment corridors identify an upper and lower limit in relationship to the capitated, episodic, or per diem payment (Figure 5–5). Differences between the payments and costs within the upper and lower limits represent either a profit or loss to the agency. "The floor plan protects the home care provider from excessive losses because of use and cost factors that could not be influenced by the provider. The floor plan guarantees the provider that the risk payments will not fall below a certain percentage of normal charges. A ceiling plan protects the HMO or PPO from overpayments and limits the profit of home care providers to an agreed upon level. The ceiling plan guarantees the payer that the risk payments will not exceed a certain percentage of the provider's normal charges."[23]

Payment floors and ceilings should be negotiated with the ability to convert to a fee-for-service payment system within 48 hours if costs exceed negotiated limits.

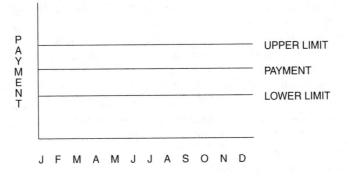

Figure 5–5 Risk Payment Corridors. Source: Reprinted from *The Managed Care Workbook: How To Get Started on the Never Ending Road to Managed Care*, p. 35, with permission of Corridor Media, © 1993.

In the event that an agency would experience profits in excess of the limits, then timing of rate negotiation or settlement should be spelled out. Integral to this negotiation is defining what constitutes direct cost. Direct cost should be all costs related to the contract. This is direct labor; employee costs or burden; and the indirect costs of providing patient care, such as case management, billing, scheduling, records management, and quality improvement. Negotiated profit margins for administrative expenses should be those administrative expenses that do not fluctuate with the provision of care and increases or decreases in patient census. Direct cost in relationship to capitated payments needs to be monitored on a daily basis. This can be accomplished through the development of a control chart that measures the relationship of actual cost to the capitated payment. Applying the negotiated floors and ceilings to the capitated payment will give an upper and lower limit to track actual costs. The control chart can be used to develop a picture of one month at a time or the entire year. Analysis of fluctuation on an annual basis will help to develop a better understanding of utilization of home health services in relationship to the population being tracked.

Whatever strategy is employed, it is important to understand how the MCO will pay for services. Cash flow can be wonderful in a capitated payment if payments are made at the beginning of the month. Payments that are made subsequent to the first of the month will increase the cost of doing business with the MCO. Verification that payments are made on a timely basis is a good strategy. If payment is not made on a timely basis, make sure that the HHA has considered alternative actions, and document what the agency's responsibilities are when the contract is terminated. What happens to the patients who remain on service, who will pay for the services that are provided?

Payments that are net of withholdings could significantly increase the cost of doing business. Withholdings will be dependent on the type of contract that is entered. If the HHA is entering into a full-service home health contract in which other providers furnish goods and services, the withholding check is designed to protect against excess utilization by the other providers. If the MCO is going to withhold money, it is important to understand what services money will be withheld for and how services can be monitored to ensure that all the withholding is returned. Make sure any withholding is clearly spelled out, and there is no possibility of retroactive adjustments to withholding. Retroactive adjustments may also apply to enrollment. Make sure that the HHA is not penalized for inconsistencies in the MCO's reporting processes.

Another factor to consider is how the other providers in the network are being incented. Home health could become a dumping ground for patients if physician groups, clinics, hospitals, and any other potential referral source transitions to a capitated status part way into the HHA's contract year. This could increase utilization exponentially. When incentives are aligned, there is a major opportunity to deliver efficient services across the entire continuum of care.

TREAD CAUTIOUSLY

Prospective payment vehicles will put agencies at risk. Agencies should take their time jumping into managed care contracts. It is important to understand each component of the process. It is also important to remember that each managed care organization will be different. There will be differences in policies and procedures, inclusion and exclusion of services, utilization patterns, reporting requirements, and payment policies. Jumping into managed care for the sake of having a managed care contract may not be a wise organizational strategy. However, entering into a managed care contract and using it as a tool for organizational learning prior to entering into additional contracts may be a prudent move.

By approaching managed care cautiously, providers have an opportunity to learn how to case manage efficiently, develop reporting systems, and train staff appropriately. Inherent in any new venture are some mistakes. It is better to make the mistakes on a small scale and recover versus potentially not recovering from a large fatal mistake. It is easier to absorb problems if a mistake represents 10 percent of the business and the balance of the business is profitable than if the mistake represents 40 percent of the business.

Another element to consider is that home health is recognized as a low-cost solution to the health care delivery system. Without common reward systems, incentives, and alliances home health could potentially be abused within the managed care network unless sufficient safeguards are built in to reward the HHA for increases in utilization beyond that on which the payment was based.

The long-run implications of managed care suggest that home care will eventually be thought of as a primary site provider instead of an alternative site provider. Home health will gain recognition as a low-cost solution across the entire continuum of care, and, as capitation moves into a global payment system, the paradigm shift will be updated to transition from an organizational perspective to a network perspective where services are actively managed for efficiency, quality, and patient outcomes.

NOTES

1. R.E. Schlenker and P.W. Shaughnessy, Medicare Home Health Reimbursement Alternatives: Access, Quality, and Cost Incentives, *Home Health Care Services Quarterly* 13, no 1/2 (1992): 91–115.

2. NAHC. 1994. *Basic Statistics about Home Care*. Washington, DC.

3. P. Boland, *Making Managed Healthcare Work: A Practical Guide to Strategies and Solutions* (Gaithersburg, MD: Aspen Publishers, 1993), 289.

4. Corridor Media, *The Managed Care Workbook: How To Get Started on the Never Ending Road to Managed Care* (Overland Park, KS: 1993), 32.

5. V.K. Saba, *Develop and Demonstrate a Method for Classifying Home Health Patients To Predict Resource Requirements and To Measure Outcomes* (Washington, DC: Georgetown University, 1991).

6. Corridor Media, *The Managed Care Workbook*, 34.

7. Corridor Media, *The Managed Care Workbook*, 35.

8. Corridor Media, *The Managed Care Workbook*, 36.

9. A.M. Kramer, et al., Assessing and Assuring the Quality of Home Health Care: A Conceptual Framework, *The Milbank Quarterly* 68, no. 3 (1990): 413–43.

10. P.W. Shaughnessy, et al., *A Study of Home Health Care Quality and Cost under Capitated and Fee-for-Service Payment Systems* (Denver: Center for Health Policy Research, 1994), v.

11. P.W. Shaughnessy, *A Study of Home Health Care Quality and Cost*, 3.1.

12. D.A. Randall, Legal Issues in Managed Care Contracting for Home Care Providers, *The Remmington Report* (August/September 1994): 43.

13. National Committee for Quality Assurance, *Accreditation Status List* (Washington, DC: September 1994), 1.

14. D.A. Randall, Legal Issues in Managed Care Contracting, 43.

15. L. Hurst, Know Your Business and Where It's Going Before Tackling Capitation, *Managed Home Care Report* 1, no. 2 (August 1994): 10.

16. D.L. Coleman, Don't Get Trapped by Managed Care Contracts, *Physician's Management* (March 1994): 52.

17. D.A. Randall, Legal Issues in Managed Care Contracting, 44.

18. H.E. Russo, Choosing a Direction for Success in Private Care, *Caring* 13, no. 6 (June 1994): 14.

19. L. Hurst, Know Your Business and Where It's Going, 10.

20. P.W. Shaughnessy, et al., *A Study of Home Health Care Quality and Cost*, 3.2.

21. L. Hurst, Know Your Business and Where It's Going, 10.
22. L. Hurst, Know Your Business and Where It's Going, 12.
23. Corridor Media, *The Managed Care Workbook*, 35.

Chapter 6

Prospective Payment Strategies

Venturing into the world of managed care will require all participants to begin to think like the customers that they serve. Customers will be a combination of patients, case managers, third-party administrators, managed care organizations (MCOs), physicians, and fee-for-service payors. Each customer will be concerned about management of care, appropriateness of services, and control of costs. From the patients' perspective, they want the necessary services to return them to their preillness condition or to obtain maximum postillness function. An agency's other customers want to see the purchaser of their health insurance (the patient) receive the necessary and appropriate services to obtain maximum outcomes given their specific situation.

Appropriateness of services may have different connotations depending on who is using the term. Appropriateness of services becomes an important concept when attempting to provide high-quality outcomes, manage outcomes, and satisfy clients. Therefore, clear communication becomes an integral component of beginning to think like the customer. Success will be due to thinking like a managed care employee, an insurer, or a case manager. The struggle will be to balance the requirements of community health nursing with the new model of managed care.

Community health nursing considers many environmental factors when developing a care plan or determining how long to leave patients on service. Services tend to have a more holistic approach; consequently, this could cause length of time on service and variety of services to be greater in a community health setting. The cost-based reimbursement system encouraged visit maximization; therefore, care plans could be developed that would provide aide services to help out with light cooking, house cleaning, grocery shopping, and trips to the drug store. Nursing services could be extended as a method of providing an external support system to a patient. Unfortunately, the paradigm shift from cost-based service provision to managed care will require reducing empathetic service provision.

In contrast, MCOs tend to be more concerned with maintenance of the physiological problems; therefore, outcomes and care management for specific physiological problems tend to be less than those in community health.[1] Furthermore, at the point services are discontinued it will be up to the patient and his or her caregiver to complete the balance of the healing process. The challenge for home health agencies (HHAs) will be to document how and why service provision made a difference in patient outcomes.

Agencies that will flourish in managed care will develop case management systems and protocols. Case management systems will determine appropriate levels of care and balance patient advocacy with the financial constraints of payors. Case management systems that utilize clinical pathways as a benchmarking device for training, continuous quality improvement, organizational learning, and negotiations will be in a better place to balance the diverse needs of all the agency's customers.

CASE MANAGEMENT

Case management is not new to home health care. Nurses manage patients/clients every day. "Inherent in the management of a client is the responsibility of the nurse to determine the type of intervention necessary and to determine when nursing service is no longer appropriate. Based on client needs and the outcome of nursing interventions, the nurse makes the decision as to whether the case remains open or is closed to nursing services."[2]

Determination of service levels, type of interventions, length of time on service, inclusion or exclusion of medical supplies, and interventions from other disciplines will affect resource consumption. Service levels will depend on the patient's physiological condition, psychosocial and environmental domain, and attitudes toward his or her own health management.[3] Every time a patient is admitted to an HHA, the assessment process includes the evaluation of multiple variables when developing a care plan. Each nurse will develop a slightly different care plan depending on his or her assessment in relationship to the agency's policies for the provision of care.

This model works well in a cost-reimbursed environment. However, with the transition into managed care, there is a need to develop consistent approaches to the delivery of care. Consistency will enable providers to measure outcomes, understand the relationships between patient requirements and costs, and analyze whether there is an opportunity to streamline the care delivery process.

One of the ways to develop consistency in clinical operations is through controlling the case management function.

> Case management can have a narrow or wide span of control. It can be a
> gatekeeping mechanism to control costs and access; it can be an advo-

cacy function to increase access to services, and navigate a confusing array of services; or it can serve a diagnostic and prescriptive function. It can be an administrative function or a service in and of itself. The most generally accepted components of case management are:

- Eligibility determination—financial, medical, or other;
- Level of care determination;
- Assessment of needs—including medical, physical, functional, psychosocial, availability of family support;
- Place of care determination;
- Care plan development;
- Service prescription or arrangement;
- Coordination of services from multiple providers;
- Budget planning for service units, time periods, episodes;
- Reassessment of needs;
- Monitoring delivery and quality; and
- Support to the family.

Other activities can also be included in the case management model. Most providers are not able to provide all services directly; thus they must develop the capacity to deal with other providers of both similar and different services. Soliciting bids, screening, hiring and monitoring service providers can be an important part of the program, even if provider based.[4]

Agencywide case management provides a mechanism to control utilization of all services provided within and throughout the agency. Case management should develop common guidelines for all of the agency's field staff to follow. Common guidelines provide an opportunity to administer consistent levels of care across all patients with similar problems. Linking case management to clinical pathways will provide HHAs with a tool to evaluate and enhance the case management process. Once clinical pathway standards are developed, case managers can be advocates for additional patient services with MCOs because they will know what services are necessary to deliver a specific outcome.

A specialized approach to case management is to designate an individual to manage chronic patients or patients who have intense service requirements. Management of these types of patients would enable the agency to maintain a close link between the patient, the family, and the payor. The agency case manager would work with the patient, family, and payor to find creative ways of providing care while attempting to control costs. Development of this type of individual provides a support mechanism for all parties, including the agency.

Another type of case management is to assign a specific nurse to a physician, hospital, or payor. The designated individual would be responsible for providing a communication link to ensure services are consistent with the objectives of the physician, hospital, or payor. This role enhances the connection between the agency and its customer and even allows for specialization and customization of services. Further specialization will occur when case management efforts are coordinated between specific teams. Inclusion of multidisciplinary teams into the case management concept will help to provide consistent services and facilitate smooth communication between all care providers.

Regardless of what approach is adopted at an agency level, the bottom line is that the case manager, case management team, or case management process must be able to assess the effect that patient problems, the patient's characteristics (age, the presence or lack of caregiver, activities of daily living, patient's home environment) will have on the amount of services a patient will require. Service levels may vary because of the required interventions, discharge patterns by physician or referral source, and the timeline for providing care. All these factors need to be considered in evaluating appropriate service levels.

Case managers who negotiate with MCOs, indemnity insurers, or other payors will need to make financial decisions based on factors other than nursing diagnosis. Therefore, it is important to understand different levels of care that may be provided within medical diagnosis classifications. Extrapolating based on primary and secondary diagnoses, other factors provided over the phone, and the agency's clinical pathway system, the case manager will be in a position to negotiate on behalf of the agency. Actual costs and service levels need to be monitored to enhance agency case management ability continually. This is especially true if the case manager will be negotiating episodic or per diem payments on behalf of the agency.

CLINICAL PATHWAYS

Clinical pathways have many names. They have been referred to as *care maps, care plans, clinical guidelines, patient management protocols,* and *care paths.* Clinical pathways are also budgets. A simple nursing clinical pathway would outline on a daily basis specific nursing interventions that are to be completed. Nursing interventions would be determined based on patient problem and designed to help patients obtain a specific outcome. Outcomes are measurable and can be determined for a specific admission and patient problem.

Understanding the frequency of visits, type of nursing interventions, and the disciplines involved will enable HHAs to examine the costs of providing care. Understanding resource consumption enhances an agency's ability to case manage. This concept is especially important in an episodic or capitated payment environment.

The measurement of resource consumption in relationship to the clinical pathway will identify how many units of service are required for a specific patient problem. Resource consumption is measured in units of service by discipline, time, and dollars. Therefore, providing more visits or interventions will increase resource consumption and the cost of providing care.

Development of clinical pathways will not take nurses' autonomy away from them when providing patient care. The clinical pathway represents an agency standard that has been developed by a multidisciplinary team. The standard provides a benchmark for developing better information about the clients who are served. Additionally, by linking costs to the clinical pathway, the agency has a tool for negotiating with an MCO for the provision of care. Armed with actual results, an agency can effectively determine whether a proposed payment will provide an adequate return based on the resources they would normally expend to provide care for a patient with a specific problem.

Other considerations to include in the negotiation process would be the amount of travel that may be required to see a patient, the timing of the referral, and the geographic location. Travel expense is a nonvalue-added expense that is incurred to provide patient care. Travel expense includes paying a provider to commute to the patient's home for actual mileage and his or her time. The timing of the referral may require the agency to bonus a nurse or a team to provide services late at night, on a weekend, or on a holiday. Geographic area may require an escort to ensure that the nurse is not harmed while seeing a patient.

Beyond negotiating, clinical pathways provide an opportunity for refinement of the care delivery process. By tracking and monitoring deviations from the clinical pathway, the HHA has an opportunity to assess whether the clinical pathway is appropriate or whether the pathway needs to be adjusted. Adjustment could be due to myriad factors. Factors could include an improper patient classification or the need to expand the clinical pathway to include another patient grouping. Adjustment could also be due to the development of a clinical pathway that was too aggressive given the patient population being served.

Development of Clinical Pathways

Clinical pathways are patient classification systems that can be used to determine resource consumption. "The elements of a patient classification system can be summarized as (a) a method for grouping patients based by disease, procedures, level of wellness, or some combination of these using either a prototype or factor design; (b) a quantification of the nursing care resources associated with each category of care; and (c) a method of calculating staffing for required nursing hours."[5]

A study conducted at Georgetown University identified that medical diagnosis is not a good indicator of resource consumption. A better indicator of resource consumption is nursing diagnosis based on patient problem. The study concluded that combining nursing diagnosis and nursing interventions was the best way of forecasting resource consumption.[6]

Therefore, clinical pathway development based on patient problem will provide agencies with the best tool for evaluating the diverse needs of the home care patient. Construction of the clinical pathway can take several forms. One form is to assemble a multidisciplinary team to develop clinical pathways based on the collective experience of the team. The cost to assemble representatives from each of the disciplines to accumulate their best guesses may be prohibitive for most agencies. A second alternative is to review existing charts and records for patients who have common characteristics. Identification of common characteristics leads to the development of homogeneous groups.

Homogeneous groups will exhibit similar characteristics. Resource consumption can be forecasted with a higher degree of accuracy. Homogeneous groups will have similar patient problems, require similar services and interventions, and lend themselves to development of a specific clinical pathway.

Once a specific homogeneous group has been targeted, results can be summarized, and the team of multidisciplinary experts can be brought back to develop the clinical pathway. Development of the clinical pathway will define the patient problem that is being addressed, the outcome to be achieved, and interventions required to achieve the desired outcome, and estimate the type and frequency of services. In reality, patients will have more than one nursing problem. The Georgetown study indicated that the average patient had three nursing diagnoses.[7] Identification of singular or groups of patient problems will identify homogeneous groups and, subsequently, clinical pathways. By grouping patients with homogeneous requirements, "variation of requirements within classes would be minimized while variation among classes would be maximized."[8]

The multidisciplinary team would summarize patient problems to determine potential clinical pathway development. Targeting of clinical pathways may be based on the frequency of a specific type of patient being admitted to the agency or a particularly high-cost problem the agency is attempting to control. The clinical pathway would identify the approximate number of visits by discipline, probable interventions for each visit, and possible outcomes for each visit. Interventions would be different by discipline, dependent on specific patient problem and whether the patient was at the beginning or end of the clinical pathway.

The oldest of the patient classification systems is the Omaha System. The Omaha system was developed over a 15-year period by the Visiting Nurse Association of Omaha beginning in 1975.

> The problem classification scheme is a listing of patient conditions or
> health problems that allows for uniform language for the collecting,

sorting, classifying, documenting, and analyzing of patient care data. The intervention scheme focuses on nursing actions or activities and provides nurses with a typology for depicting the services offered by a community agency. The intervention scheme consists of three levels of abstraction: 1) categories; 2) targets; and 3) client-specific information. Four intervention categories make up the first level of the intervention scheme: 1) health teaching, guidance, and counseling; 2) treatments and procedures; 3) case management; and 4) surveillance. The second level in the intervention scheme is called targets, which are objects of nursing interventions or nursing activities. This level of abstraction is used to further describe a plan or intervention category that is specific to a patient's problem. The third level of the intervention scheme is devoted to the listing of client-specific data, and makes up the detailed portion of the care plan for a specific patient problem or nursing diagnoses.[9]

The ability of the Omaha System to characterize large aggregate populations across different agencies has great potential for future research. Administrators, practitioners, and policy makers can use aggregate data as a basis for examining the client case mix and relating that mix to specific nursing diagnoses, interventions, and client outcomes. Furthermore, the cost-effectiveness of such relationships can be evaluated, an action that is of increasing interest to policy makers. Changes in client's knowledge, behavior, and status outcome ratings between admission and dismissal in such a large sample strongly suggest that home health service does make a difference.[10]

Inclusion of a standardized intervention scheme will enhance the development and measurement processes. From a development perspective, all clinical pathways will use a common system. This system, once adopted, would provide a consistent way of determining specific interventions to apply to patient problems. Interventions could then be evaluated to determine effectiveness. Interventions from a measurement perspective could be evaluated to determine whether they were accomplishing the intended outcome and whether combining interventions or increasing the frequency of interventions would have a material effect on patient outcomes.

The clinical pathway can have two types of outcomes. The first outcome is codeveloped with the patient. This outcome is for the total episode of care. An example of an outcome would be that a wound is healed or the patient is pain-free. Outcomes will take different forms depending on specific patient problems.

"By negotiating outcomes with clients at the start of care, both client and care manager are clear about the purpose of the service."[11] This is an especially powerful consideration in the managed care environment. First, codevelopment of outcomes enhances patient accountability. Patient accountability should help in meeting the clinical pathway objective on time. If the objective is not met on time, and it is due to noncompliance, it may make it easier for the nurse/case manager to close down the case.[12]

The second set of outcomes is at the intervention level. Outcomes at the intervention level would represent targets for anticipated levels of patient progress. Each level of progress or lack of progress represents a choice point for the multidisciplinary team that is providing patient care. The clinical pathway can then be altered accordingly based on the team's assessment of how the patient is doing along the pathway.

Evaluation of Actual Results against Clinical Pathways

Clinical pathways represent an internal standard based on agency protocols. The standard can serve as a tool to assist clinicians in the development of care plans. Care plan development should use the clinical pathway as a guide; however, every patient is unique, thus requiring customization to meet specific needs. Variation from the clinical pathway can then be used to learn more about the population that the agency serves. For instance, variation could be due to the fact that there is no caregiver present to help a patient practice ambulating; therefore, a physical therapist is ordered.

Variation could result from the development of the clinical pathway for one specific patient problem and the patient had three problems. An example would be if the clinical pathway was developed for an open surgical wound, but the actual patient problem was an open surgical wound that included the additional problems of pain and nutrition. In this situation, there are two homogeneous groups: one group for open surgical wounds only and the other group for the three patient problems of wounds, pain, and nutrition. On recognition of another homogeneous group, the agency can choose to develop another clinical pathway or continue to analyze variances due to the lack of homogeneity in its classification system.

Clinical pathways will provide an agency with an internal benchmarking system. This is extremely important for several reasons. The first is that home health currently has no national standards. The second is that by developing an internal benchmarking system, the agency can use its own standards to improve its processes. Process improvement using an internal benchmarking system ensures that there is consistency in measurement and populations being measured. Use of a national or regional standard may have major differences in the population being measured. Differences in age, sex, rehabilitative practices, and discharge practices could significantly affect national or regional results. Until there is a way to minimize the effect of patient and practice variation, the internal benchmark provides the best tool for continuous quality improvement efforts.

Variation could be measured in terms of units, hours, dollars, or outcomes. Variation from the internal benchmark could be used as a source of organizational learning. Understanding why the variance took place will help to build appropriate clinical pathways. Inherent in the construction of clinical pathways is the goal of building efficiencies into the care delivery process. Efficiencies can be built into the process by understanding the relationships between patient problems, visit requirements, frequency of visits, and visit interventions. Clinical pathways are evolutionary, and, by experimenting with the mix of visits, the frequency of visits, and the combining of interventions, economies can be gained.

Analysis of outcomes can become a source of organizational learning as well. Outcome measurement can take five forms: outcomes can be (1) met, (2) met early, (3) met late, (4) never met, or (5) changed. If outcomes are met early, it is important to understand whether this is attributable to specific patient characteristics, a specific team, an acceleration of visits, or inclusion of aide services. Analysis of the met late outcome may uncover that patients in this category never received visits from a specialist, because of noncompliance or because the team provided substandard care. Additionally, attaching a reason to the outcomes of changed or never met will help to improve the learning process.

Variance analysis will also identify differences in resource requirements because of specific patient characteristics. For instance, service intensity can be very different based on the type of physiological problem that a patient may have. Service intensity can be compounded by the patient's home environment because of architectural barriers, psychosocial problems, or the patient's role as primary caregiver for another individual. Many variables are considered in the actual management of patient problems. Therefore, a good patient classification system will consider the same variables when estimating resource consumption and use the initial assessment as a base for the development of a clinical pathway.

Continuous Quality Improvement

Continuous quality improvement (CQI) occurs through developing an internal standard, plan, or benchmark. Once the benchmark has been developed, nurses and field staff would be trained in its use. Actual results would be monitored against the standard, and variances could be analyzed. Findings from the analysis process would cause the standards to be revised. Revision of the standards would require updating staff on changes in the standard, and the monitoring and analysis would resume using the revised standard.

This approach to quality improvement is a little different from the medical model of quality assurance. Quality assurance is a retrospective process. Charts and records were reviewed to assess whether the care that was provided was sufficient given the nurse's assessment. One of the paramount concerns was to support reimbursement levels. Often quality assurance was performed weeks or months after the care had been provided, so when mistakes were found, the efforts of the quality assurance department could be in vain because of the amount of time that had transpired between actual service and opportunity identification.

The other end of the quality improvement spectrum is a process that is assessment focused. When quality improvement initiatives are built into the assessment process and taken into consideration while developing clinical pathways, then outcomes and the quality improvement process become dynamic. Each point along the clinical pathway actually becomes an opportunity for the nurse, therapist, aide, or patient to assess how he or she is progressing against the standard. Positive variances may provide an opportunity to enhance outcomes or reduce costs. Negative variances may provide opportunities to identify different approaches in care delivery. Changing an agency's CQI process to an outcome-oriented, assessment-based system will enhance the perception of quality in the eyes of the patient, community, and payor.

An assessment-driven CQI process also focuses on the management of quality outcomes. This concept looks at each point along the clinical pathway as a choice point. Choice points allow providers, patients, and patients' caregivers an opportunity to assess how they are doing in relation to the codeveloped outcomes that were selected on admission into the home health program. Choice allows for different strategies to obtain desired outcomes or possibly changing outcomes if circumstances change. This approach is more dynamic than outcome measurement in that it is based entirely on two points in time: (1) admission and (2) discharge.

Combining multidisciplinary teams with a CQI program that builds on assessments could have far-reaching effects for creating efficiencies in the care delivery process. Assuming that the goal of the team is greater than the goal of any one discipline, by experimenting with frequency of visits and the combination of interventions, there may be an opportunity to increase patient outcomes and lower agency cost. Sharing the results of combined efforts with each team may spark some healthy internal competition to enhance team and agency performance continually.

Actual results could then be used as a marketing tool for the agency. For instance, if results indicated that 98 percent of patients who were admitted because of a surgical wound achieved their goals within 9 visits, then these results could be shared with managed care providers, the community, and other payors. It would also be possible to say that the agency can guarantee these results for $630. Additionally, the results of patient satisfaction surveys could be linked to these results.

Outcomes

Outcomes are the natural evolution of the CQI process that places emphasis on actual performance by identifying where changes are needed. Patient outcomes when linked to clinical pathways and the case management process can provide an agency with a powerful tool for assessing the quality and value of services. When viewed from a systems orientation, outcomes provide a target to achieve. Agency processes are then designed to achieve that outcome. Outcome obtainment is the result of agency processes with respect to patients characteristics, such as their physiological and psychosocial problems, their home environment, and how their particular service requirements may have been influenced by physician or payor practices. Other inputs would include team members; how well team members relate to the patient; and inclusion or exclusion of medicines, medical supplies, equipment, and therapies.

Process would look at how the inputs mesh to accomplish actual results. The overall process includes many interventions. Interventions could be actual visits or telephone contact. Interventions would depend on patient problems and would vary depending on where the patient was on the clinical pathway. The cumulative result of many interventions and the patient's own healing represents the process. Process approaches will be different by agency, and, therefore, the results or outcomes will differentiate providers.

Patient progress will be measured in relationship to the desired outcomes. Patient outcomes will be a reflection of the level of care that an agency is providing, patient problems, and how well the care delivery team and patient work to accomplish mutually determined outcomes. This information is extremely important to patients, payors, accrediting agencies, and MCOs. MCOs have a responsibility to the purchasers of their products to deliver high-quality services. When contracting with an MCO, this responsibility is delegated to the HHA for providing high-quality care and measurable outcomes.

Patient Satisfaction Surveys

Another responsibility that is transferred from the MCO to the HHA is the monitoring of patient satisfaction. Patient satisfaction is a necessary component for the MCO's accreditation process and necessary to ensure that employers, groups, and individuals will continue to purchase their health insurance from the plan. Linking outcomes and patient survey results allow the agency and the MCO to market their services.

It is up to the agency to choose how to perform patient surveys. Monitoring survey results may indicate that a higher success rate occurs when the survey is performed by phone, a day after discharge, instead of mailing the survey to the patient's home after he or she has been discharged. The National Association of Medical Equipment Suppliers had the following recommendations for developing patient surveys[13]:

- *Standardize Questions*—Each participant should use the same survey tool and ask the same questions.

- *Standardize Scale*—Each participant should establish a consistent scale. The five-point scale provides the greatest variation without being too difficult for the customer.
- *Analyze Distribution Method*—The specific delivery or distribution method should be reviewed; each provider should maintain a consistent method.
- *Standardize Data Collection*—Data collection should be standardized to reduce the variations seen in the quality of the data analysis. The initial data should be designated to allow for classification by these factors: location, month, question, percentage response, and rate of return.
- *Differentiate Product Line*—Additional consideration should be given to methods to differentiate the information received by product or service-specific answers.

Development of specific questions would depend on what the agency was attempting to measure and what services were being provided. Development of questions should be designed to provide benchmarks for the agency to understand how it can improve its services. Question design should encompass administrative and clinical aspects of the care delivery process.

Payor-dependent Clinical Pathways

Development of multiple clinical pathways to maximize reimbursement could cause problems with operational efficiency. Clinical pathways that are designed to take advantage of different nuances in payment systems hypothetically could have different service levels for similar patient problems. This concept creates organizational inefficiencies by having different procedures, protocols, and review processes for each payor. This process adds a layer of complexity at the provider level, requiring field staff to keep track of what type of insurance the patient has instead of focusing on providing high-quality, outcome-oriented care. Furthermore, CQI processes would be duplicative and potentially ineffective.

A potential solution lies in the ability of the agency's case management system. Case managers can help to adjust service levels if they have an understanding of the agency's contractual obligations and the payment mechanisms of each contract. For instance, the agency may be in a fully capitated arrangement for nursing services but can bill the MCO for equipment ordered for the patient. Therefore, through ordering equipment that will enhance the healing processes, the agency can adhere to its clinical pathway and meet all of its patients' needs.

Population-dependent Clinical Pathways

Population-dependent clinical pathways will help the HHA reduce the risk of excess utilization in a managed care environment. MCOs commonly develop risk pools based on characteristics of the covered lives within the risk pool. For instance, one pool may be for a population in excess of 65 years of age. This population would require a different level of services than a working population with grown children or a working population with infants. Understanding the differences in populations can help the HHA develop specialized clinical pathways or build efficiencies into the clinical pathway because there is a higher probability of having alternate caregivers at home in a working population in contrast to an elderly population.

Reports

Results reporting will be critical in monitoring the provision of services in the managed care environment. Reporting needs to focus on utilization by contract, physician, hospital, employer group, or any other potential referral source. From a clinical pathway perspective, actual costs should be compared against the agency standard. All variances should be explained. Table 6–1 is a report that compares actual costs against the agency standard. The clinical pathway has been broken down into the two components of intermittent services and medical supplies. Variances are tracked against each.

In this situation, the aggregate number of intermittent service units is exactly as planned; however, the mix of services is different. Nursing substituted the services of a registered nurse (RN) for those of a licensed practical nurse (LPN). Total service units were the same; however, cost was less. The next step of the variance analysis would be to determine whether outcomes were positively or negatively affected by the change in service mix. It may be that by substituting a lower priced service (the LPN), the same outcome was achieved but at a lower agency cost.

Other reports could look at the composition of patient problems. Patient problems can be singular or multiple. Groupings of patient problems represent homogeneous groups that may require development of a specific clinical pathway. Patient problem identification can also be done within the major groupings of medical diagnoses. Grouping within medical diagnosis categories will assist the provider in determining the range of services that could fall within a medical diagnosis. This could provide a valuable insight into negotiating with MCOs that only have data based on disposition at the time of discharge from a hospital.

Additional reports could include an analysis of outcomes by patient problems. This report would identify the total admissions that an agency had for a particular patient problem, the percentage of admissions that achieved a specific outcome, and what the cost was to achieve a specific outcome. Cost analysis should identify low cost, median cost, mode cost, average cost, and maximum cost. Understanding how costs fluctuate by cost classification and outcome within a patient problem classification will enable an agency to link the care delivery processes to CQI and costing.

Table 6–1 Illustrative Clinical Pathway Cost Variance Analysis Format

Any Home Health Agency
Clinical Pathway Analysis: Actual vs. Standard

	Clinical pathway		Actual cost		Variance	
	Units	Cost ($)	Units	Cost ($)	Units	Cost ($)
Intermittent services						
Nursing	5.00	326.25	4.00	261.00	1.00	65.25
Nutrition	1.00	73.00	1.00	73.00		
LPN	____	____	1.00	33.86	(1.00)	(33.86)
Subtotal	6.00	399.25	6.00	367.86	0	31.39
Medical supplies						
Box of 4 × 4's	1.00	4.15	1.00	4.15		
Roll of tape	1.00	0.89	1.00	0.89		
Box of gauze	1.00	1.95	1.00	1.95		
Subtotal	3.00	6.99	3.00	6.99		
Grand total	9.00	406.24	9.00	374.85	0	31.39

Note: Clinical pathway developed for patient problem: integument impairment and nutritional deficit. Desired outcome to be achieved in five nursing and one nutrition visit. Stated outcome: wound is healed; patient is nourished.

Report definition would depend on who was to receive the report. If the report was for internal purposes, it may want to identify every patient who was admitted on a daily basis by patient problem and estimate total units of service that would be required prior to discharge. A report looking at discharged patients may focus on variances. Variances could be due to the initial estimate of total units being less or greater than actual requirements. Another discharge report may want to focus solely on patient outcomes. Reports for external purposes may display patient names, identification numbers, and all services that were provided to the patient during the reporting period. Another external report may look at the results of the patient survey results.

Attaching Cost to the Clinical Pathway

A great deal of time was spent on developing the concept of case management and clinical pathways. This is because one of the largest consumers of resources in an agency is the provision of patient care. Management of the care delivery process can be accomplished by using clinical pathways. Clinical pathways provide an estimate of resources that will be consumed depending on a specific patient problem. Clinical pathway estimates provide a standard for the entire agency, thus providing the agency with a standard or benchmark for managing the care delivery process. Deviations from the original estimate can be monitored against outcomes to determine whether there is a more efficient or economical way of providing care. Deviations will also indicate trends that are occurring within the community. These trends may require that the agency go back to the MCO and renegotiate.

Provision of patient care is the direct labor for the nurse, therapist, or aide to visit a patient, make telephone contact, or interact with other team members for case management purposes. Direct labor cost is incurred for travel to the patient's home, preparation for the visit, treatment time, documentation of the visit, and case management. In addition to direct labor cost is the employer cost, which is directly attributable to an employee. This cost would include payroll taxes, workers' compensation, health benefits, paid time off, possibly pension contributions, and continuing education. In addition to the direct labor and related overhead is the cost of materials and supplies. Materials and supplies include equipment, medical supplies, and infusion therapies.

The costs identified above represent resources that, when consumed, can be matched to a specific patient. Direct cost represents anywhere from 40 percent to 70 percent of an agency's revenue. Management of the direct cost of patient care represents an opportunity for HHAs to flourish in the managed care environment. Management of the direct cost of providing patient care should be done on a daily basis. This is very important for the management of risk-based contracts.

Assignment of costs to a clinical pathway provides an opportunity to develop a cost profile by clinical pathway. This profile can be used to assist in negotiations when the MCO calls and asks whether a particular patient can be accepted. Armed with good cost data, the agency can decide whether it is in its financial interest or political interest to accept this patient. Beyond specific patient identification, the cost profile can be used to determine whether lines of service should be continued or discontinued.

BUILDING EFFICIENCIES INTO THE PATIENT CARE DELIVERY PROCESS

Cost containment is central to success in a managed care environment. Cost containment usually has a negative connotation; however, when transitioning from a cost-reimbursed environment to a managed care environment, the meaning implies the need to build efficiencies into the care delivery system. Efficiencies are critical when the agency is receiving an episodic or capitated payment for services that it provides.

The actual cost of providing care represents a significant portion of an HHA's cost. (See Table 6–2.) When viewed as a percentage of revenue, the range will fluctuate depending on the payment system and the costs associated with providing care. For instance, if the HHA's normal charge for a nursing visit was $100,

Table 6–2 Cost of Service in a Fee-for-Service Environment

Rate	Cost	Percent
100.00	40.55	41
90.00	40.55	45
80.00	40.55	51
70.00	40.55	58
60.00	40.55	68

paid on average $33.79 for a nursing visit, and benefits ran approximately 20 percent, then it would have a patient care cost of 41 percent. The patient care cost would increase dramatically as the agency began to enter into discounted fee-for-service arrangements. The same nursing visit would have a 68 percent patient care cost if the discounted rate were $60.

To gain efficiencies in the provision of patient care, agencies need to get the unit cost of a nursing, therapy, or aide visit down as low as possible. The agency will need to consider how to build economies into the care delivery process. One of the best ways to decrease per unit cost is to look at agencywide productivity and how it relates to the cost per unit. Cost per unit will vary based on whether the agency pays its field nurses on a salary basis, hourly basis, or per visit. Cost will fluctuate because of different benefit packages for full-time versus part-time staff.

Every HHA will have a different strategy when it comes to recruitment, retention, and payment of its field staff. An approach that is useful in determining the most effective payment method for an agency to utilize for its field staff is to contrast the cost of the different payment methodologies. Table 6–3 illustrates how a per visit rate would be calculated for a salaried nurse. The calculation begins by determining the total amount of direct care time that a nurse would have available. This is calculated by subtracting nonpatient-care time from the total number of weeks in the year. Nonpatient-care time depends on agency policy. Policies could differ based on education, seniority, work experience, or technical qualifications. Typical nonpatient-care time includes vacation, sick time, personal time, time allotted for continuing education, and paid holidays.

To determine the number of visits that a salaried nurse can do in a year requires multiplying the average number of visits per day by the number of days in the work week, and then by the number of patient care weeks. This result will be divided into the nurse's annual salary expense. In Table 6–3, a minimum and maximum salary were used and increased by a factor of 20 percent for benefits.[14] Benefits would include health insurance, pension contribution, life insurance, employer payroll taxes, and workers' compensation insurance.

Table 6–4 indicates the range of per visit cost that could occur with a salaried employee. Fluctuations in per visit cost could be due to inefficiencies in the sched-

Table 6–3 Cost per Visit Calculation for a Salaried Nurse

	Minimum	Maximum
Total annual weeks	52	52
Less:		
Vacation	3	3
Paid holidays	1	1
Sick	1	1
Personal/education	1	1
Total nonpatient time (weeks)	6	6
Direct care work weeks	46	46
Visits per week @ 5.0	25	25
Total annual visits	1,150.00	1,150.00
Salary cost	$31,022.00	$38.723.00
Assume 20% benefit factor	6,204.40	7,744.60
Total salary cost	$37,226.40	$46,467.60
Per visit cost	$ 32.37	$ 40.41

uling of visits requiring the nurse to spend large amounts of time traveling between clients. Other factors could include meeting time, extended visit time, or poor management of organizational resources.

The 1994 National Association of Home Care *Basic Statistics about Home Care* indicates that the minimum and maximum per visit rates according to its survey were $25.83 and $33.79, respectively.[15] These rates did not include benefits. When increased for an estimated 20 percent benefit factor, the minimum and maximum rates are $31.00 and $40.55, respectively. Using the results in Table 6–4, this would indicate that the nurses in most agencies do approximately five visits per day.

However, by building efficiencies into the scheduling process, there may be a way to get an average of 6 visits per day from salaried nurses. The difference of $5.39 ($32.37 – $26.98) using the minimum pay scale, and $6.74 ($40.41 – $33.67) using the maximum pay scale across 20,000 annual nursing visits would provide the agency with significant savings in its patient care cost for nursing. The annual savings in the minimum pay range would equal $107,800 ($5.39 × 20,000 visits) and $134,800 ($6.74 × 20,000 visits) in the maximum pay range.

Efficiencies could be built into the scheduling process by analyzing the geographic area that the agency serves. Teams could be assigned to specific locations, blocks, ZIP codes, counties, or even apartment buildings. Assignment of providers or teams to specific locations should help to reduce nonvalue-added activities such as travel. If an agency is expanding its geographic area, it may want to consider paying staff on a salary basis for visits in tight geographic areas and utilizing

Table 6–4 Cost per Visit Fluctuation Based on Average Annual Visits

Visits per week	Cost per visit	Cost per visit
3.0	53.95	67.34
3.5	46.24	57.72
4.0	40.46	50.51
4.5	35.97	44.90
5.0	32.37	40.41
5.5	29.43	36.73
6.0	26.98	33.67
6.5	24.90	31.08
7.0	23.12	28.86

a per visit mechanism for the outliers. However, careful planning would be required to prevent discrimination problems.

Another cost to consider in analyzing salary versus per visit cost is the concept of replacement cost. Replacement cost is the cost of providing care when an employee is using company-provided benefits such as vacation, sick, personal, or education time. These employees will be paid for their time even though they are not providing patient care. However, care will still need to be provided in their absence. In effect, agencies will experience a higher cost of service in those periods when employees are using company-provided benefits.

When an agency transitions from a fee-for-service or a discounted fee-for-service environment to an episodic, per diem, or capitated payment system, the approach to building efficiencies into the system needs to be expanded. Service delivery will need to be evaluated in the context of the tools outlined above: case management, clinical pathways, and the relationship of care to quality and cost.

Efficiencies could be gained by simply combining skilled interventions that had once been separated into two distinct visits. This will create a longer visit; however, if the savings are greater than the increase in per visit cost, then there is an economic savings to the HHA. Using the average per visit cost from Table 6–4, a simplified example can be constructed to demonstrate this concept. If an agency is able to reduce two visits for every patient who enters the agency by combining skilled interventions, it would save $32.37 per patient assuming a productivity of 5 patients per day. Additionally, for purposes of illustration, if visits were combined, it may cause a shift in agency productivity from 5 visits per day to 4.5 visits per day, and the agency would experience an average cost increase per visit from $32.37 to $35.97 for all nursing visits.

Table 6–5 illustrates the possible savings that would accrue to an agency by combining skilled interventions and reducing the total number of visits. Additional savings would occur through the reduction of administrative costs related to the provision of patient care, such as travel. In Table 6–5, it was estimated that on

Table 6–5 Illustration of Agency Savings if Visits Are Decreased by Combining Interventions

	Patients	Visits per patient	Total RN visits	Per visit cost ($)	Total ($)
Original agency cost	2,000	10	20,000	32.37	647,400
Revised agency cost	2,000	8	16,000	35.97	575,520
Savings in direct care					71,880
Expense decrease in travel	(10 – 8) × 2,000 = 4,000 visits; 15 miles/visit @ 0.29				17,400
					89,280

average 15 miles were traveled for every nursing visit. Reducing total visits by 4,000 saved the agency approximately $17,400. Included in the reduction of travel expense are the savings in travel time, documentation time, and preparation time that would occur by reducing the number of visits. This would offset the reduction in daily productivity.

Transferring of responsibilities to informal caregivers can also reduce patient care expense. Duties that can be transferred are functions that would be performed by an aide, such as light meal preparation; shopping; and assistance with activities of daily living, such as bathing, transferring, eating, and toileting. Additionally, assistance with ambulation could reduce the need for physical therapy visits.

Additional economies can be built into an agency's patient care delivery system by developing an internal case management system that focuses on contact time instead of visit time. Development of an internal monitoring system that utilizes the telephone will enable an agency to save money. Contact can be made to the patient, the patient's caregiver, or even the patient's neighbor. The purpose of the contact would be to evaluate the patient's condition and assess whether there was a need for a professional visit or whether an intervention could be conducted over the phone. It may be that by walking a patient or caregiver through the steps of administering medication or changing a dressing, the patient will remain on target with his or her healing process, and the agency would not incur the cost of an additional visit.

Using the example in Table 6–5, if an internal case management system is developed that saves on average 1 nursing visit per patient annually, as a result of a 5- to 10-minute phone call, the agency would save approximately $64,740 (2,000 × $32.37). Depending on the agency's structure, this could either be a net savings or offset by the cost of an individual whose sole responsibility is to provide case management support. This function will also serve to provide an agency support system for patients and their caregivers. It may also help to enhance communications between the agency and its other clients, such as physicians, payors, and managed care case managers.

Table 6–6 Illustration of Agency Savings if LPN Services Are Substituted for RN Services

	Patients	Visits per patient	Total RN visits	Per visit cost ($)	Total ($)
Original agency cost	2,000	10	20,000	32.37	647,400
Revised agency cost					
RN	2,000	8	16,000	32.37	517,920
LPN	2,000	2	4,000	17.34	69,360
Revised agency cost					587,280
Decrease through service substitution					60,120

Substitution of services can be an important source of efficiencies to the HHA in an episodic or capitated payment system. Table 6–6 illustrates that an agency provides on average 10 nursing visits to the 2,000 patients that it serves on an annual basis. Two of the ten visits have interventions that can be performed by an LPN. This would provide the HHA with an annual savings of $60,120. Service substitution could be accomplished by utilizing any lower cost service as long as the managed care contract permitted substitution, and the substituted services were performing services for which they were trained and qualified. This concept would potentially enable LPNs, home health aides, and physical therapy assistants to be substituted for more costly services.

Technology

Advances in technology will enable HHAs to build efficiencies into the care delivery process. Efficiencies can be gained by decreasing the amount of time that is spent doing documentation, filing, retrieving records, and satisfying reporting requirements. Documentation is a required part of the home health process. Traditionally, nurses have scribbled notes concerning the patients who were seen onto a notebook, index card, or some other paper medium. Notes were then rewritten into an agency-specified format for inclusion in the patient record. This process created work and consumed time. In addition, notes were often illegible, slow to be submitted to the office, lost in the mail, or lost within the agency. This required rewriting and possibly caused delays in the billing process.

Some agencies developed transcription systems to get around this problem. Nurses, therapists, and aides were provided with hand-held tape recorders to document their visits. Documentation followed a predescribed format to ensure consistency. Tapes could then be mailed into the office for transcription. Although this process helped to streamline the documentation process, it still had major inefficiencies. Inefficiencies resulted from an additional layer of staff to transcribe notes into either hardcopy for the patient's records or directly into the internal clinical system.

Advances in technology and falling prices have enabled HHAs to invest in portable computers for agency staff to use when making visits. The portable computer allows nurses, therapists, and aides to enter documentation directly into a mask or predefined format that can then be transferred directly into the agency's information system. The provider can complete documentation either directly in the home or in his or her car prior to proceeding to the next client. Updating the agency's computer system could be accomplished by transferring data via a modem during the documentation process, saving to disk, and mailing the disk to the agency, or transferring data at night.

Utilization of computer systems assists the agency in collecting more data, collecting data quicker, and receiving data in a consistent format. Collection of data concurrent with the actual visit potentially enhances collection of patient data by not relying on a provider's memory or translation of scribbled notes. Additionally, concurrent documentation may increase the agency's ability to identify the amount of medical supplies that is used at the patient level.

Medical supply cost will be very important to control in a noncost-reimbursed environment. Medical supplies represent a cost of doing business; however, HHAs have never had to implement inventory control systems because of the reimbursement environment. Supplies were taken out of medical supply closets by nurses and placed in their trunks for convenience; however, this led to spoilage and waste if the supplies were not used in time. Spoilage could occur because the supplies' useful life expired, a change in weather conditions caused the supply to freeze and break or to melt, or they became damaged in the car. Advances in information systems will facilitate the tracking of supplies by nurse, therapist, or aide. Actually supply usage can be reconciled to draws from inventory, and costly or abusive practices can be halted.

Initially, there may be some reluctance to use the portable computer, but in the long run, it should increase morale by simplifying the task of documentation. If simplification of the documentation task can increase productivity from 5 visits per day to 5.25 visits per day, the cost of the lap-top has been paid for in 1 year.

Reductions in Travel Costs

A prospective payment environment requires that agencies manage all costs. Costs that are variable will fluctuate directly with the amount of services that are provided by the HHA. Management of the provision of care along the clinical pathway will help agencies to control their direct costs. A large element of direct cost is a nonvalue-added administrative expense known as travel expense.

Travel expense has two components: (1) actual travel time and (2) the cost of traveling to the patient's home. An analysis of the total miles an agency travels will reveal a substantial administrative component in the provision of patient care. In Table 6–5, an assumption was made that the average mileage per nursing visit was 15 miles. If an agency reimburses its field employees at the federal limit of $.29 for 1995, then it will be incurring an additional $4.35 cost per visit. Extending this amount by 5 visits per day would cause an agency to incur an average annual travel expense per nurse of $5,002.50 (1,150 visits × $4.35).

An alternative to paying travel expenses is to explore the purchase of an automobile for the nurse to use when providing nursing visits. Purchasing a car would be warranted if the monthly expense for the purchase, maintenance, fuel, license and registration, and insurance was less than the average monthly reimbursement that an agency would incur when reimbursing at $.29 per mile.

Besides possible economic advantages that would accrue to the agency, there is an opportunity for some less quantifiable events to take place. First, the nurse, therapist, or aide will have dependable transportation to visit patients. Field staff who have undependable personal vehicles may not be able to provide timely visits to the agency's clients. Additionally, providing cars to field staff could boost morale or help with retention. Another advantage that could accrue to the HHA is using the automobiles as a marketing tool. Painting all agency automobiles with the HHA's logo, name, address, and telephone number will help with name recognition and potentially generate additional business for the agency. Furthermore, by purchasing tape players for the automobiles, field staff could take advantage of travel time to work on their continuing education credits.

Other Administrative Costs

Direct patient care is supported by many processes that go on within the agency. These processes could include intake, records management, scheduling, billing, and case management. These costs will fluctuate indirectly with patient care. Cost fluctuation will depend on the volume of activities performed during the month, the number of patients on service, and how many activities are not automated.

Indirect costs are a very real cost of managed care and should be included in the calculation of the direct cost of a managed care contract. Often indirect costs are ignored and treated as part of the fixed costs of an agency. Ignoring indirect costs when negotiating with an MCO will distort the true cost of the managed care contract. Additionally, it will make it more difficult to determine what the necessary return needs to be to remain financially viable.

Dissection of the Patient Care Delivery Process and Additional Opportunities

Review of all elements of the patient care delivery process will identify additional areas for reducing direct and administrative costs. Cost reduction could be a result of looking at each type of expense and asking what if we changed the way we did things, is there a more efficient or economical way of providing care, and who will benefit by the proposed changes? Will the proposed changes enhance the communication processes with the MCO, will the patient benefit, will the employees benefit, or will the agency benefit?

Process review could be very specific or global. In either case, defining the outcome is a necessary ingredient. If the outcome is to reduce administrative expenses related to the provision of patient care, then that goal needs to be paramount to individual team members; otherwise, the process will not work. Process analysis requires participants to be critical thinkers and to question whether a process adds value to the agency or simply cost. Services that add only cost need to be evaluated in light of the agency's quest for financial viability in an environment that is no longer cost-reimbursed and in which revenue streams are flat.

BUNDLING MULTIPLE SERVICES INTO THE CLINICAL PATHWAY

Up to this point, the discussion has centered primarily on inclusion of the six main disciplines into the clinical pathway. Combining other services may offer the HHA an opportunity to generate a higher return than may have been possible if each were priced separately. This strategy may be difficult, given the agency's organizational design. If the HHA developed separate companies to maximize reimbursement, then it may have difficulty blending different product lines or services together to determine whether a bundled pricing methodology would make sense.

A bundled pricing methodology is nothing more than combining skilled intermittent services with private duty, home infusion, and home medical equipment. An agency may provide all of these services or only one. If, however, it provides all of these services, an opportunity exists for creative pricing of a full range of services. Pricing could be determined in an episodic fashion for a particular patient problem or in a hybrid fashion.

A hybrid fashion may offer a flat price for intermittent services and medical supplies, but private duty, home medical equipment, and home infusion would be priced in a fee-for-service fashion. The pricing decision may be to price one service at cost, while all other services provide a healthy return. Service packages could also be developed for a specific referral source, physician group, or payor.

One strategy would be to analyze patient activity to determine if there is a particularly high-volume patient problem that could be addressed by the agency. The analysis would then combine the agency's actual results to develop a bundled critical pathway. Once the pathway is developed, the agency could look at different pricing scenarios and offer them to the payor or whoever was interested in controlling costs. This approach could also help the agency to enter into a specific niche that had been occupied by a competitor.

Creativity really becomes the bottom line in negotiating with MCOs. HHAs that are willing to break out of the fragmented payment system concept and bundle services together have an opportunity to capture managed care contracts. MCOs would prefer to deal with one contractor for home health services instead of four because it reduces their administrative burden.

Bundling of services can be targeted to a specific referral source. Clinical pathways can be designed to focus on the specific needs of that referral source. Efficiencies that are built into the care delivery process may save the MCO hundreds of thousands of dollars. This kind of success could certainly warrant sharing in some of the savings with the HHA. In either event, the goal for the HHA should be to meet or surpass the expectations of the MCO, the patient, the physician, and any other client of the HHA. Goals will be surpassed by continually providing high-quality care and outcomes and demonstrating cost-effectiveness. Cost-effectiveness can be enhanced by working within an integrated delivery system. This is accomplished by having a common goal instead of fragmented goals.

NOTES

1. P.W. Shaughnessy, et al., *A Study for Home Health Care Quality and Cost under Capitated and Fee-for-Service Payment Systems* (Denver: Center for Health Policy Research, 1994), vi.

2. C. Feldman, Decision Making in Case Management of Home Healthcare Clients, *Journal of Nursing Administration* 23 (January 1993): 33.

3. D.A. Peters, Development of a Community Health Intensity Rating Scale, *Nursing Research* 37, no. 4 (July/August 1988): 204.

4. J.K. Williams, Case Management: Opportunities for Service Providers, *Home Health Care Services Quarterly* 14, no. 1 (1993): 7.

5. Peters, Development of a Community Health Intensity Rating Scale, 203.

6. V.K. Saba, *Develop and Demonstrate a Method for Classifying Home Health Patients To Predict Resource Requirements and Measure Outcomes* (Washington, DC: Georgetown University, 1991), vii.

7. *Ibid.*

8. *Ibid.*

9. S.A. Moorhead, et al., Nursing Interventions Classification: A Comparison with the Omaha System and the Home Healthcare Classification, *Journal of Nursing Administration* 23, no. 10 (October 1993): 25.

10. K.S. Martin, et al., Home Health Clients: Characteristics, Outcomes of Care, and Nursing Interventions, *American Journal of Public Health* 83, no. 12 (1993): 1,734.

11. D.A. Peters, Strategic Directions for Using Outcomes, *The Remmington Report* (June/July 1994): 9.

12. C. Feldman, Decision Making in Case Management, 37.

13. Healthcare Quality Management, *Quality HME Services: Measuring the Benefits, Phase 2 Report: Measuring Outcomes* (Yuba, CA: 1994), 20–21.

14. NAHC, *Basic Statistics about Home Care 1994* (Washington, DC: National Association of Home Care, 1994), 7.

15. *Ibid.*

Part III

Cost Accounting

185

Chapter 7

Cost Accounting Basics

The focus of this chapter is to develop several different concepts related to the organizational expenses of a home health agency (HHA). The chapter will begin with the development of cost accounting terms and definitions. Once the foundation has been developed, the discussion will transition to the differences between cost reporting and cost accounting. The chapter will conclude with the need to develop a cost accounting system using realistic indicators of how costs follow activities.

Cost accounting is different from financial accounting. Financial accounting measures the results of operations to identify how well an organization performs over a defined period of time. The purpose of financial accounting is to present the results of operation in a consistent format with common terminology for internal and external evaluation. The output of the financial accounting process is the financial statement. The financial statement is a summary of revenues and expenditures for the current period (income statement); accumulation of assets, liabilities, and owners' equity since inception (the balance sheet); and a summary of how cash was generated and applied (statement of cash flow). However, the financial statement does not help management understand the relationship of costs to revenues.

This is the purpose of cost accounting. Cost accounting provides a bridge between financial reporting and the needs of management. Management supplements the financial statements with graphs, charts, and additional reports that enhance the meaning of the financial statements. The discipline of cost accounting enables the measurement process to be quantified in terms that measure tangible activities within the agency. Cost accounting provides managers with a tool to explain deviations because of fluctuations in price, volume, productivity, cost base, or changes in corporate overhead.

Cost accounting also provides a base for making informed decisions about operations. Decisions could be short term (tactical) or long term (strategic). Typically, cost accounting provides a tool to measure the profitability of services. The measurement of services could be done for a single encounter, such as a nursing visit or a private-duty shift. Measurement can also be done on the aggregate of a grouping of similar services. Frequently, groupings are referred to as *product lines*. Product lines are specific services that are offered by an HHA and generally targeted toward a subset of the customer base. Product lines could include skilled intermittent services, continuous care, adult, pediatric, hospice, infusion therapies, or home medical equipment.

Product lines will vary by agency. One agency's strategy may be to offer a single product line, whereas another agency may choose to offer multiple product lines. One agency may choose to offer multiple product lines from one company, whereas another agency may separate each product line into a separate legal entity. Regardless of what strategy is employed, agencies must understand their costs to survive in the managed care arena.

One of the paradigms regarding managed care is this: knowledge is power. Knowledge of an organization's cost structure and how costs fluctuate with service requirements, volume, changes in patient problems, and organizational structure will provide management with a competitive advantage when bidding, pricing, and evaluating strategies for competing in the dynamic health care delivery system.

COST CONCEPTS

The measurement of costs provides managers with a tool for planning, managing, and controlling their organizations. From a planning perspective, if managers understand how costs will vary because of a decision that they make, then they are able to make their decisions knowing the risks, implications, and benefits that a course of action will bring to the agency. Cost measurement also provides a tool for continuous feedback regarding actual operational results. Feedback will depend on what the agency chooses to monitor, how the plan was initially developed, and what the agency chooses to do with the results once they are obtained. Costs can also be used as a method to control spending within an organization, monitor profitability, forecast cash requirements, and provide a solid base for modeling. Use of actual agency results provides a firm foundation for the analysis of prospective opportunities that an agency may choose to ignore or take. Crucial to this process is understanding how costs respond to different service levels. A key to understanding is provided by how easily costs can be traced to a specific activity or service. Costs can either fluctuate directly or indirectly with service provision.

Direct Costs

Direct costs are incurred every time a unit of service is provided. Direct cost includes labor, materials, and an administrative-type expense such as travel. Labor is the cost of an employee or subcontractor to provide an intermittent visit, private-duty shift, or an administrative activity. The direct labor cost will vary depending on the pay scale of the employee. For instance, the average hourly compensation of HHA caregivers according to a *Home Health Agency Compensation Survey Report* from the National Association of Home Care as of July 1993 is listed in Table 7–1.[1]

Table 7–1 indicates some of the differences that can occur in the direct cost of a visit. Direct cost will vary by discipline. Differences in rates reflect the amount of training, education, and responsibility that is required of the employee. Differences between minimum and average levels will depend on geographic area, seniority, technical skill level, resource availability, and service requirements.

Direct labor cost will also depend on how the agency chooses to pay its field staff. An agency that pays on an hourly basis could compute the cost of one visit by multiplying the actual amount of time that it took to perform the visit by the employee's rate of pay (Table 7–2). Differences in practices will cause many different rates to be assigned to the cost of that visit.

One agency may pay its hourly nurses for an 8-hour day. If the nurse performs 5 visits during the day, the cost per visit is $25.60. However, the actual time spent for each one of the patients seen during the day varied. In this example, visit time fluctuated between a low of 1 hour to visit Patient B, and 1.75 hours to visit Patient E. Visit cost was $16.00 and $28.00, respectively. This is an illustration of how direct cost can become overcosted (Patient B) or undercosted (Patient E) if an average cost of $25.60 is assigned to each visit.

Table 7–1 Comparison of Minimum and Average Rates by Discipline on a Visit and Hourly Basis

	Per visit		Per hour	
	Minimum	Average	Minimum	Average
Registered nurses	25.83	33.79	14.31	18.21
Licensed practical nurses	18.54	21.53	10.07	12.69
Physical therapists	39.51	44.86	19.93	24.82
Occupational therapists	39.78	43.66	18.44	23.23
Speech therapists	40.73	44.25	20.00	24.34
Medical social workers	40.38	45.44	15.15	19.08
Home health aides	11.70	13.52	6.52	8.55

Source: Reprinted from *Basic Statistics about Home Care*, p. 7, with permission of the National Association of Home Care, © 1994.

Table 7–2 Comparison of Cost per Visit Using Average Number of Visits versus Actual Cost on an Hourly Basis

Average	Specific	Hours	Rate ($)	Cost ($)
8 Hours	Patient A	1.25	16.00	20.00
$ 16.00 Rate	Patient B	1.00	16.00	16.00
$128.00 Cost per day	Patient C	1.50	16.00	24.00
	Patient D	1.35	16.00	21.60
5 Visits	Patient E	1.75	16.00	28.00
$ 25.60 Cost per visit		6.85		109.60
	Administrative	1.15	16.00	18.40
	Total	8.00		128.00

Furthermore, direct cost can either be variable or fixed. A variable cost is one that will fluctuate with every unit of service that is provided. An employee who is paid on a per visit basis is an excellent example of a variable cost. The employee will not be paid unless he or she visits one of the agency's patients. An employee who receives a salary is an example of a fixed expense. This employee will receive the same paycheck regardless of whether he or she does one visit or seven visits during the course of the day. This is demonstrated by Table 7–3.

Direct labor cost is influenced by the length of the visit. Visit length is determined by the composition of the visit components. Visit components include travel time to and from the patient's home, actual treatment time, planning and preparation for the visit, documentation, and follow-up. Planning and preparation could consist of speaking to the patient's case manager, reviewing the patient's medical record, or requesting appropriate supplies from inventory. Documentation and follow-up could be passing results on to team members, updating the patient's chart or automated record, or coordinating future activities with the case management team members.

Table 7–3 Productivity and Cost per Visit

Hours	Rate	Daily pay ($)	Visits	Cost/visit ($)
8	16.00	128.00	3	42.67
8	16.00	128.00	4	32.00
8	16.00	128.00	5	25.60
8	16.00	128.00	6	21.33
8	16.00	128.00	7	18.29

In addition to labor, direct cost also includes materials. Materials could be patient supplies such as bandages, alcohol swabs, gloves, or catheters. Materials can also include medications, home medical equipment, and intravenous (IV) therapies. Direct labor and materials are traceable to a specific patient. Costs that are direct will have a positive correlation to every unit of service that is provided. In other words, direct cost is a variable cost. Variable costs are incurred with every unit of service provided. Service provision may generate a billable activity in a fee-for-service environment or represent an additional cost in a capitated payment system.

Direct labor and materials are referred to as *prime cost*. Prime cost does not include the cost of employee benefits; however, to ignore this cost from the calculation of direct cost would significantly undervalue the cost of a unit of service. Employee benefits represent a cost to an employer. In relationship to prime cost, benefits represent overhead or burden to the service delivery process. Perhaps a way to differentiate is the following. If an HHA contracts with a temporary agency to provide therapy services, the cost per unit of labor is whatever the agency is willing to pay. When calculating the cost per unit of labor for an employee, the agency must add actual payroll cost plus benefit cost to determine the true cost per visit.

Benefits are used as a tool to recruit and retain competent staff. Employee benefits will vary by agency, seniority, job classification, and region. Employee benefits can include paid time off, such as vacation, personal, and sick time. Other benefits could include health insurance, employer's contribution toward the employee's social security, life insurance, pension contributions, tuition reimbursement, auto allowances, and myriad other perquisites.

Employee benefits as a percentage of an employee's salary will also vary. Table 7–4 demonstrates this phenomenon. Two types of employees are listed: (1) a nurse and (2) a home health aide. Rates were from those listed in Table 7–1. The illustration assumes that both the nurse and the aide will receive 2 weeks of vacation, 3 sick days, 2 personal days, employer-purchased health insurance costing $1,500, and the employer's contribution toward the employee's social security retirement benefits.

Both employees received the same benefits; however as a percentage of salary, they had different rates. The nurse had an 18 percent benefit rate, and the aide had a 23 percent benefit rate. Use of an average benefit rate will result in an under- and overcosting effect similar to the cost per visit calculation illustrated in Table 7–2. Additionally, benefit percentages will fluctuate because of different employee classifications and perquisites.

In addition to employee benefits, burden also includes the cost of an employer's obligations. An employer is obligated for payroll taxes for unemployment insurance and workers' compensation. Additional employer costs would include mal-

Table 7–4 Comparison of Benefit Factors between Nurse and Home Health Aide

	Weeks	Hours	Rate ($)	Total ($)
Salary				
Nurse	49	40	18.21	35,692
Home health aide	49	40	8.55	16,758
Benefit calculation				
Paid time off				
Nurse	3	40	18.21	2,185
Home health aide	3	40	8.55	1,026
Health benefits				1,500
Payroll taxes				
Nurse	37,877	7.56%		2,863
Home health aide	17,784	7.56%		1,344

Summary	Nurse	Home health aide
Salary	35,692	16,758
Paid time off	2,185	1,026
Health benefits	1,500	1,500
Payroll taxes	2,863	1,344
Total benefits	$ 6,548	$ 3,870
Benefit percentage	18%	23%

practice insurance because of the litigious nature of society and compensation for employee travel expenses. Employer payroll taxes are required by federal and state statutes. Rates are consistent across all employee classifications. Workers' compensation rates depend on job classification. Rates are lower for administrative employees and increase as the probability for a job-related injury increases. Home health aides typically have the highest rate assigned to their job classification because of the potential for a job-related injury. Injury could occur because of back strain or slipping when assisting a patient in transferring.

Table 7–5 illustrates the computation of workers' compensation expense and how burden affects each class of employee. In this example, nurses have a workers' compensation rate of $5 for every $100 of payroll. Home health aides have a rate of $14 for every $100 of payroll. When workers' compensation is added to the overhead calculation for benefits, it increases the burden significantly.

Other direct costs include travel expenses. Travel expenses represent a significant cost to the HHA. Travel requirements will vary depending on whether the HHA is located in an urban, suburban, or rural area. Travel includes the cost of paying the home health caregiver to commute to the patient's home plus reimbursing him or her for wear and tear on his or her automobile. If an agency provides

Table 7–5 Comparison of the Workers' Compensation Burden Differentials for Nurses and Home Health Aides

	Nurse	Home health aide
Workers' compensation rate	$ 5.00	$ 14.00
Salary + paid time off	$37,877.00	$17,784.00
Workers' compensation expense	$1,893.84	$ 2,489.76
Burden percentage	24%	38%

automobiles for its staff to utilize for the provision of patient care, then the cost of repairs, maintenance, and depreciation would be calculated into the direct cost of a patient visit. Identification of other direct costs associated with equipment, supplies, and IV therapies would include the cost of delivery to the patient's home, labor cost of the delivery, labor cost of mixing the IV, cost of capital, and inventory cost.

Other costs that could be considered direct costs would be phone contact with the patient. Phone contact may be done in place of a visit. Identification of contact time by patient represents a direct cost of patient care. Identification of phone call cost to a specific patient represents a direct cost of the agency. This could be the cost of the call placed from the agency or a car phone.

Indirect Costs

In the above section, direct costs were addressed. Indirect costs are all costs that are not direct. Indirect costs can be either variable or fixed. These costs are incurred to support the primary purpose of the agency. If the primary purpose of the agency is to provide skilled intermittent visits, then indirect costs are incurred to support the provision of skilled intermittent visits. Indirect cost is also incurred to support the administrative requirements of the agency.

Indirect costs do not fluctuate directly with volume and tend to be either fixed or semifixed. A fixed cost remains the same regardless of the number of visits or continuous care hours an agency provides. A semifixed cost remains fixed at certain volume levels. Once volume increases beyond a certain point, semifixed costs will increase. The semifixed cost will then remain fixed until volume rises to the next level, thus requiring more cost to be incurred. These types of costs can also be referred to as *step-variable* or *step-fixed*.

Semifixed costs are illustrated by Figure 7–1. An example of a semifixed expense would be a biller. A biller is hired when volume is minimal and will be able to satisfy the HHA's billing requirements up to a certain level. Once visit volume reaches a point where a single biller is not able to satisfy the job requirements, an agency is faced with a decision. It can either allow work to slip, hire a part-time employee, get assistance from another department, or hire a second full-time

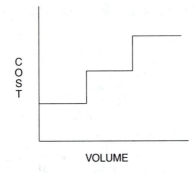

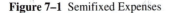

Figure 7–1 Semifixed Expenses

biller. If the latter is chosen, costs will increase in a step fashion up to a certain volume level, at which point the agency will be faced with the decision of whether to hire another employee. Inherent in the concept of step costs is a relevant range. The relevant range is the volume over which the cost is expected to remain fixed.

Indirect costs that are semifixed will fluctuate with agency volume. These costs are predominantly labor costs for support activities such as data entry, records management, scheduling, billing, quality improvement, and administrative job functions. Not all indirect costs exhibit the characteristics of step costs.

Some indirect costs will have a fixed component and fluctuate with usage. Figure 7–2 illustrates the cost of a car phone. A car phone has a fixed-cost component, the monthly service fee, and a variable cost component that is based on usage. An outside payroll service will exhibit the same cost characteristics. Factors that will cause indirect expenses to fluctuate include the number of employees that an agency has, the number of visits, seasonality, the number of patients on service, weather conditions, type and complexity of services that are offered, and the capabilities of in-house staff and systems.

Costs that do not increase or decrease with volume are known as *fixed costs* (Figure 7–3). Fixed costs generally remain constant. Rent and the chief executive officer's (CEO's) salary are good examples of fixed expenses. Indirect expenses are also referred to as *overhead*. Overhead is the total of all indirect expenses regardless of whether they are semifixed or fixed.

Some costs will remain fixed for a specified range of time. Depreciation is an example of costs that remain fixed for a year at a time. Purchases of new fixed assets would increase the total depreciation expense; however, depreciation expense for the old assets would remain constant. This example could also apply to rent expense. Rent expense remains fixed until the agency needs to find new space. Rent will increase or decrease and then remain flat for the duration of the lease.

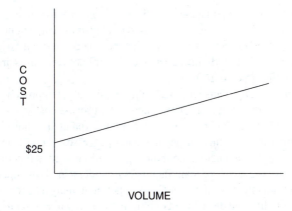

Figure 7–2 Variable Cost that Has a Fixed Element

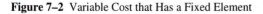

Accountability

Understanding cost behavior and the how and why of cost fluctuation is an important step in managing the home health operation. This is a two-step process. The first step is the measurement of costs. Cost measurement provides a framework for managers to make sound business decisions. The second step is ownership or accountability. Without accountability, no one will own the results that appear in the financial statements.

Accountability will vary at different levels within the management structure. Ultimately, the CEO is responsible to shareholders or the board of directors for the

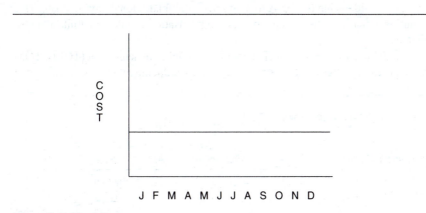

Figure 7–3 Fixed Cost

results of the HHA. Other managers will be responsible for their departments only. Costs within a department are composed of controllable and noncontrollable expenses. Controllable expenses are expenses that the department heads or managers can directly or indirectly influence. Noncontrollable expenses are expenses over which they have no control.

This has caused many managers to adopt an input/output approach to management of costs. Unfortunately, this does not consider process cost across functional boundaries. When managers have an opportunity to expand their horizons beyond the scope of their departments, or departmental processes, there is an enormous opportunity to build efficiencies into their organizations. Cross-functional analysis of costs allows managers or team members to understand how inputs and outputs affect each member of the team. Cross-functional analysis encourages a departure from an individual department or empire mentality to embracing the larger process.

Avoidable Costs

Avoidable costs are costs that an agency would never incur if it chose an alternate path. Avoidable costs are usually identified as part of an analysis or a pro-forma regarding a possible direction for the agency to pursue. The agency may choose to pursue a direction because it will provide a source of revenue in the future, or, conversely, an agency may choose not to pursue a new venture because of the risk and costs that are associated with it. By avoiding a course of action, the agency can prevent incurring unnecessary costs.

An example of avoidable cost is choosing to increase salaries of all employees from 4 percent to 7 percent. Table 7–6 illustrates that choosing an increase of 4 percent would enable the HHA to avoid $16,148 in additional payroll costs. This figure is actually higher when workers' compensation is calculated into the cost increase.

Avoidable costs are also an element of total quality management (TQM). TQM attempts to do things right the first time, thereby reducing redundancy, waste, and

Table 7–6 Calculation of Avoidable Cost

Salaries ($)	Rate	Increase ($)	Federal Insurance Contributions Act (FICA) ($)	Total ($)	
500,000	7%	35,000	2,678	37,678	
500,000	4%	20,000	1,530	21,530	
				16,148	Avoidable cost

errors. Redundancy, waste, and errors are avoidable costs. Costs can be avoided by taking the time on the front end to think and do the task properly in order to prevent doing it over. Avoidance of costs can also be accomplished by building efficiencies into the system. This is an especially important concept when re-sources are becoming scarce.

Future Costs

Future costs take into consideration events that will cause changes to take place. An example of this would be when a new contract is being considered. In the event that the contract was awarded to the agency, future costs would be incurred to handle increases in volume (direct costs), recruitment of additional staff, and many other indirect administrative costs. Analysis of future costs should consider changes in an agency's cost structure due to the regulatory environment, inflation, and resource availability.

Analysis of future costs is important when considering new acquisitions. Acquisition costs have current and future components. The current component is the actual outlay for the object being acquired, such as a new computer system. The new computer system may have a defined charge for hardware and software; how-ever, a hidden cost may include wiring of the facility, conversion of data from the old system to the new system, training, and delivery costs. Future costs may in-clude the cost of new personnel to run the system, training of existing staff, hard-ware repairs or replacements, and the creation of new reports. Future costs could also include a planned maintenance program that considers replacing equipment when it approaches a certain age.

Incremental Costs

Incremental cost represents additional cost to an HHA. The additional cost is normally the result of an expansionary action, such as taking on a new managed care contract. Incremental cost would include the direct cost associated with the new contract and any indirect costs. Indirect costs that would be considered incre-mental would depend on the service level required in the new contract. Typically, incremental cost would be the cost of support services to meet the requirements of providing patient care, billing, reporting, and case management of the managed care organization's (MCO's) patients. In addition, if the contract required that a home health coordinator be placed at a physician's office, clinic, or hospital, then this would be an incremental cost to the agency. If the agency had to rent addi-tional office space, this would also be considered an incremental cost of the con-tract.

Opportunity Costs

Opportunity costs are a measure of missed opportunities as a result of a chosen path. HHAs have limited resources. Resources are time and money. Directions are chosen, and the resources of time and money are directed toward their pursuit. Many opportunities may arise that could provide a greater return than the one selected, thus increasing the cost of the venture or chosen direction.

Opportunity cost can also be viewed in relationship to visit volume. If an agency has resources to perform 20,000 visits, and its payor mix consists of 90 percent cost-based payors and 10 percent commercial payors, then opportunity cost would be calculated as the difference in revenue streams between the cost-based payor and the commercial payor. Therefore, if the agency can shift to an 80/20 payor mix, the agency will increase its bottom line.

COST REPORTING

Cost reporting is different from cost accounting. Cost reporting is a process that was designed by the Health Care Financing Administration (HCFA) to reimburse HHAs for reasonable costs in the provision of patient care. The cost report's sole purpose is to determine reimbursement, not to serve as a tool for cost accounting. The cost report assumes that all visits are of equal duration, that every payor has similar requirements, and that indirect costs of the HHA should be shared equally among all providers. Consequently, cost per visit is the same across multiple payors.

The cost per visit calculation is the result of a cost step-down process. Costs are initially classified as either salary, employee benefits, transportation, contracted services, or other costs. Using the five classification categories, costs are then grouped into general service cost centers, HHA reimbursable service centers, HHA nonreimbursable services, or other costs. The process of cost finding then allocates general service costs to reimbursable and nonreimbursable cost centers.

The general service cost centers allocate costs assigned to them in sequence. Providers have an opportunity to choose an allocation process that provides for a more exact cost-finding process. Several methods can be used to allocate general service costs to reimbursable and nonreimbursable cost centers. For purposes of this discussion, costs will be allocated using the accumulated cost method.

The process of allocating general service cost begins by summarizing expenses as salary, employee benefits, transportation, contracted services, or other costs within the reimbursable and nonreimbursable sections as direct expenses. General service cost is treated as an indirect expense (unless an alternative cost-finding method is used), and the indirect cost is allocated to the reimbursable and nonreimbursable cost centers.

Table 7–7 Assignment of Overhead Using Medicare Methodology

	Direct ($)	Indirect ($)	Total cost ($)	Visits	Per visit ($)
Administrative and general	721,325				
Skilled nursing	774,499	413,668	1,188,167	14,813	80.21
Physical therapy	185,407	99,028	284,435	3,686	77.17
Occupational therapy	26,795	14,312	41,107	565	72.75
Speech therapy	12,286	6,562	18,848	249	75.70
Medical social services	14,008	7,482	21,490	124	173.31
Home health aide	290,375	155,092	445,467	9,164	48.61
Supplies	47,145	25,181	72,326		
Total	1,350,515	721,325	2,071,840	28,601	72.44

The allocation process calculates the total of the direct expenses listed in the reimbursable and nonreimbursable cost centers and then pro-rates indirect expenses on the relationship of the total direct cost per cost center to the aggregate cost. In the example illustrated by Table 7–7, the total of reimbursable and nonreimbursable expenses is $1,350,515, so skilled nursing would have $413,668 worth of indirect expenses assigned to the cost center ($413,668 = 721,325 × (774,499/1,350,515)).

This process assumes that all services and cost related to the provision of services are homogeneous. Homogeneity crosses payors, product lines, programs, employee pay classifications, and service requirements. The result is to arrive at an average cost per visit. Average cost implies that for every visit that was performed, the amount of resources that was consumed was consistent across total visits for that discipline.

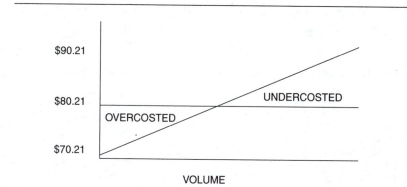

Figure 7–4 Under- and Overcosting Cost per Visit

Figure 7–4 illustrates this phenomenon. The development of an average cost using the Medicare cost report ignores events that take place within an agency. For instance, the discipline of skilled nursing could include routine nursing, high-technology visits, and admission visits. Each visit has a different cost associated with it because of the element of time. Additionally, the agency compensated its nursing professional higher for admission and high-technology nursing visits because of the increased time element and technical skills, respectively. Assuming that the routine visit had a cost of $70.21, then the cost of that visit was overstated by $10.00, and the high-technology nursing visit was understated by $10.00 because its actual cost was $90.21. Use of average costs ignores seasonality, differences in productivity between caregivers, compensation levels, and the element of time.

The application of indirect expenses in a uniform format causes each cost center to bear an equal amount of overhead. However, the cost report allocates overhead using accumulated cost. The accumulated cost method causes a higher proportion of indirect expenses to be assigned to the nursing cost center. This is because nursing has a higher volume of services than other disciplines and a higher hourly or per visit cost attached to it.

Table 7–8 illustrates the percentage of overhead that was assigned to each of the reimbursable cost centers. Nursing received 57 percent of the indirect cost; however, nursing was only responsible for 52 percent of the visit volume. An inverse relationship existed for home health aides. Only 22 percent of the overhead was applied to this cost center; however, the home health aides were responsible for 32 percent of the volume. Application of overhead will affect an agency's cost per visit. Use of the Medicare cost report will lead to visits being over- and undercosted. Table 7–9 demonstrates the inequities that this type of costing method will cause.

Indirect costs will vary depending on an agency's administrative structure. Administrative structures will depend on the type of services that an agency provides, how efficient its processes are, and its organizational design and philosophy. Indirect costs incurred by an agency may be for a particular payor, because of a spe-

Table 7–8 Comparison of Overhead Assignment Using a Single Allocation Base

	Visits (%)	Accumulated cost (%)
Skilled nursing	52	57
Physical therapy	13	14
Occupational therapy	2	2
Speech therapy	1	1
Medical social services	0	1
Home health aide	32	22
Supplies		3

Table 7–9 Average Cost per Visit Using Medicare Methodology

	Direct ($)	Indirect ($)	Total cost ($)
Skilled nursing	52.29	27.93	80.22
Physical therapy	50.30	26.87	77.17
Occupational therapy	47.42	25.33	72.75
Speech therapy	49.34	26.35	75.69
Medical social services	112.97	60.34	173.31
Home health aide	31.69	16.92	48.61

cific technical skill requirement to service a group of patients, or because of a community requirement. The cost report ignores the reason that the cost was incurred when calculating an average cost. From a payor or program perspective, this represents a cross-subsidization of expenses. This is analogous to the over-/undercosting scenario illustrated in Figure 7–4.

Reimbursement for medical supplies makes the same assumption regarding the application of overhead; however, medical supply reimbursement goes one step further. Reimbursement is calculated on the ratio of cost to charges. Total medical supply cost is calculated by taking direct expenses for medical supplies, adding indirect expenses as part of the step-down function, and then calculating the ratio of total cost to total charges for medical supplies. Once the cost-to-charge ratio is calculated, then Medicare supply charges are broken out, the ratio is applied to total charges, and the cost of Medicare supplies is calculated. This process assumes that medical supplies should receive a pro-rated amount of indirect costs and that there is a linear relationship between charges and actual resources consumed.

The Medicare program has recognized that the cost-finding process may not be reimbursing providers correctly for services provided. Use of unique cost centers, discrete costing, and the home office will help providers receive more appropriate reimbursement for services provided. However, these methods and the cost report in general do not meet management's needs for cost measurement and management of costs. Cost measurement will be especially critical in a managed care environment.

COST ACCOUNTING

Cost accounting is a process of cost assignment and allocation. Cost assignment is the matching of costs to specific activities. Allocation is spreading costs based on an arbitrary base. Allocation of indirect costs to cost centers enables managers to determine total costs of providing services. The difficulty for HHAs is developing a cost allocation process that considers the complexity of services and allocates a fair portion of overhead to those services. The preceding section focused on one of the purposes of cost accounting: reimbursement. Other purposes include the valuation of inventories for financial reporting purposes, managerial purposes, and use as a tool for motivation of employees and CQI.

Cost accounting from the perspective of inventory valuation seeks to assign all period costs to the cost of goods sold. Assignment of costs includes salaries, benefits, carrying cost, and other related costs of operation. Inventory is also costed for purposes of valuation for financial and tax purposes. Different inventory valuation practices will yield different costs of goods sold and ending inventory.

Cost accounting for management purposes attempts to measure, control, and determine profitability by payor line, program, and patient. This function has always been important but has taken a back seat to reimbursement issues. The paradigm shift to set payment systems prospectively has created a need for cost accounting systems that enable management staff to understand whether they are over- or undercosting their products and services. Without the availability of timely information, management will be operating in the dark.

A third function of the cost accounting system is to provide managers with tools to evaluate the productivity of their employees, departments, and teams. Understanding the relationships between input and output provides a tool to design efficient and economical health care delivery systems. Evaluation of services is another integral component. Managers need to be able to measure patient satisfaction, caregiver burden (both in the home and the field employee), and patient outcomes; analyze variances from agency standards of care; and estimate resource consumption requirements based on patient problems.

There are several concepts that are especially pertinent to good cost accounting systems. The first is the human element. Home health is a very labor-intensive business. Employees are usually very conscientious, caring, and interested in doing a good job. A cost accounting system could present a threat to them if they believe the sole purpose is to measure their output in relationship to agency-defined standards. However, if employees are encouraged to use the cost accounting system as a tool for organizational learning, job enhancement, and proper pricing of services, then the cost accounting system belongs to them. It is no longer management's, and data can be used as a tool instead of a club. Additionally, a byproduct of pricing services properly is continued employment.

Another concept that can make or break a good cost accounting system is the cost of data collection. Collection of data is an expensive proposition, and if the cost of data collection outweighs the benefits, then this is a cost to be avoided. Advances in information technology will enable HHAs to collect large amounts of data that previously would have been prohibitive to collect. This is especially important in a managed care environment where knowledge is power. Additionally, data collection is one of the many hidden costs of managed care.

A Historical Perspective

Managers have recognized that the cost report serves one purpose only: reimbursement. However, the format has caused managers to remain within the cost-reporting box. The box has caused many managers to attempt to identify different bases to allocate indirect expenses to arrive at a per visit cost by discipline. Every cost analysis will have a different purpose. One cost analysis may look at cost per visit across the agency; another, profitability by payor; a third, cost per visit by payor; and a fourth might attempt to identify profitability by product line.

The allocation of indirect expenses may have used several different allocation bases. Possible allocation bases could include hours, visits, accumulated cost, duplicated patient count, or charges. Table 7–10 illustrates several different alloca-

Table 7–10 Comparison of Overhead Assignment Using Different Allocation Bases

	Hours	Visits	Accumulated cost	Duplicate patient count	Charges
Base					
Skilled nursing	8,641	14,813	$774,499	1,030	$1,844,515
Physical therapy	3,686	3,686	185,407	367	368,600
Occupational therapy	706	565	26,795	28	53,675
Speech therapy	249	249	12,286	121	23,655
Medical social services	186	124	14,008	67	11,780
Home health aide	16,037	9,164	290,375	313	504,020
Supplies			47,145		
Total	29,505	28,601	$1,350,515	1,926	$2,806,245
Allocation					
Skilled nursing	211,248	373,588	$ 413,668	385,755	$ 474,119
Physical therapy	90,113	92,962	99,028	137,449	94,746
Occupational therapy	17,266	14,249	14,312	10,487	13,797
Speech therapy	6,087	6,280	6,562	45,317	6,080
Medical social services	4,547	3,127	7,482	25,093	3,028
Home health aide	392,063	231,119	155,092	117,225	129,555
Supplies			25,181		
Total	721,324	721,325	$ 721,326	721,326	$ 721,325
Percent applied					
Skilled nursing	29%	52%	57%	55%	66%
Physical therapy	13%	13%	14%	19%	13%
Occupational therapy	2%	2%	2%	1%	2%
Speech therapy	1%	1%	1%	6%	1%
Medical social services	1%	0%	1%	4%	0%
Home health aide	54%	32%	22%	16%	18%
Supplies	0%	0%	3%	0%	0%
Total	100%	100%	100%	100%	100%

tion bases. Utilizing the cost report approach from Table 7–7, the $721,325 of general and administrative costs were allocated using different allocation bases.

Each allocation base will produce different results. Five different allocation bases were used to allocate indirect costs to direct visit costs. For instance, the use of hours resulted in 29 percent of the overhead being applied to nursing; however, when charges were used, 66 percent of the overhead was applied to nursing. Depending on which allocation base is chosen, some very significant cost per discipline swings occur.

Attempting to bid on managed care contracts using volatile information such as shown in Table 7–11 could make the agency a big winner or a big loser. The spread of nursing cost using charges as an allocation base versus hours is $17.74 ($84.29 – $66.55). This differential could cause the agency to over- or underbid the contract by $262,782 ($17.74 × 14,813 visits).

Application of overhead causes a major problem when using the cost-reporting framework to cost services. Perhaps the largest problem is the costing of direct cost per visit. Table 7–9 identified a direct cost per visit for a skilled nursing visit of $52.29. To arrive at this figure, the cost report aggregated nursing salaries, employee benefits, transportation, contracted services, and other. This methodology assumes that all visits have an equal cost. However, there are many different types of nursing visits that are combined. Included in the combination of costs are different payment methodologies (per visit, salary, or hourly), differences in employee cost versus contracted cost, and payor differences.

Use of an average cost per visit methodology for direct cost ignores different types of nursing services, such as admission visits, routine nursing visits, supervisory visits, extended nursing visits, or high-technology visits. Visit cost could also be identified as treatment time, travel time, documentation time, preparation time, and case management. Table 7–12 illustrates differences that could occur using direct costs as identified in the cost report model.

Identification of costs in this format is better than using the average cost method of $52.29 for every nursing visit. By isolating the different types of activities that are performed within an agency, managers have an opportunity to make better

---

Table 7–11 Comparison of Average Cost per Visit Using Different Allocation Bases

	Hours ($)	Visits ($)	Accumulated cost ($)	Dup/count ($)	Charges ($)
Skilled nursing	66.55	77.51	80.21	78.33	84.29
Physical therapy	74.75	75.52	77.17	87.59	76.00
Occupational therapy	77.98	72.65	72.75	65.99	71.84
Speech therapy	73.79	74.56	75.70	231.34	73.76
Medical social services	149.64	138.19	173.31	315.33	137.39
Home health aide	74.47	56.91	48.61	44.48	45.82

Table 7–12 Comparison of Different Types of Visits and Their Respective Costs

	Cost ($)	Visits	Cost/visit ($)
Admission visit	91,328	1,030	88.67
Routine visit	437,351	10,908	40.09
Supervisory visit	16,029	350	45.80
Extended visit	160,197	1,675	95.64
High-technology visit	69,594	850	81.88
	774,499	14,813	52.29
Employee	668,749	12,463	53.66
Contractor	105,750	2,350	45.00
	774,499	14,813	52.29

pricing decisions and management decisions. For instance, a manager may look at this analysis and decide that he or she needs to increase the agency pricing structure for high-technology nursing services because it is costing twice as much as a routine nursing visit. A second manager may decide that he or she can reduce agency operating expenses by utilizing independent contractors to handle patients in remote geographic areas. A third manager may want to understand how much down time or administrative cost is included in this classification.

The point is that managers need timely, valid, and correct information to make decisions. To understand agency costs will require adopting a cost accounting system that is based on activities and assigns costs in a fashion that portrays actual resource consumption instead of an arbitrary application.

ACTIVITY-BASED COSTING

Activity-based costing (ABC) is a cost accounting methodology that matches the cost of resources to activities. Activities are then linked to cost objects. What this means is that a causal relationship is identified between how resources were used to accomplish the objectives of the organization. Financial accounting categorizes resource consumption (total payroll cost). ABC summarizes the resources that were consumed by activities. This approach is action-oriented. By understanding what actions are occurring within an organization and how these actions affect an HHA's prices, productivity, and competitive advantage, managers can then make sound business decisions. ABC is not a quick fix but part of an evolutionary process. The process begins with changing what information is collected, determining what outcomes are to be measured, and then using the collected information as a tool to shape or shift the organization.

"From a historical perspective, ABC was used first to describe improved product costing. Professors Robert S. Kaplan and Robin Cooper of the Harvard Business School became leading spokesmen by articulating in business periodicals how grotesque misallocations of overhead could distort the true costs of products."[2] Allocations that used a one-stage allocation process distorted product costs. This is similar to the cost report. The cost report uses a one-stage allocation process based on accumulated costs. "Misallocation occurs because the variability of indirect and overhead costs is not always in proportion to the allocation base."[3] This is evidenced by Table 7–11, where cost per visit fluctuates based on the allocation base that was used.

ABC, on the other hand, utilizes a two-stage allocation process (Figure 7–5). The first stage develops a relationship between costs and activities. This relationship is referred to as *resource drivers*. Resource drivers enable the grouping of common activities into a cost center or cost pools through identification of activities that consume resources. Activities can be general or very specific. Either approach will help to quantify the relationship between activities and resource consumption. Examples of activities, at a gross level, are the functions of billing, scheduling, provision of patient care, recruitment, quality improvement, accounting, and records management. Within each of these aggregate groupings are specific activities.

The second stage is the assignment of activities to products, or cost objects. Cost objects could be products, customers, payors, product lines, or programs. Activities are assigned to cost objects using activity drivers. If the cost object is

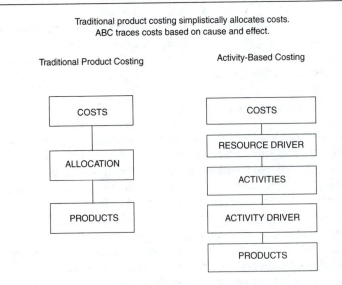

Figure 7–5 Comparison of Traditional and ABC Methodologies. Source: Reprinted with permission from *Emerging Practices in Cost Management* by B.J. Brinker, p. A5-1, © 1993, Warren, Gorham & Lamont, 31 St. James Avenue, Boston, MA 02116. All rights reserved.

the payor, and the activity is the billing process, then the activity driver could be the number of claims by payor. The final result is analysis-dependent and will be determined by what an agency's needs are. Assignment of activities to a customer group would be based on the requirements of the customer group. An example of this process is demonstrated by the concept of the billing department. Table 7–13 illustrates how the process works with payor designated as the cost object.

Costs are accumulated in the general ledger for the billing department. The billing department estimates or tracks the activities that it performs for each payor. In this situation, the billing department has two primary activities: (1) billing and (2)

Table 7–13 ABC Cost Assignment Principles

		Total
General ledger costs		
Payroll		22,000
Taxes		1,760
Health benefits		1,500
Workers' compensation		216
Supplies		345
Phone		777
Postage		335
Depreciation		740
Rent		1,974
Utilities		502
		30,149
	Effort	*Total*
Activities		
Billing	0.75	22,611
Collections	0.25	7,537
		30,149
	Claims	*Billing*
Cost objects		
Medicare	1,345	10,271
HMO	1,000	7,636
Medicaid	235	1,795
Commercial	381	2,909
		22,611
	Effort	*Collections*
Cost objects		
Medicare	15%	1,131
HMO	5%	377
Medicaid	60%	4,522
Commercial	20%	1,507
	100%	7,537

collections. The billing department estimates that 75 percent of its time is spent performing billing activities, and the balance, or 25 percent, is spent on collection activities. Therefore, the resource driver is time or effort.

Once activities have been identified, then activity drivers need to be identified to assign activity cost to the cost object. In this case, activity cost is being assigned to a specific payor. The cost drivers are the number of claims that were processed during the period and the amount of time spent resolving collection problems. Therefore, the activity of billing is assigned to the different payors using the number of claims as a cost driver, and the activity of collections is assigned to the different payors using the amount of actual effort expended for each payor.

AN APPROACH TO ABC

The following model demonstrates a simplified approach to how ABC could be applied in the home health setting. The objective of the analysis is to obtain better discipline costs by payor. To obtain better information will require capturing general ledger costs by discipline, payor, and department.

Table 7–14 illustrates an agency whose expenses have been categorized by departmental classifications, and where operational cost has been accumulated by discipline and by payor. This is illustrated by Table 7–15. Billing, scheduling, records management, and administration have been identified as the primary activities. For ease of presentation, no secondary activities have been addressed.

Proper identification of activity cost requires the assignment of all administrative expenses that support the activities of billing, scheduling, records management, and administration. To begin, the administrative expenses of recruitment, postage, depreciation, telephone, rent, and utilities were targeted. These expenses support the billing, payroll, scheduling, office, records, operations, and administrative departments. To assign the targeted expenses to the primary activities will require identifying resource drivers. Resource drivers establish a causal relationship between raw resource cost and activities. Tables 7–16 through 7–20 illustrate the allocation of each expense category using its respective resource driver. The following resource drivers were identified:

- for recruitment, number of new hires;
- for postage, actual usage;
- for depreciation, departments where equipment was used;
- for telephone, number of extensions for base charge and actual usage;
- for rent, square footage; and
- for utilities, square footage.

Table 7–21 illustrates the assignment of administrative expenses to the billing, payroll, scheduling, office, records, operations, and administrative departments.

Table 7–14 Departmental Costs in Dollars

	Operations	Billing	Schedule	Payroll	Office	Records	Administrative	Total
Salaries	844,000	22,000	21,500	26,000	74,500	18,000	321,000	1,327,000
Payroll taxes	67,520	1,760	1,720	2,080	5,960	1,440	25,680	106,160
Health benefits	18,000	1,500	1,500	1,500	4,500	1,500	12,000	40,500
Workers' compensation	75,960	216	215	260	745	180	3,336	80,912
Contract labor	213,000						15,000	228,000
Supplies—medical	47,145							47,145
Auto reimbursement	83,000				347		3,200	86,547
Insurance—malpractice							8,500	8,500
Insurance—general							2,000	2,000
Computer support							3,600	3,600
Computer supplies							1,800	1,800
Office supplies		345		537		238	11,431	12,551
Education	1,455			250			850	2,555
Beepers	435						185	620
Interest							15,000	15,000
Dues							4,300	4,300
Accounting							8,500	8,500
Legal							15,000	15,000
Recruitment							2,300	2,300
Postage							3,350	3,350
Depreciation							3,700	3,700
Telephone							18,500	18,500
Rent							42,500	42,500
Utilities							10,800	10,800
Total	1,350,515	25,821	24,935	30,627	86,052	21,358	532,532	2,071,840

Table 7–15 Direct Cost in Dollars by Payor and Discipline

	Medicare	HMO	Medicaid	Commercial	Total
Nursing	454,734	220,376	62,900	36,489	774,499
Physical therapy	99,256	50,981	16,250	18,920	185,407
Occupational therapy	15,050	8,602	663	2,480	26,795
Speech therapy	8,496	2,651	97	1,042	12,286
Medical social services	11,663	1,604		741	14,008
Home health aide	205,747	69,426	4,941	10,261	290,375
Supplies	31,025	8,676	3,410	4,034	47,145
Administrative	1,890				1,890
Total	827,861	362,316	88,261	73,967	1,352,405

Note: HMO = health maintenance organization.

Table 7–16 Assignment of Rent and Utilities Using Square Feet as the Cost Driver

	Sq. ft.	Rent	Utilities
Billing	150	1,974	502
Payroll	100	1,316	334
Scheduling	100	1,316	334
Office	500	6,579	1,672
Records	80	1,053	267
Operations	800	10,526	2,675
Administration	1,500	19,736	5,016
Total	3,230	42,500	10,800

Table 7–17 Assignment of Telephone Using Number of Extensions and Actual Usage

	# of Extensions	Usage (%)	Base ($)	Usage ($)	Total ($)
Billing	1	4	133	644	777
Payroll	1	2	133	322	455
Scheduling	1	17	133	2,737	2,870
Office	4	10	533	1,610	2,143
Records	1	1	133	161	294
Operations	4	41	533	6,601	7,134
Administration	6	25	802	4,025	4,827
Total	18	100	2,400	16,100	18,500

Table 7–18 Assignment of Postage Using Actual Usage

	Usage (%)	Postage ($)
Billing	10	335
Payroll	8	268
Scheduling	0	
Office	25	838
Records	1	34
Operations	20	670
Administration	36	1,205
Total	100	3,350

Table 7–19 Assignment of Depreciation Based on Departmental Usage

	Equipment (%)	Depreciation ($)
Billing	20	740
Payroll	10	370
Scheduling	5	185
Office	25	925
Records	2	74
Operations	10	370
Administration	28	1,036
Total	100	3,700

Table 7–20 Assignment of Recruitment Cost Based on the Number of New Hires

	New Hires	Recruitment
Billing		
Payroll		
Scheduling		
Office	1	383
Records		
Operations	5	1,917
Administration		
Total	6	2,300

Table 7–21 Summary of Traceable and Assignable Departmental Cost in Dollars

	Traceable	Recruitment	Postage	Depreciation	Phone	Rent	Utilities	Total
Billing	25,821		335	740	777	1,974	502	30,149
Payroll	30,627		268	370	455	1,316	334	33,370
Scheduling	24,935			185	2,870	1,316	334	29,640
Office	86,052	383	838	925	2,143	6,579	1,672	98,592
Records	21,358		34	74	294	1,053	267	23,080
Operations	1,350,515	1,917	670	370	7,134	10,526	2,675	1,373,807
Administration*	451,382		1,205	1,036	4,827	19,736	5,016	483,202
	1,990,690	2,300	3,350	3,700	18,500	42,500	10,800	2,071,840

Recruitment	2,300
Postage	3,350
Depreciation	3,700
Telephone	18,500
Rent	42,500
Utilities	10,800
	81,150

*Less assigned cost.

Costs listed as traceable were identified specifically at the time of posting operating expenses to the general ledger. To complete the first stage of the allocation process requires allocating the cost of the payroll and office departments to the primary activities.

Payroll and office are support departments. They support the primary activities that take place within an HHA. Included in the office cost center is the receptionist, office manager, and an individual whose primary purpose is to handle personnel issues. Office costs will be allocated based on the number of full-time employees in the HHA. The payroll cost center consists of one individual whose primary obligation is to handle the payroll process. Costs within this department will be allocated to the other departments based on the number of checks that were issued to each department during the course of the year. The allocation is illustrated by Tables 7–22 and 7–23.

The allocation of the office and payroll costs is added to the cost of the billing, scheduling, records, operations, and administrative departments (Table 7–24). At this point, total activity cost has been identified, and it is time to use activity drivers to allocate cost to the cost objects or payors.

Table 7–22 Assignment of Pooled Payroll Cost to Higher Level Support Departments

	Paychecks	Payroll ($)
Billing	26	1,357
Payroll		
Scheduling	26	1,357
Office	0	
Records	26	1,357
Operations	432	22,549
Administration	208	10,857
Total	718	37,477

Table 7–23 Assignment of Office Management Costs to Higher Level Departments

	Full-time equivalents	Office
Billing	1	4,108
Payroll	1	4,108
Scheduling	1	4,108
Office	0	
Records	1	4,108
Operations	12	49,296
Administration	8	32,864
Total	24	98,592

Table 7–24 Cost Structure after the Reassignment of the Payroll and Office Cost Pools

	Traceable	Assigned	Sub–1	Office	Sub–2	Payroll	Sub–3
Billing	25,821	4,328	30,149	4,108	34,257	1,358	35,615
Payroll	30,627	2,743	33,370	4,108	37,478		
Scheduling	24,935	4,705	29,640	4,108	33,748	1,357	35,105
Office	86,052	12,540	98,592				
Records	21,358	1,722	23,080	4,108	27,188	1,357	28,545
Operations	1,350,515	23,292	1,373,807	49,296	1,423,103	22,549	1,445,652
Administration	451,382	31,820	483,202	32,864	516,066	10,857	526,923
Total	1,990,690	81,150	2,071,840	98,592	2,071,840	37,478	2,071,840

Table 7–25 illustrates the four activity drivers that will be used. The billing function will be assigned to each payor based on the number of claims that were generated during the year. The activity driver for scheduling will be based on actual effort. Records management will use the activity driver of total patients by payor, and operational and administrative expenses will use the activity driver of visits by payor. Actual results of the cost assignment are illustrated in Table 7–26.

Table 7–27 illustrates the results of the analysis. The ABC model identified different average costs by payor because of the amount of effort that each payor required. The above results indicate that patients with Medicaid consume more resources than patients who have commercial insurance. Managers may know this

Table 7–25 Activity Drivers

	Claims	Effort	Patients	Visits
Medicare	1,345	40%	1,115	17,094
HMO	1,000	28%	951	7,918
Medicaid	235	22%	162	1,784
Commercial	381	10%	381	1,805
Total	2,961	100%	2,609	28,601

Table 7–26 Activities Assigned to Payors (Cost Objectives)

	Medicare	HMO	Medicaid	Commercial	Total
Direct costs	827,861	362,316	88,261	73,967	1,352,405
Billing	16,178	12,027	2,828	4,581	35,614
Scheduling	14,042	9,829	7,723	3,511	35,105
Records	12,199	10,405	1,772	4,169	28,545
Administrative	370,658	171,691	38,683	39,139	620,171
	1,240,938	566,268	139,267	125,367	2,071,840

Table 7–27 Cost per Visit Calculation

	Cost	Visits	Cost/visit
Medicare	1,240,938	17,094	72.59
HMO	566,268	7,918	71.52
Medicaid	139,267	1,784	78.06
Commercial	125,367	1,805	69.46
	2,071,840	28,601	72.44

Table 7–28 Cost per Visit—Medicare

	Direct	Supplies	Indirect	Total	Visits	Cost/Visit
Nursing	454,734	20,000	203,494	678,228	8,421	80.54
Physical therapy	99,256	1,890	45,817	146,963	1,896	77.51
Occupational therapy	15,050		7,274	22,324	301	74.17
Speech therapy	8,496		4,155	12,651	172	73.56
Medical social services	11,663		2,441	14,104	101	139.64
Home health aide	205,747	11,025	149,896	366,668	6,203	59.11
	794,946	32,915	413,077	1,240,938	17,094	72.59

Table 7–29 Cost per Visit—HMO

	Direct	Supplies	Indirect	Total	Visits	Cost/Visit
Nursing	220,376	6,075	109,163	335,614	4,238	79.19
Physical therapy		50,981	25,449	76,430	988	77.36
Occupational therapy		8,602	4,817	13,419	187	71.76
Speech therapy		2,651	1,364	4,015	53	75.75
Medical social services		1,604	412	2,016	16	126.00
Home health aide	69,426	2,601	62,747	134,774	2,436	55.33
	353,640	8,676	203,952	566,268	7,918	71.52

intuitively; however, if they relied on the results of the Medicare model, they would assume that every payor had an average visit cost of $72.44, as illustrated in Table 7–7. Tables 7–28 and 7–29 illustrate differences in the cost per visit by discipline for two payors. Table 7–28 illustrates cost per visit for Medicare, and Table 7–29 illustrates it for a health maintenance organization.

CONCLUSION

Activity-based costing (ABC) has been widely heralded as a better ap-proach (or family of approaches) than traditional costing methods for identifying the cost of various activities within business organizations. ABC is particularly useful in companies with multiple products or services, because product or service complexity usually requires expensive overhead support activities, which need careful cost management. Simplistic volume-based allocation methods used by conventional costing systems often produce distorted unit costs for products and services.[4]

ABC will provide HHAs with a tool to measure accurately the cost of providing services. However, like most tools, there is a cost attached to it. The cost is due to data collection. To obtain better information will require an investment in determining what information needs to be captured, development of the tools to capture data, and the enlistment of employees and support for data collection.

Once data have been input into the system, the uses are basically unlimited. However, a word of caution needs to be mentioned in relationship to the new data that will be available. Data should be used as a tool to advance organizational learning instead of how they have been used historically. Historically, data have been used as an "I got you" instrument. Use of data in this fashion does not foster team growth, and it certainly will not help in the identification of how much effort goes into a particular activity, especially if the employee feels that the data will be used against him or her.

Included in the paradigm shift of using data as a tool instead of "I got you" is beginning to think about activities from an outcome perspective. Do the activities that are being performed achieve a specific outcome? Is this outcome consistent with the organization's values and mission? If the answer is no, then ask why not. Understanding how actions and activities relate to an organization's mission will accomplish many things. One result is understanding how much cost is attached to achieving an outcome but more important is the determination of whether an outcome can be enhanced. Is the activity and related outcome an investment in the present or future or purely a cost that needs to be avoided?

Understanding costs by activity and outcome can enhance team and organizational performance. These considerations are extremely important in light of managed care, increased competition, and shrinking margins. Enhanced organizational performance leads to financial viability, job security, and an organization that values the relationship and contributions of all members of its team.

NOTES

1. National Association of Home Care. 1994. *Basic Statistics about Home Care*, Washington, DC: 7.
2. G. Cokins, *An ABC Manager's Primer* (Montvale, NJ: Institute of Management Accountants, 1993), 4.
3. *Ibid.*, 11.
4. B.J. Brinker, *Emerging Practices in Cost Management* (Boston: Warren, Gorham & Lamont, 1993), A5-1.

Chapter 8

Design of an Activity-Based Costing System

The previous chapter identified basic concepts that management should consider when making financial decisions. The chapter concluded with an introduction of the concepts and uses for activity-based costing (ABC). Activity-based costing could be viewed as another cost accounting vehicle solely for the benefit of the accounting department. However, this would be extremely limiting. This narrow view would limit the design of the system, the input into the system, and the benefits that would accrue to the agency.

An ABC system can be a powerful tool if implemented and used properly. Benefits range from improved product costing to operational efficiency. Understanding product cost is a basic requirement for survival in a prospective payment or managed care environment. Operational efficiency becomes a multifaceted opportunity when an ABC system is employed to gather data to evaluate cross-functional activities, organizational outcome measurement, and the cost of quality. "Probably the most exciting difference between traditional product costing and ABC is the direct influence ABC can have on nonfinancial operations management. The notion that managing activities efficiently will reduce total costs is fundamental to ABC."[1]

The critical success factors from an ABC implementation perspective are understanding what outcomes the agency wants to achieve, establishing what data are critical to measure and evaluate to monitor desired outcomes, and enlisting the support of everyone in the organization to assist in data collection requirements. The ABC project should also have a driving force behind implementation and its ongoing use. The success of the ABC system will require someone from senior management to champion the ABC system.

Involvement of senior management is critical for several reasons. First, ABC represents a change management system. Change management occurs because everyone in the organization will become involved with the process of data collection. Data collection will cross all departments and functional boundaries. Senior management must be able to overcome organizational barriers that would exist if ABC were viewed as being initiated by accounting for the sole benefit of accounting. Beyond collection, senior management can help the organization move from analysis into action. Action is using the results of the ABC system to make sound business decisions.

> A lack of commitment on the part of top management may be indicated by the conduct of business as usual and the delegation of ABC implementation to others. When top management has a history of not being involved in change or of grasping at every new fad that comes on the scene without following through, employees will conclude that "this, too, will pass." Management at the highest levels of a company must show commitment to ABC in ways that are visible to subordinates. Management can show support for ABC by actively participating in ABC implementation; attending training sessions; actively using the ABC system or methodology; and establishing performance measures that are realistic, measurable, and published internally.[2]

WHAT OUTCOMES DO YOU WANT FROM YOUR ABC SYSTEM?

Outcome management is the best place to begin in designing an ABC system. By articulating and prioritizing outcomes, an agency can then determine what data collection requirements are necessary to evaluate specific outcomes. Implementation begins by developing a team to begin the outcome identification process. Senior representatives from operations, quality improvement, accounting, human resources, information systems, and administration should participate on the team during this process. Representatives will target outcomes within their departments as well as across the organization. Additionally, "when the CEO serves as project advocate and sponsor, and senior operating managers are the project targets, the transition between analysis process—getting to the numbers—and the action process—making significant organizational or strategic changes—can be smooth and rapid."[3]

Specific outcomes will depend on the complexity of the agency. A small agency may only have one product line such as skilled intermittent visits or personal care, while a larger agency may have multiple product lines that serve multiple locations. In either case, the scope of the ABC implementation should be identified. Scope is determined by how the project is defined. A project could be very specific and target one specific department or process, or it could be a global project and target agencywide processes. Obviously, a smaller project will require less time and resources than a global project; however, the answer depends on what the goals are of the individual who is championing the ABC implementation. The other thing to keep in mind is that this will be an evolutionary process, and initial outcomes and activities may change as the organization begins to gather data.

One outcome that could be chosen from this process is to determine accurate costs for the provision of care. This is a broad topic with several different approaches that then need to be answered by the team members as they begin to design the data collection tools. These questions are listed below:

- Do costs need to be identified on a payor-specific basis?
- Is cost identification for direct costs only, or should all indirect costs be included?
- What is the group's definition of direct expenses to be included?
- Are direct costs to be identified by discipline?
- Are direct costs differentiated by labor, materials, and burden?
- Are labor costs to be identified by activity?
- What is the group's definition of indirect expenses to be included?
- Are indirect costs to be identified by department or activity?
- Do costs differ by product line or program?
- Do services add value or simply add cost?
- What is the cost per clinical outcome?

The answer to these questions will help the team become clear on what information will need to be collected. The scope of the ABC project will be defined depending on how the project team answers the above questions.

Another goal of the ABC system implementation could be to determine specific objectives that an agency will want to monitor. Objective identification can be purely clinical, administrative, or both, and can be as simple as having a tool to monitor the factors that an agency deems critical to successful operations. Examples of objectives, or critical success factors, as they apply to the accurate determination of costs in the provision of care could include the following:

- unit cost for sensitivity analysis;
- identification of a profit margin by payor, product, or service line;
- identification of a financially viable payor mix;
- appropriate mix of services for a particular clinical pathway;
- identification of the cost per activity by payor;
- meeting time;
- productive versus nonproductive time across all classes of employees;
- identification of the cost per activity for the entire agency;
- determination of step levels for adding employees by job function;
- identification of departmental outcomes;

- cost of turnover versus retention;
- linkage of information into continuous quality improvement processes; and
- use of results as part of the employee evaluation process.

IS THE CURRENT PROCESS KNOWN BY ALL TEAM MEMBERS?

Do all of the team members who have been assembled have a clear picture of the processes that take place within a home health agency (HHA)? Does everyone receive financial statements that reflect departmental costs and operational results? Before the employees can be educated to the change management process, the project team must understand the processes that take place within the agency.

A logical place to begin is with the financial statements, statistics regarding previous operations and forecasted operations, budgets, organizational charts, and future plans. This grouping of information provides a starting point for understanding operations from a global perspective. Each team member would then be able to identify specific activity for which he or she is responsible. Eventually, activity identification will begin to identify cross-functional processes.

Identification of cross-functional activities enables management to understand activities within major processes. Cross-functional analysis also allows managers to take into account "the interconnectivity and mutual dependencies among their departments."[4] Listed in Exhibit 8–1 are several activities related to the primary process of billing. Each secondary process is completed by different departments within the HHA.

Furthermore, identification of activities from a cross-functional perspective illustrates the concept of internal customers within the agency. In this illustration, each successive step will be affected by how well the prior activity was performed. Costs can then be attached to each activity, and changes that are made within the system can then be quantified to measure improvements resulting from continuous quality improvement efforts.

Exhibit 8–1 Activities that Comprise the Main Process of Billing

Activity	Department
Documentation of field visit	Field staff
Data entry of field activity	Billing or data entry staff
Prebill review	Quality assurance
Run submission of bills	Billing
Review submission of bills	Accounting or operations management

One of the ways to trace processes is through the use of a flow chart. A flow chart is a picture of how data flow within an organization that identifies inputs, processes, and outputs. Data are traced through every process across organizational boundaries and, therefore, provide a good visual tool to illustrate the concept of cross-functional processes.

Understanding of the processes that take place within an agency will enable managers to determine whether they want to target one specific primary process or multiple processes. Each process will have a different relationship to cost and to the objectives determined by the project management team. Each process will be composed of multiple activities and cross-functional boundaries.

DEVELOPMENT OF COMMON TERMINOLOGY

Common terminology will be critical in getting everyone into the ABC system mode. Common terminology can be as basic as defining the different types of services that are offered by an agency. Service definition can then be expanded into alternative classifications based on whether the agency offers multiple product lines or programs. This classification depends on whether the agency is tracking the different types of service that it provides and whether these distinctions are clear to all customers and employees.

ABC systems have developed their own terminology. This change in terminology is different from the way managers and employees have been educated in the past. Financial reporting systems have focused on the management of total expenditures by expense category. Cost accounting systems have focused on controllable versus noncontrollable expenses. An ABC system focuses on activities.

Activities are the events that consume the work day. Therefore, the cost of activities represents how resources are consumed, and activities are then matched to the

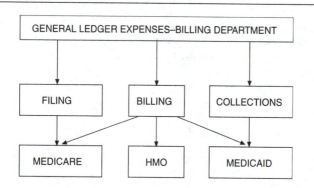

Figure 8–1 The ABC Framework for Cost Assignment

customers, products, or services that are provided by an agency. "Resource costs represent people, computers, technology, equipment, machines, supplies, and other factors. These factors allow productive activity and the serving of customers, whether internal or external."[5] The ABC framework is illustrated by Figure 8–1.

In this example, the billing department's expenses would be classified in the general ledger. Direct expenses for the billing department would include salaries, payroll taxes, health benefits, workers' compensation, and supplies. These expenses would then be assigned to activities using resource drivers. Resource drivers establish a link between the activities performed by the employees of the billing department and the cost of the billing department identified within the general ledger. The activities in this example are filing, billing, and collections. Resource drivers in this situation could be based on a time study conducted by the employee or an estimate determined by the employee(s). Managers or a member of the project team can also interview employees for their estimates of how they spend their time.

Filing, billing, and collections represent activity cost pools. Activity cost pools are composed of cost elements. Cost elements are the percentage of general ledger expenses attributable to each activity. Table 8–1 illustrates the resummarization of general ledger cost into activities using resource drivers. Table 8–2 illustrates the cost elements of each activity.

Activities are then assigned to cost objects. The cost object in Figure 8–1 is payors. Activity cost is assigned to cost objects using activity drivers. In this ex-

---

Table 8–1 Resummarization of General Ledger Cost into Activities Using Resource Drivers

General ledger	
Payroll	$22,000
Payroll taxes	1,716
Health benefits	1,500
Workers' compensation	220
	$25,436
Resource driver	
Filing	20%
Billing	45%
Collections	35%
	100%
Activities	
Filing	$ 5,087
Billing	11,446
Collections	8,903
	$25,436

Table 8–2 Cost Elements of Each Activity

	Filing ($)	Billing ($)	Collections ($)	Total ($)
Payroll	4,400	9,900	7,700	22,000
Payroll taxes	343	772	601	1,716
Health benefits	300	675	525	1,500
Workers' compensation	44	99	77	220
	5,087	11,446	8,903	25,436

ample, three different cost drivers were used. The cost driver for billing was the number of claims by payor. The cost driver for collections was actual effort. Effort was determined by keeping a time record. The cost driver was based on a weighted average using the number of claims. The agency's billers estimated that they spent three times as much effort on Medicare claims and two times as much effort for Medicaid claims as they did for health maintenance organization (HMO) claims. Table 8–3 illustrates the assignment of activities to payors using cost drivers. "The more accurate a company wants its reported costs to be, the more activity drivers the company will need to achieve that accuracy."[6] However, increasing the number of cost drivers will also increase data collection costs.

The education process begins with senior managers and then progresses through each level of the agency. If everyone understands the process, then it will make it easier to implement. It is also important for managers to understand that this is a management process and not an accounting process.

EDUCATION OF EMPLOYEES

Education of staff is critical to the success of an ABC implementation. Employees will be responsible for capturing data in new formats. This represents a change to the employee and, depending on how it was explained to the employee, will determine his or her willingness to assist in obtaining management's new goals. Care should be taken in sharing the purpose of an ABC system, how data will be used, and how they will affect the employees who are gathering the data. "For example, if a biller is asked to participate in time studies or interviewed about the activities of the billing operation, the employee may slant his answers to match what he sees as a threat to his job ('Yes boss, it takes me fifteen minutes to package the bills for shipment.'). The employee might also tell the interviewer what he thinks the interviewer wants to hear ('Yes, it takes me five minutes to package those bills for shipment.')."[7]

The above example demonstrates that employees can view the implementation of an ABC system as a threat to their jobs, especially if the project is presented as a way to reduce expenses. The other point that the above example illustrates is

Table 8–3 Assignment of Activity Cost to Payors Using Cost Drivers

	Cost drivers			Activity cost by payor			
	Claims	Effort	Average	Filing	Billing	Collections	Total
Medicare	35	30%	105	3,735	6,359	2,671	12,765
HMO	10	20%	20	711	1,817	1,781	4,309
Medicaid	18	50%	18	641	3,270	4,451	8,362
	63	100%	143	5,087	11,446	8,903	25,436

employees may give answers based on what they think someone wants to hear instead of the facts. Being up front with all of the employees that one of the goals of the ABC system is to help make employees more effective will achieve better results. This can be accomplished by explaining that management needs to understand the processes that occur within each department. Process identification will require understanding activities by payors, product lines, and programs. Once activities are identified by the amount of time that each activity requires, the frequency with which the activity takes place, and the sequence of a particular activity within the processing chain, then management can identify alternative actions to improve organizational efficiency. "For example, the interviewer might say that the company is looking for ways to improve profitability by managing activities, thus making employees more effective in their jobs. In this way, the biller is more likely to give an unbiased answer ('Yes boss, it takes me about 10 minutes to get the bills prepared for mailing . . . but we could eliminate this step if we went to electronic billing.')."[8]

Management needs to be clear how it will use the results of the ABC process. If the intention is to use data to eliminate positions, then this needs to be stated. Otherwise, there will be a creditability issue, and employees' fears will be realized. Additionally, data can be used as a tool for organizational learning. Organizational learning can benefit all members of the organization if this is the intent of management. If the intent of management is to continue to use data in the old paradigm of "I got you," then some of the potential benefits will never accrue to the users of the ABC system.

DATA COLLECTION

Data collection requirements will vary depending on the decisions of the project team. Data collection requirements may be targeted to a specific function, outcome, or agencywide activities. Regardless of the scope of the ABC implementation, the project team will need the support of all employees of the agency. The project team may also require the support of individuals or organizations that are providing services on behalf of the agency.

There are several ways to determine the primary and secondary processes within an agency and the activities that support them. As discussed earlier, a review of the financial statements, budgets, organizational charts, and policies and procedures will provide an overview of the activities within the agency. To gain a more in-depth understanding will require gathering information from employees at all levels within the agency.

One way to gather information is to observe activities. This can be accomplished by walking around, asking questions, and participating in meetings. Another approach is to interview employees. As suggested above, interviewers are more likely to obtain accurate information if they are up front about the purpose of the ABC system and what will be required of everyone in the data collection and analysis processes.

The process of interviewing is expensive because it requires the time of the interviewer and the interviewee. Interviewing can be done on a one-to-one basis using structured or unstructured interview techniques. A structured interview technique is a predetermined list of questions. An unstructured interview builds on the previous questions and answers. Probably the most efficient way to determine activities is to do the interviewing process as part of a departmental meeting. The departmental meeting will have all players present and should begin by developing common terminology and educating everyone on the purpose of the ABC system and the intent of management.

Processes and activities can be identified for the group or for individual employees. The objective of the manager is to take notes of all activities being identified. The manager or interviewer should also help to prompt the departmental players with "what about this" or "what about that" questions. This process should also coach employees to think about what factors (resource drivers) would cause them to spend more time at one particular activity versus another activity, whether the activities are routine or nonroutine, the amount of time each activity requires, and the frequency of the activity.

Concurrently, the interviewer would have employees identify where their particular activities are in relation to the total process. Is the department solely responsible for an activity or process, or does it process the output from another department's process, or do departmental processes or activities become another department's input? "To expand upon this, a process is a series of activities that are linked to perform a specific goal. Each activity is a customer of another activity and, in turn, has its own customers. In short, activities are all part of a customer chain, with all activities working together to provide value to the outside customer."[9] Figure 8–2 illustrates the concept of internal customers. Exhibit 8–1 identified how the billing process crosses several departments, and, within each

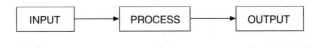

Figure 8–2 Process Flow

department, there are secondary processes or activities related to the primary process of billing.

Activities can then be summarized and prioritized. Summarization and prioritization would be based on how the departmental employees saw their efforts rolling up into activities. The follow-up to the initial meeting will require the manager or the interviewer to document the results and forward them to the participating employees for their review. The process of establishing activities could also use employee job descriptions as a starting point. This, of course, assumes that job descriptions were designed based on activities.

The next step would be to determine how activities relate to the cost objects being studied by the agency. These questions ask, "How is the output of our activities used?" "What does it look like?" "How can it be measured?" The answers will identify activity drivers. Employees may or may not know how each successive step in the process is used by the next customer in the chain. In a simplified example, if the objective was to determine the activity driver for the billing process in order to assign costs to each payor, then the number of claims by payor could be used.

If a department is a link in the processing chain, it may not know how its particular process fits into the cost object being measured. However, it needs to know how its particular process fits into each subsequent element of the entire process. Understanding how each activity interrelates to the next and previous activity will enable employees and managers to eliminate waste and redundancy and improve the process. Hopefully, "the ABC approach can even develop into a management style or strategy for continuous quality improvement by focusing the attention of managers and employees towards resource allocation at the activity level."[10]

Time studies are another method of data collection. Time studies can be either continuous or for selected intervals. Use of time studies will help management to identify activities by employee or by department based on the activities and processes identified above. A sample data collection form is at the end of the chapter. Categories can be added or changed depending on organizational requirements.

A key element of data collection will be an agency's information system. Understanding what information is already being collected and what will need to be collected will help to measure the cost of data collection. Data collection will be enhanced if the information system can be adapted or modified to meet the needs of the agency. Otherwise, the agency will need to employ a spreadsheet application like LOTUS 1-2-3 to price its cost objectives properly.

MANUAL SYSTEMS

Manual systems will make it relatively difficult, but not impossible, to gather information for ABC purposes. The agency will need to realize that data collection for the purpose of determining better product costs and improving organizational efficiency will cost money. The following is an example of the steps that the accounting department would have to go through in order to determine an accurate cost for the provision of patient care.

An agency may require accounting to classify all activities by payor classification. This may require accounting to change its chart of accounts to accommodate the increased data collection requirements. Beyond changing the chart of accounts, the accounting staff will need to identify all services by payor. Accounting may be able to use the billing system to summarize this information, or it will need to find an alternative method.

At a minimum, accounting will need to determine total activity for the period in question by payor classification. This activity will need to be identified by patient to determine his or her payor classification, then matched to the nurse, therapist, or aide who provided the service. Once the agency's caregiver is known, then accounting has the task of attaching a cost to the visit that was performed. This information will come from either of two places: (1) payroll or (2) accounts payable. Furthermore, depending on how the agency chooses to pay its caregivers, accounting may be able to identify a generic visit rate or be forced to analyze each patient visit to identify whether the visit received a premium rate. This process is further complicated by employees who are paid salaries. This will require determining the number of patients seen by the employee in the pay period and calculating an average cost per visit. Calculation of an actual cost per visit based on time is possible with a manual system; however, the labor cost would probably exceed any benefit the agency would receive.

Once the direct cost per visit is determined, then accounting would need to apply burden to each one of the visits. Burden represents payroll taxes, health insurance, paid time off, workers' compensation, and any other employee benefit. These costs would need to be pro-rated to the direct visit cost. Application of burden would need to be employee-specific. Additionally, care would need to be taken to consider how payroll accruals will affect the costing process, because the payroll periods will not coincide neatly with the analysis period. Beyond labor cost, materials will also need to be identified by patient in order to assign the actual cost to payors.

If the objective is to assign both direct and indirect costs to payors, then the next step for accounting is to go through all of the payroll earnings of the support departments and assign costs to activities using resource drivers. Costs can be aggregated by department, by employee, or by other common activity or function for assignment to cost objects. Overhead expenses will also need to be assigned.

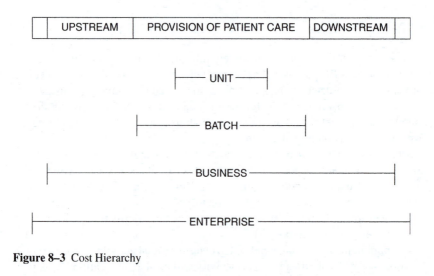

Figure 8–3 Cost Hierarchy

Once all of the agency's costs have been assigned to cost objectives, a cost per unit can be calculated by payor. The process that is outlined is an overview of the process that would be required if an agency implemented an ABC system in a manual accounting environment. An obvious cost of implementation would be the time of the accounting staff to accumulate costs in a different format. Cost will increase with the complexity of the organization. This may require hiring an individual for this sole purpose.

BEHAVIOR OF COST

Costs exhibit a hierarchical behavior (Figure 8–3). Activities and, therefore, costs exhibit different behaviors within an agency. Behavior depends on the complexity of the agency, the customer and payor requirements, and how services are provided. At the lowest possible level is unit cost. This is a direct cost to the agency and will fluctuate with every unit of service provided. Unit cost is identifiable as part of the provision of care. The next level within the cost hierarchy is batch-related activities. Batch-related activities support the provision of patient care from intake through discharge. Batch costs will be an indirect cost of patient care and a combination of fixed and variable expenses that will fluctuate with volume. The third level of the cost hierarchy is business-related expenses to a specific product line, program, or customer base. These costs are indirect and will fluctuate minimally with volume. The last level of the cost hierarchy is the enterprise or facility level. These costs remain fixed regardless of the number of product lines or volume of services.

Unit-level costs are materials, labor, and burden. Material cost is identifiable on a patient-specific basis. Material cost can include supplies provided by the agency, supplies ordered by the agency, medical equipment ordered for the patient, intravenous (IV) therapies, and other medications. Labor is the cost of having an employee, contractor, or subcontracted individual provide patient care. The cost of labor will fluctuate based on how much time was spent by the provider when supplying patient services. If the provider is an employee of the agency, then labor cost will depend on how the agency is paying its employees.

Visit time is the best indicator of resource consumption. Identification of visit time will provide agencies with a better cost per visit than using an average cost per visit methodology. Tracking total visit and support time provides a mechanism to measure total cost of providing patient care. Cost per visit is an activity within the primary process of providing patient care. Telephone support time is another activity cost within the primary process of providing patient care.

Depending on an agency's payment methodology, cost per visit can be separated into micro activities. Assuming that an agency pays on a per visit basis, the secondary activities represent travel time, documentation time, preparation time, treatment time, and possibly case management/conference time. If an agency pays for an eight-hour day or a salaried work week, then administrative cost becomes another element of the micro activities. Understanding the cost attached to these activities will enable agencies to measure resource consumption better at a unit cost level and help to quantify opportunities to build efficiencies into the delivery of patient care.

Burden at a unit cost level represents the benefits that are paid to field staff and anyone who has direct patient contact. Burden is the aggregation of employer taxes and employee benefits. The unit cost for burden will depend on how the agency has defined its programs and how well it monitors the relationship between patient care time and administrative time. Generally, the greater the amount of administrative time in relationship to patient care time, the higher the cost per unit.

Costs that are classified as batch costs support the primary activity of providing patient care from intake to discharge. Unlike unit costs, batch costs do not fluctuate directly with volume. This is because of their nature. A batch activity is intake and discharge, scheduling, billing, records management, and case management. These activities can support many units of service. Additionally, these activities will not be identifiable at a patient level; however, they will be identifiable at a customer or payor level, a program level, or a product-line level.

Understanding the primary and secondary activities at a batch level will help managers understand the different levels of indirect costs that are directly related to a specific contract. When batch activities are added to unit costs at an activity level, management will have a tool to evaluate profitability on a contract-by-contract basis. Use of this type of information may enable managers to renegotiate contracts based on actual effort and activities provided on behalf of a managed care organization.

Identification of batch-level costs also serves another purpose. Batch-level costs will fluctuate indirectly or in a step fashion with volume. Therefore, when performing an incremental analysis that looks at possible increases or decreases in volume, the analysis can be expanded to include support staff activities in addition to unit costs.

The third level of the cost hierarchy is business-related costs. These costs are specific to a product line, program, or operation. Costs at this level are insensitive to fluctuations in volume and are typically incurred to support business activities. Examples of business-related cost would be a manager who is hired for a particular product line, marketing, customer service, and interest expense.

These expenses exhibit an upstream, downstream, and overview quality. This is illustrated by Figure 8–3. The upstream element would be cost incurred through marketing the services of an HHA to a managed care organization prior to being awarded a contract, development of policies and procedures, and development of a product line. Overview costs would be the ongoing maintenance of the program or product line, and downstream costs would be the measurement of actual results, interest expense for receivables, and client surveys. This type of cost is traceable to specific programs or product lines. Therefore, to charge it to every program or product line would cause individual costs to be overstated or understated.

From an analytical perspective, costs at this level are sensitive to management discretion. Costs will depend on how an agency chooses to develop and maintain the services that it offers. For instance, one agency may have three separate product lines: skilled intermittent services, private duty, and hospice. This agency may choose to have a separate manager over each product line. A second agency may only have one manager over all three product lines but plan on adding an additional manager to assist the primary manager. Therefore, these types of decisions can be built into any analyses or costing studies that the agency may perform.

The final level of cost is enterprise or facility costs. This is the cost of supporting the entire operation. Costs at this level have little bearing on the number of services offered and the volume of services within each product line. Costs at this level are rent, utilities, the chief executive officer's (CEO's) salary, and general office insurance.

Cost identification at the unit, batch, business, and enterprise level can begin through assignment in the general ledger at a payor, program, or product-line

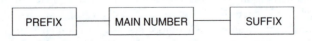

Figure 8–4 Simplified General Ledger Number

level. Cost identification through either direct identification or measurement of time spent on various activities will enhance the cost measurement process.

DEVELOPMENT OF THE CHART OF ACCOUNTS

The chart of accounts provides one of the keys to cost classification for purposes of ABC. The chart of accounts is a listing of all accounts that are used by an HHA's general ledger system. The chart of accounts is a series of numbers that has been designated to represent accounts for purposes of financial reporting. Generally, the chart of accounts begins with assets and concludes with the expenses of the organization. The assignment of specific numbers is usually done in groups; for example, the account numbers ranging from 1,000 to 1,999 represent an organization's assets, 2,000 to 2,999 represent an organization's liabilities, revenues are lumped together, cost of services are lumped together, and so forth.

Assignment of account numbers allows the HHA's accounting staff to identify expenses within each of these macro categories. Identification of expenses using a four-digit account number can become unwieldy as the complexity of an agency increases. To begin with, an agency may set up an account for each of the six disciplines. To differentiate cost between employee and contracted services would require setting up six additional accounts. If the HHA decided that it was interested in understanding discipline cost by payor, and it served five payors, then the 12 accounts would mushroom to 60 accounts, and so forth.

Therefore, charts of accounts were designed using prefixes and suffixes. A prefix would attach to the front of the account number, and a suffix would follow the account number. By utilizing prefixes and suffixes, the design of the chart of accounts will be more efficient. Figure 8–4 illustrates the concept of prefixes and suffixes. Prefixes and suffixes can consist of single digits or multiple digits.

The design of the account number can take different shapes because of the number of digits assigned to each prefix, main number, and suffix. The account can also have multiple prefix and suffix classifications. This depends on the design of the accounting system. Figure 8–5 illustrates the addition of two other prefixes and suffixes.

Prefixes and suffixes enable the chart of accounts to capture more information for purposes of ABC and financial reporting. Design of the chart of accounts should consider what the reporting goals of the organization are. An HHA that is only worried about financial reporting and completion of the Medicare cost report

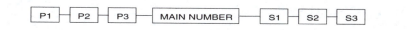

Figure 8–5 Complex General Ledger Number

will have less requirements than an agency that is interested in managing organizational expenses through monitoring activities. Other considerations will include whether the HHA has multiple companies or branches and what its organizational design entails. A consistent account design across multiple companies will enhance consolidated reporting efforts and enable reporting operational results in a hierarchical fashion.

Chart of accounts design will depend on the desired outcome an agency hopes to achieve and its accounting system. If the outcome is to combine costs for consolidated reporting purposes, then the establishment of a numbering scheme that considers company is important. Every outcome should be considered and evaluated for practicality. This is due to a limitation imposed by manual systems and systems that do not capture costs in a format that will achieve the desired outcome.

One agency may choose to identify costs by payor or by contract, while another agency is interested in cost by program or product line, and a third agency is interested in cost by branch and by department. The design of the chart of accounts should accommodate these factors. Further classification could include identification of costs by activity and for purposes of measuring quality. The measurement of quality could differentiate between accounts that add value to the provision of patient care or merely add cost.

Numbering schemes can be devised that do not rely on three different prefix categories and three different suffix categories. If the information system that is in use constrains the general ledger account number to a two-digit prefix, a four-character main number, and a four-digit suffix, then the account number can be designed to work within this constraint. There may be a need for the agency to prioritize what information it wants to collect until it can get an information system that meets all of its needs.

An approach to designing an account number when the number of digits is limited is the following: Each digit represents a different cost characteristic that the agency wants to document. For instance, the prefix may use the first digit to represent company, and the second digit of the prefix may represent branch. This way, accounts could be coded to reflect differences by company and division. The only drawback is that coding is limited to nine possibilities. The same approach can be used for the four-digit suffix. The first digit could represent product line; the second, program; the third, payor; and the fourth, department. Although at first glance, this may seem awkward, it enables the agency to define costs in an interrelated order. The main number can remain constant for major classifications of expenses and revenues.

ACTIVITY ANALYSIS

Once the data collection process has been completed, the project team should be able to compile a listing of activities to begin to determine resource centers and

Exhibit 8–2 Possible Resource Pools and Resource Drivers

Resource pool	Resource driver
Human resources	The number of full-time equivalents
Payroll	The number of paychecks
Financial reporting	The number of financial statements
Information systems	Departmental effort
Receptionist	The number of phone calls
Facility expenses	Square feet
Administrative expenses	Departmental consumption
Administrative expenses	No relation to activities
Billing	The billing activities
Scheduling	The scheduling activities

activity centers. The general ledger can provide the starting point by grouping costs by departmental classification into resource centers that can then be traced directly or through a causal relationship to activities. The ultimate goal is to trace as many costs as possible directly to the activity and to the cost objective. The second preferred method is through the use of resource drivers and activity drivers that develop a causal relationship between the activities that consume resources and the cost objects or customers that consume activities. The final method is allocation. A partial listing of resource pools is presented in Exhibit 8–2.

"The next step is to inventory all activities that are performed in an activity unit (center). A major benefit of the inventory of activities is that it provides a basis for focusing upon non-value-added activities, and, you can determine if the activity is primary or secondary. Primary activities are normally related to the organizational unit's mission, while secondary activities support primary activities."[11]

Exhibit 8–1 illustrated a process flow for the billing department. Exhibit 8–3 expands the flow of secondary activities to include classification based on value-added activities or activities that purely add cost. The five activities related to the process of billing have varying degrees of value. For instance, documentation of the field visit could be considered a value-added activity. This activity would add value because it provides information of current and future use to the agency, the payor, and other providers that will base their clinical decisions on actions and interventions that have taken place.

Data entry, on the other hand, is a cost. It adds no value to the provision of patient care. This is a cost that could be eliminated when transferring to a pen-based system or a documentation system that allows the field provider's notes to be updated into the system automatically. The third activity, prebill review, could be viewed from either perspective. This activity could be viewed as a value-added activity to prevent internal documentation problems from being communicated to payors or clients. However, this is a cost that in theory could be prevented with proper training of field staff and a system of checks and balances within the infor-

Exhibit 8–3 The Concept of Activity Attributes

Activity	Department	Value or cost
Documentation of field visit	Field staff	Value
Data entry of field activity	Billing or data entry staff	Cost
Prebill review	Quality assurance	Value/cost
Run submission of bills	Billing	Cost
Review submission of bills	Accounting or operations management	Value/cost

mation system. The fourth activity performed by the billing department is an administrative cost of doing business. This cost could be minimized through information system enhancements. The last step is another step similar to quality assurance that is intended to provide value, but if all inputs were correct on the front end, then this step would not be necessary.

Once primary activities have been defined, then activity drivers should be identified. "The team also must avoid combining activities from different levels of the variable and cost-intensive activity hierarchy, for example, combining unit-level activities and batch-level activities. If the team traces an activity to a cost object using an incongruent activity driver, the team is still spreading costs the traditional way and is continuing to introduce distortion error."[12] "Users will likely want to start with only a limited number of cost drivers so that they will not be overwhelmed with complexity. Cost drivers can be added later as the need becomes apparent."[13]

This is an evolutionary process, and, unless the software is already in place to accomplish ABC, the measurement process could become rather expensive. If a manual model is employed, the agency may want to consider fewer activity drivers to begin with and add additional drivers as the perceived benefits begin to justify the increased time and effort required to obtain better results. Exhibit 8–4 lists several primary activities and their possible activity drivers.

THE EVOLUTION OF THE COST ACCOUNTING SYSTEM

Robert Kaplan, the leading guru on cost accounting, identified four stages that organizations go through in the evolution of their cost accounting systems. "The stage one level of poor data quality is generally found in new organizations. The data are not compiled accurately, resulting in data errors, math errors, large variances, and significant year-end adjustments."[14] Many agencies are clinically driven. The owners are nursing entrepreneurs who have placed all of their energies into developing high-quality service provision, and the "back office" activities have not received the same amount of attention. This was a workable strategy in a cost-reimbursed payment system, especially through the use of consultants to come in quarterly or at year end to clean up financial statements and produce a cost report.

Exhibit 8–4 Primary Activities and Possible Activity Drivers

Primary activity	*Activity driver*
Provision of patient care—labor	Unit cost identified at the patient level
Provision of patient care—materials	Unit cost identified at the patient level
Billing	Number of claims
Scheduling	Number of patients on service
Logistics	Travel requirements
Records management	Number of charts
Administration*	Effort
Customer service	The number of complaints
Recruitment/retention	The number of new hires

*Administration could be expanded to quality improvement, nursing management, and administration. Expansion of the primary activity into smaller subsets would require the identification of additional activity drivers.

As agencies grew, many began to hire accounting personnel to manage the financial operations. This is characterized by Kaplan's Stage 2.

Stage 2, with its focus on external reporting, is generally represented by competent data collection. Data are not overly error-prone and tend to meet the standards and requirements for the various required external reports. At one time, costing systems may have been designed to provide management information, but as external reporting requirements have increased, over time, the systems have been modified to meet external needs. According to Kaplan, today such systems tend to have serious limitations with respect to product costing and profitability analysis.

Specifically, Kaplan feels that such systems are not timely, are overly aggregated, and are contaminated by cost allocations. Reporting on a month's operating results several weeks after the month ended is too slow, according to Kaplan. Modern computer information systems should allow for a much more continuous flow of data needed for control actions. The departmental approach to costing yields too little information on what is happening with respect to each of the organization's product lines. This is not to say that departmental information is not valuable, just that it is not sufficient. Allocations of cost, although often needed for external reporting, serve little purpose but obfuscation when they are assigned to products or units that have no control over them.

Not only do allocations interfere with effective evaluation of units and managers, they create significant problems with the decisions that managers must make about individual products or product lines. This is especially true when costs vary in some way other than described by the cost allocations being used.[15]

This is exactly why HHAs need to consider ABC systems. No longer can the Medicare cost reporting methodology be employed as a tool to evaluate profitability. The allocation principles distort costs causing managers to make poor decisions. Moreover, Stage 2 is aggravated by information system vendors that are employing old technology in their system architecture, financial reporting systems that are not integrated, and systems that depend on the flow of paperwork from the field.

Reporting the financial results of operation several weeks after the month end has closed can be especially detrimental in a managed care environment where an HHA has entered into a risk-based contract. Providers need to monitor service utilization and costs on a daily basis, and if utilization or costs exceed prenegotiated risk corridors, then they need to go back to the managed care organization (MCO) and renegotiate the contract or convert to a fee-for-service arrangement.

> Kaplan's Stage 3 is a transitional, evolutionary stage. In this stage, all of the information from Stage 2 would be retained. External reporting would continue using the same information in an uninterrupted manner. However, an added focus would be placed on product costing with an activity-based cost system and on operational control with development of an operational performance measurement system.
>
> Stage 3 has a focus on direct measures of operations such as quality, timeliness, flexibility, and customer service. Information is available on a more current and frequent basis. Information is presented in graphs rather than numbers. According to Kaplan, the goal of these short run financial summaries is not to control employees but to provide information to guide their learning and improvement activities.[16]

This is a major paradigm shift regarding the use of information. This says that agencies value their employees and know that if they have better information available to them, they will be able to help enhance organizational efficiencies. This goes hand in hand with the concept of empowering employees and organizational learning. "Stage 4 is one of integration. In this future stage, the old costing systems of Stage 2 would be phased out. Data collected under Stage 3 primarily for management purposes would be reconciled to generate the external reports. In Kaplan's vision, this will be a reversal of the current situation. Costing now collects data for external reporting. Managers try to squeeze relevant information from that data. In Stage 4, costing will collect information for managers. External reports will be made by modifying the managerial data as best as possible."[17]

ABC reports would be the primary reports that would be used by management. Reports would be activity oriented and could look something like Table 8–4.

Table 8–4 Example of an Activity-based Management Report

Any Home Health Agency
For the month ended June 199X

Revenue	$150,000
Provision of patient care	
Travel	5,200
Treatment time	54,590
Telephone contact	2,350
Documentation time	1,300
Case conference	1,650
Billing	
Data entry	1,350
Quality assurance review	250
Submission of bills	185

↓ ↓

Administration	
Meetings	8,500
Conflict resolution	2,300
Total activities	145,675
Net income	$ 4,325
Revenue	$150,000
Value-added activities	72,354
Nonvalue-added activities	73,321
Net income	$ 4,325

AUTOMATED SYSTEMS

The benefits that will accrue to an HHA through ABC systems will be significantly enhanced by automated information systems that employ a relational database methodology. The relational database methodology will allow data to be extracted from a common database, thus facilitating the blending of clinical and financial activities to monitor the costs of providing services. These data can be enhanced if activities are also identified and tracked as part of the daily processing. The relational database methodology enables users to extract data easily once they are in the system.

The question becomes this: Is the process of activity identification viewed as a valuable activity, or is it solely a cumbersome process that employees would rather not have to do? The answer to that is management dependent. However, it needs to be noted that information systems are evolving to enable agencies to develop sophisticated ABC systems. These systems will enable managers to manage the processes of the agency and, through understanding the processes, use them for the competitive advantage of the agency. Without sophisticated measurement systems, management will continue to be operating in the dark, thus putting the agency at a competitive disadvantage in an era where low-cost, high-quality providers will be the winners.

One of the ways to become a low-cost provider is to measure the services that are being provided. Measurement entails understanding what the processes and activities are, establishing outcomes for those activities, and then designing systems to enhance organizational efficiency. One of the tools that will help providers with this task is the information system. A sophisticated information system will eliminate many nonvalue-added tasks. For instance, the process of documentation requires entry into the information system. This only needs to be done once, not repeatedly by different departments that need the same information.

From an ABC perspective, resource and activity drivers could be automatically calculated from information within the system. Actual effort could be tracked as part of the payroll process and the results monitored on a monthly basis. Another positive outcome of an integrated system would enable management to measure performance results across all functions within the agency.

PERFORMANCE MEASUREMENT

Performance measurement is another benefit that will accrue to an agency beyond better cost information. Performance measurement enables users to consider the efficiency of an operation and the quality of services being provided by the agency, and develops a time and money relationship. An example of efficiency would be monitoring actual results against plan. The plan called for 1,000 nursing visits to be performed in the month at an average cost of $40 per visit. Actual results indicated 1,050 visits at a per visit cost of $41. Table 8–5 illustrates an operational efficiency analysis.

Actual results indicated a $3,100 negative variance from plan. The analysis indicates that this variance is due to two elements: (1) volume and (2) price. The volume element of the analysis indicates that 50 more visits were performed than originally anticipated; therefore, $2,050 of the variance is attributable to increased volume. The price element of the efficiency analysis indicates that the average cost per visit was $1 higher than originally planned. One dollar multiplied by the actual volume indicates that $1,050 of the variance is attributable to the higher price.

Once the first level of the analysis is completed, then the second part of the analysis requires explaining whether the volume and price had a positive effect on the agency. The second part of the analysis requires looking at the composition of the actual payor mix. Was the increase of 50 visits beneficial to the agency? This

Table 8–5 Variance Analysis To Determine Operational Efficiency

	Plan	Actual	Variance
Visits	1,000	1,050	50
Rate	$ 41	$ 42	$ 1
Cost	$41,000	$44,100	$3,100

Volume		Price	
Actual	1,050	Actual	$42
Plan	1,000	Plan	41
Increase in visits	50	Increase in visits	$1
Plan rate	× $41	Actual volume	×1,050
Volume difference	$2,050	Volume difference	1,050

will depend on whether the increase in visits was attributable to a cost-based payor, a fee-for-service payor, or an episodic or capitated payment structure. If the increase was for the last, then this will be a negative variance. If the increase is for a fee-for-service payor, then as long as the revenue on a per visit basis was in excess of the direct and indirect costs of providing care (unit and batch costs), then this would represent a positive variance. An increase or decrease in the cost-based payor would only matter if the agency was very close to the limits and needed additional volume to lower costs below the limits or the increase caused a dilution of the interim rate.

Included in the second part of the analysis is determining why the average cost of a nursing visit increased from $41 to $42. An increase in cost could be attributable to a change in the mix of nursing personnel. Table 8–6 indicates that the original plan used 80 percent employees and 20 percent contracted nursing services to meet its anticipated volume requirements.

Table 8–6 Variance Analysis To Determine Volume Fluctuations

Plan	Visits	Rate ($)	Cost ($)
Employees (80%)	800	40.00	32,000
Contract (20%)	200	45.00	9,000
	1,000		41,000
Actual			
Employees (67%)	700	40.50	28,350
Contract (33%)	350	45.00	15,750
	1,050		44,100

Exhibit 8–5 Data Collection Form To Analyze Activities

Data Collection Form—Administrative Employee

Employee name:

Time	Process	Activity	Payor	Program	Service Line	Company	Location
8:00–8:15							
8:15–8:30							
8:30–8:45							
8:45–9:00							
9:00–9:15							
9:15–9:30							
9:30–9:45							
9:45–10:00							
10:00–10:15							
10:15–10:30							
10:30–10:45							
10:45–11:00							
11:00–11:15							
11:15–11:30							
11:30–11:45							
11:45–12:00							
12:00–12:15							
12:15–12:30							
12:30–12:45							
12:45–1:00							
1:00–1:15							
1:15–1:30							
1:30–1:45							
1:45–2:00							
2:00–2:15							
2:15–2:30							
2:30–2:45							
2:45–3:00							
3:00–3:15							
3:15–3:30							
3:30–3:45							
3:45–4:00							
4:00–4:15							
4:15–4:30							
4:30–4:45							
4:45–5:00							

Total by Code

Process Code
A. Payroll
B. Accounting
C. Billing
D. Collections

Activity Code
1. Collect and total time sheets
2. Enter payroll data
3. Review payroll
4. Prepare quarterly payroll taxes
5. Prepare checks for distribution
6. Write up journal entries

Location
a. Main office
b. Branch office

Company
I. Private duty company
II. Certified HHA

The actual plan indicates that a larger quantity of the more expensive contracted services was used. Additionally, the average cost of an employee visit increased by $.50. Further investigation may reveal that full-time staff were on vacation, employees were scheduled ineffectively, or employee productivity was up, but the employees were assigned more labor-intensive cases than the contractors. Understanding why both results occurred will provide management with an understanding of the dynamics of the underlying processes.

Efficiency can also be viewed from the concept of capacity. If an employee is paid for a 40-hour week, and he or she is productive 30 out of the 40 hours, then there is an unused capacity of 10 hours. On review of the individual's time records, management may find that he or she was in meetings, on vacation, doing rework of another department's output, waiting for work, or performing busy work to appear busy. This type of analysis can lead to better ways of utilizing an agency's expensive labor force. Exhibit 8–5 shows a sample data collection form to analyze activities.

"To recap, the ABC process view provides operational intelligence about the work going on in a company. This includes information about the external factors determining how often the activity is performed and the effort required to carry it out. Operational intelligence also includes information about the performance of an activity, such as its efficiency, the time it takes to perform the activity, and the quality with which it is carried out."[18] The use of activity-based costing systems will be addressed in further detail in the following section on activity-based management.

NOTES

1. B.J. Brinker, *Emerging Practices in Cost Management* (Boston: Warren, Gorham & Lamont: 1993), A4-3.

2. *Ibid.*, A4-1.

3. R. Cooper, et al., *Implementing Activity-Based Cost Management: Moving from Analysis to Action* (Montvale, NJ: Institute of Management Accountants, 1992), 314.

4. G. Cokins, et al., *An ABC Manager's Primer* (Montvale, NJ: Institute of Management Accountants, 1993), 3.

5. *Ibid.*, 8.

6. American Institute of CPAs, *Activity-Based Costing* (New York: American Institute of CPAs, 1992), 2–5.

7. Adapted from: I.K. Kleinsorge and R.D. Tanner, Activity-Based Costing: Eight Questions To Answer Before You Implement, *Journal of Cost Management*, Fall 1991, 84–88.

8. *Ibid.*

9. B.J. Brinker, Emerging Practices, A1–4.

10. Adapted from: J.B. MacArthur, Activity-Based Costing: How Many Cost Drivers Do You Want?, *Journal of Cost Management*, Fall 1992, 37–41.

11. AICPA, *Strategy for Success: Implementing an Activity-Based Costing System* (New York: American Institute of CPAs, 1994), 4–6.

12. G. Cokins, *An ABC Manager's Primer*, 19.

13. J.B. MacArthur, Activity-Based Costing, 37–41.

14. S.A. Finkler, *Cost Accounting for Health Care Organizations* (Gaithersburg, MD: Aspen Publishers, 1994), 614.

15. *Ibid.*

16. *Ibid.*

17. *Ibid.*

18. P.B.B. Turney, "What an Activity-Based Cost Model Looks Like," *Journal of Cost Management,* Winter 1992, 54–60.

Chapter 9

Activity-Based Management

The previous chapter developed the concepts behind activity-based costing (ABC). Activity-based management (ABM) goes one step further than activity-based costing by analyzing activities from a business process perspective. A visual representation would view activity-based costing in a vertical framework where inputs of resources are traced to activities, and the activities are then matched to outputs, or cost objects. The primary concern of activity-based costing is to cost services properly by matching resource consumption to services.

Activity-based management looks at activities and their related costs cross-functionally, or horizontally. This horizontal view seeks to identify why activities took place and how they relate to business processes across the agency. The goal of activity-based management is to focus on customer expectations, both internal and external, with the ending result being an increase in perceived value by the customer. This is accomplished by questioning why activities are performed; that is whether activities are related to meeting customer expectations or the objectives of the organization.

Figure 9–1 shows the vertical and horizontal nature of ABC and ABM, respectively.

ORGANIZATIONAL COST DRIVERS

Once activities have been identified cross-functionally, then data can begin to be captured to begin the management process. Cost-driver identification reveals factors that affect the cost of an activity and the amount of time required to perform an activity. The concept of a cost driver differs from that of an activity driver. "Activity drivers are consequences of what has happened, whereas operational cost drivers reveal what is making it happen. Costs tend to be incurred at the process level, not at the activity level. Operational cost drivers are factors that influ-

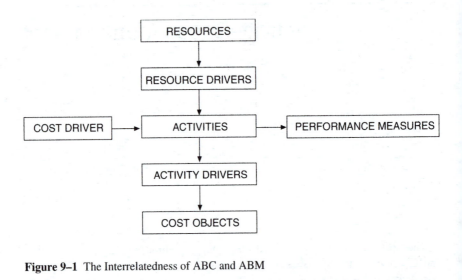

Figure 9–1 The Interrelatedness of ABC and ABM

---

ence a change in cost of several related activities, whereas activity cost drivers measure the frequency and intensity of the demands placed on activities by output-oriented cost objects."[1]

Operational cost drivers look at what the root cause is of the activity. Root cause analysis questions whether the activity is a continuation of an existing process that was started in a previous department. If the following sequence of events represent an agency's billing process, it is easy to identify the activity triggers for each department's contribution to the billing process.

In Exhibit 9–1, the billing activity begins with the submission of nursing documentation. The root cause of this activity is the completion of the nursing visit and the summarization of nursing activities so the agency can be paid for the visit to the patient's home. Completion and submission of nursing documentation would be the activity trigger or root cause of the billing or data entry staff's entry of field activity into the billing system. A workload indicator would be the number of patients on service, the ratio of visits to patients, and the complexity of services provided. Performance measures would be the quality and timeliness of the incoming documentation. The root cause or activity driver for the quality assurance department would be the output of the billing or data entry department. The workload indicator would be the number of patients on service, and the performance measure could be the number of data entry errors.

Tracing of activities cross-functionally enables managers to identify opportunities for process improvement, determining whether activities are contributing to customer expectations or whether activities do nothing more than add cost. Activi-

Exhibit 9–1 Activity Flow through Departments

Activity	*Department*
Document field visit	Field staff
Perform data entry of field activity	Billing or data entry staff
Perform prebill review	Quality assurance
Run bills for submission	Billing
Review bills before submission	Accounting or operations management

ties that add cost should be eliminated, and those activities that provide value to the customer should be enhanced. Process improvement is a way to enhance customer and organizational value. All activities within the organization should be geared toward enhancing customer value and organizational value.

PERFORMANCE MEASUREMENT

Performance measurements are a way to quantify the amount of effort by activity that goes into every service that is offered by an agency. "Performance measures mark the effectiveness of newly developed activities, close the gap between the customer and the organization, integrate the organization internally and with its partners, and ensure behavioral change. They are the means to creating the horizontal organization. Performance measures must achieve the following: encourage the achievement of strategic objectives; focus on the future activities of the organization, not past results; be nonfinancial as well as financial; and create a common language between operations and finance."[2] Performance measurements evaluate organizational quality, service, and cost from the customer's perspective.

Quality is defined from the customer's perspective, so at a minimum, internally developed performance measures should be developed that meet the customer's expectations. However, the real goal is to exceed the customer's expectations. Additional measures of quality from a performance measurement perspective are the accuracy of the activity and the presence of innovation in service delivery. These two measures increase perceived value from the customer's viewpoint.

Service measurement is the second element of performance measurement. Service measurement incorporates the elements of time, volume, and rate. These measures answer the question of whether process output is produced on time and in a sufficient quantity to keep downstream processes moving (just-in-time mentality) and how fluctuations in volume affect the flow of process output. Additionally, do changes in volume or timeliness have an impact on the quality of the services being provided? Will an agency still be able to perform initial visits 12 hours after the referral is made by a managed care organization (MCO) if the MCO has referred 20 other patients in the same day, or will clinical outcomes still be achievable if a hospital changes its discharge practice?

Cost measurement determines the cost of the activity and calculates a per unit cost for labor, material, and indirect expenses. Costs are calculated in relationship to service measurement criteria such as process time and volume. Costs are also compared to the quality of the output and changes in the delivery process.

Linking of operational drivers to activity cost, service volume and time, and quality enables managers to perform process value analysis, define internal benchmarks, and reengineer processes. "Process value analysis using activity based management data provides managers with a framework and a systematic approach for planning, predicting, and influencing cost. This approach focuses management attention on the interdependency between departments and functional activities. Also, by analyzing the cost drivers of activities within business processes, managers can understand and act on the causes of cost, not their symptoms."[3] Furthermore, "multiple cost drivers can be associated with an activity. A performance measure is an indicator of the work performed and the results achieved in an activity, process, or organizational unit. Performance measures may be financial or non-financial."[4]

PERFORMANCE MEASURE DEVELOPMENT

The following steps can be followed to develop performance measures[5]:

1. Identify the key products/outputs that the customer wants. This requires understanding what a managed care organization expects from the home health agency with which it contracts. What outcomes does it expect for the patient population that the agency serves? Will this be different by diagnosis or referral source? What kind of reporting, follow-up, and communications will be expected of the agency?

   From an internal customer perspective, does every department within the activity process chain understand how their department's output will be used by subsequent departments? Does every department know when subsequent departments need information, what form it should be in, and why they are involved in the process?

2. Identify the customer's requirements for the outputs in terms of quality, price, design, and function. This is the ability to tell the MCO how much it will cost if it refers a patient to the agency who has no caregiver at home, multiple activities of daily living (ADL) requirements, and comorbidities. Beyond pricing, can the agency state that 80 percent of the patients who

have similar requirements have been able to achieve the outcome of independence in 7 days and that they will require the following mix of services, supplies, and home medical equipment?

Internally provided services can be evaluated to determine whether they are meeting the needs of the departments that receive the services. Perhaps the time to produce monthly financial statements is too long; then the process could be redesigned to meet the needs of the users of the financial statements by providing them with a flash report that estimates where the agency is on a daily and month-to-date basis. This process requires understanding the needs of the customers, current processing requirements, and a willingness to adapt to the needs of the customer.

3. Identify the organization's and the industry's benchmarks for the outputs. Development of organizational benchmarks may be easier than reliance on information that is available publicly through the Freedom of Information Act. Unless every agency has developed an ABM system, it will be impossible to measure internal benchmarks against external benchmarks.

   However, there are exceptions. Some of the exceptions could include ranges of cost and units of service by nursing diagnosis, number of days in accounts receivable by payor classification, average age of payables, productivity figures for field staff, and costs associated with quality.

   From a continuous quality improvement process, the development of internal standards will provide a meaningful benchmark because the processes are known. Refinement of the activities that support the larger processes will establish quantifiable process improvement results.

4. Develop performance measures for the outputs that take into account customer wants and requirements and identify benchmarks. This is the development of the performance measure to evaluate how well the internal processes are doing against the customer's wants and requirements. Performance measures will identify the quality, service, and cost requirements.

5. Map the organization's processes as they are now understood; identify problems; and then fix the problems by eliminating, simplifying, and focusing the processes. This is the relationship of activities to departments, each department's contributions to the process, and the end result or departmental output. Visually, this is illustrated by Figure 9–2. Each activity is traced across many departments, and total activity cost is the sum of each department's efforts. Additionally, each activity identifies a workload measure such as visits, patients, accounts analyzed, reports produced, and so forth.

6. Identify the industry benchmarks for processes. These will develop over time.

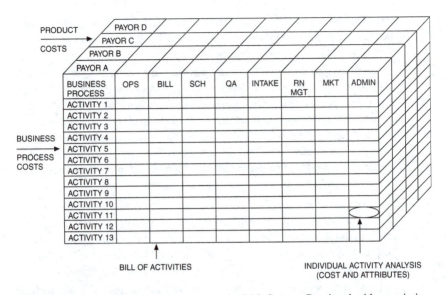

Figure 9–2 Three-dimensional Illustration of ABM. Source: Reprinted with permission from *Emerging Practices in Cost Management* by B.J. Brinker, p. B6-5, © 1993, Warren, Gorham & Lamont, 31 St. James Avenue, Boston, MA 02116. All rights reserved.

ACTIVITIES

"The What" section of ABM, as shown in Figure 9–3, consists of activities. This is the common link between cost objects (the vertical element) and business processes (the horizontal view). Identification of activities through the assignment of different attributes such as time, cost, value-added or nonvalue-added costs (quality), workload indicators, responsiveness, and ranking of customer expectations will add another dimension to an ABM system. When managers have an opportunity to review the output of their activity analysis, results can be used to effect change management because now managers will understand all of the activities that go into accomplishing a process aimed at obtaining a specific goal. This approach provides a tool for proactive management that was never available using after-the-fact financial statements that explained how resources had been consumed by expense classification but had no relationship to activities or the organizational mission. Figure 9–2 provides a visual example of how costs become three dimensional in an ABM environment.

As discussed in Chapter 8, resources are consumed by different processes within the agency. In this example, operations, billing, scheduling, quality assurance, intake, nursing management, marketing, and administration represent the main processes. Each one of these processes performs many different activities related to each of an agency's cost objects. In this example, the cost objects are

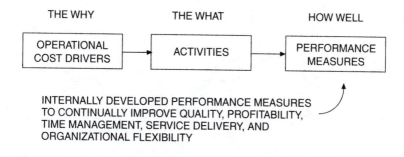

Figure 9–3 ABM: The Horizontal View. Source: Reprinted from *An ABC Manager's Primer* by G. Cokins, A. Stratton, and J. Helbling, p. 27, with permission of the Institute of Management Accountants, © 1993.

---

payors. Payors could be substituted for product lines, contracts, programs, or other costing objectives.

Business process costs are illustrated in Figure 9–2 as Activities 1 through 13. Activity identification would be dependent on the objectives of the ABM system. If the objectives were strategic in nature, the number of activities would be small and at a summary level. If the objective was to understand all of the activities within the agency, then there would be many activities listed under business processes.

An easy way to think of this is in relationship to the bill of activities (see Exhibit 9–2). The bill of activities is a listing of all of the activities and their related costs that would be assigned to a department or a payor. The bill of activities can either be at a summary level listing primary activities or at a detailed level listing primary and secondary activities.

Individual activity analysis will identify how costs are incurred cross-functionally throughout the organization and whether activities are primary, secondary, or project related. Identification of duplicative efforts, waste, and other nonvalue-added activities becomes easier when viewed in this type of format. Furthermore, "the cross-functional aspects are especially important because many decisions in an organization affect the activities performed by people in other parts of the organization. Many impacts of a decision are unknown and are not intended by the decision maker."[6] An example of this would be when there is a decision to offer another service, open a branch office, or pursue another business venture. Most managers do not consider the ripple effect that decisions will have on an organization and the resources that get consumed in planning, analysis, and implementation of management decisions. Tracking activity cost helps to quantify the opportunity cost of management decisions.

Exhibit 9–2 A Listing of Activities

Bill of Activities
I. Direct costs
    A. Nursing
        1. Treatment time
        2. Travel time
        3. Travel cost
        4. Supplies
        5. Case conference
    B. Therapies
    C. Home health aide
II. Billing
III. Scheduling
IV. Records
V. Marketing
VI. Nursing management
VII. Administration

Activity Analysis

When determining what activities to analyze, managers must first determine what outcome they are interested in obtaining from their ABM system. In Chapter 8, activities were analyzed for purposes of product costing. Activities are now identified within the context of processes across the entire organization. Some questions that would be raised are the following[7]:

- What activities do we perform, and what do they cost?
- What or who drives the need for the activities?
- Are the activities value-added or redundant?
- What is the cost of waste, meetings, and complexity?
- Of what business processes are the activities a part?
- How do product costs change under an ABM system?
- What product lines or contracts do the activities support?
- What other cost objectives do the activities affect?
- How do costs fluctuate within cost hierarchy levels?
- How can the activities be improved or eliminated?
- What relationships exist between volume and full-time equivalents?
- What potential cost savings are possible through automation?

Questions will be determined by management's intent. If management's intent is solely to reduce costs, then questions will focus on the elimination of activities, potential cost savings, and ways to make activities more efficient. If management's intent is to look at measuring quality improvement efforts, then the questions would be geared toward what activities need to be measured. ABM lends itself to many process improvement activities because it links processes and costs together cross-functionally. Furthermore, ABM is a tool to enhance the outcome measurement process. Outcome measurement when reduced to dollars provides a common ground for evaluating all quality improvement efforts between internal and external customers. Dollars will become the lowest common denominator and more meaningful for trend analysis than a host of quality metrics. An improvement in visit volume may be attributable to increasing the length of each visit; however, from an aggregate cost perspective there has been no improvement.

An activity analysis looks at each activity by department across the entire organization. Figure 9–4 identifies the concept of a process orientation. The analysis defines activities on a departmental basis. Activities are normally action oriented and are prefaced by a verb. An example could be "recruit employees" or "prepare financial statements." Where the activity is performed will determine the series of inputs, processes, and outputs that will take place departmentally. Activity placement will also determine performance measures, such as what is expected from the receivers of a department's output. Departmental output could be going directly to a customer of the agency or to an internal customer. When the activity analysis is linked to performance and workload criteria, then activities can be analyzed from the viewpoint of "what we do and why we do it" to determine whether they are meeting the organization's objectives (Figure 9–5).

Assignment of Attributes to Activities

Assignment of attributes to activities provides a mechanism to classify and summarize activities and their related costs for further analysis. Assignment of attributes adds another dimension to the ABM process. First, departmental costs and organizational costs can be summarized by activity. Second, by assigning an attribute to every activity as either value-added or nonvalue-added, it is possible to quantify how much effort and resources are spent toward one type of value attribute or the other.

A third attribute could be determined by the performance measure(s) assigned to the activity. Aggregation of costs by performance measure will enable managers to calculate a cost per unit. Subsequent process improvement efforts can be measured against previously calculated cost per units to quantify improvement efforts. An example would be determining the cost of producing financial statements in 11 days after the month has ended. If total activity cost is $2,500 and the cost of producing financial statements in 8 days after the month has ended is

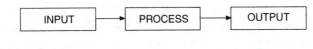

Figure 9–4 Process Flow

$3,500, then management can determine whether $1,000 additional cost on a monthly basis is worth having financial statements 3 days earlier.

Analysis of process cost could be broken down into the activities that are part of the larger process. Analysis of individual activities may determine where further reductions in cycle time could occur.

Many costs within an agency are not assignable to a specific payor. These costs are administrative in nature and are incurred to comply with regulatory requirements; to provide feedback to management, bankers, and third parties; and basically to support the organization. Activity attributes can be established to separate costs between those that are directly related to cost objects, such as a payor, and those activities that are not attributable to a payor. This classification method helps to identify costs that are controllable by administration and operations. Ac-

---

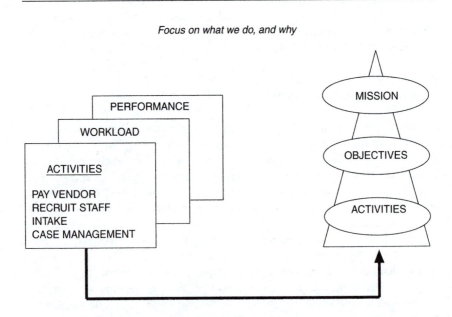

Figure 9–5 Linking ABM to Organizational Objectives. Source: Reprinted with permission from *Handbook of Cost Management* by B.J. Brinker, p. C1-7, © 1994, Warren, Gorham & Lamont, 31 St. James Avenue, Boston, MA 02116. All rights reserved.

tivity attributes can be further enhanced by determining whether costs are fixed, semifixed, or variable. This latter enhancement enables ABM results to be used as input for sensitivity analysis.

A fourth attribute category would be the assignment of patient-related classifications to activities. Attributes in this category would permit additional analysis of patient care costs. For instance, attributes could include patient problem for outcome measurement; outcome; physician; referral source; primary medical diagnosis; secondary diagnoses; case manager; payor; sex; type of visit; date and time of intake; time of admission visit; amount of time spent on patient care, travel, or documentation; or supply usage.

Performance measures could then be developed using planned outcome in respect to actual outcome for a specific patient problem. Analysis of variance would provide insight into whether the clinical pathway was too aggressive, whether teaching methods were noneffective, or whether variances were caused by the physician or patient. Aggregation of common patient problems would indicate the cost per unit for labor and materials and could then be used for episodic pricing or bidding on capitated contracts.

Use of the type of visit, date and time of intake, and time of admission visit attributes would facilitate aggregating all admission visits. The agency could then determine the cost of an admission visit and the number of visits that conformed to the performance measure if all admission visits would be performed within 12 hours of intake. Analysis of the results would lead to continuous quality improvement activities.

VALUE-ADDED VERSUS NONVALUE-ADDED COSTS

Aggregation of costs by primary or macro activity will identify the total amount of resources that was consumed for a specific activity. Identification of activities through the use of a value attribute will enable aggregate activity cost to be defined by whether it adds value to the agency or purely cost. Figure 9–6 illustrates how costs could be summarized by macro activities.

The quantification of value-added versus nonvalue-added activities enables managers to determine how they want to proceed in their continuous quality improvement efforts. Activities will cross many functional boundaries and, therefore, will require the support of all managers in accomplishing the larger task of continuous quality improvement. Continuous quality improvement efforts may require someone to champion improvement efforts for each one of the activities.

Efficiencies and reduction of nonvalue-added activities can occur through the simplification of processes and procedures. Processes that have multiple steps are a source of nonvalue-added activities. Exhibit 9–1 identified several possible steps in a billing process. Each step was questionable as to whether a payor would view it as a value-added step in order to receive correct bills and supporting documenta-

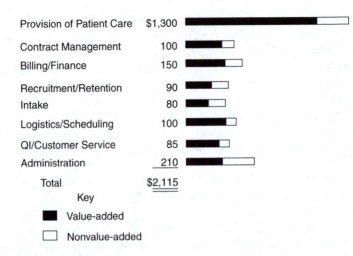

Figure 9–6 Value Analysis Using Activity Attributes. Source: Adapted with permission from *Handbook of Cost Management* by B.J. Brinker, p. B4-19, © 1994, Warren, Gorham & Lamont, 31 St. James Avenue, Boston, MA 02116. All rights reserved.

tion for the services that were provided. Furthermore, each step had multiple opportunities to create errors (nonvalue-added activity) that would need to be corrected prior to the submission of invoices to the payor (customer). Figure 9–7 illustrates possible approaches for activity improvement.

Prior to advances in technology and declining computer costs, the nurse, therapist, or aide scribbled notes down on a piece of paper to be transcribed later. During the time between the actual visit and the completion of the documentation, facts could have been forgotten, notes lost, or combined with other patients'. Once the documentation was completed, it would need to be submitted and entered into the billing system. Incorrect entry of data could occur because of not being able to read the notes, not understanding terminology in context of the patient's problems, or just plain making transcription errors.

Simplification of the process in Exhibit 9–1 could occur through having patient documentation entered directly by the nurse, therapist, or aide. Entry of documentation could be accomplished by entering data into a lap-top computer and transmitting the data immediately, after hours, or by dropping off a data disk at the agency. Further enhancements to the process would eliminate the prebilling process by moving quality assurance into a proactive stance by educating and training teams of care providers in the use of clinical pathways and contract parameters and developing guidelines so that everyone is responsible for the quality of the information going into and out of the system.

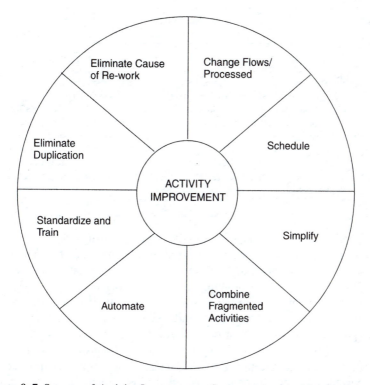

Figure 9–7 Sources of Activity Improvement. Source: Adapted with permission from *Handbook of Cost Management* by B.J. Brinker, p. B4-23, © 1994, Warren, Gorham & Lamont, 31 St. James Avenue, Boston, MA 02116.

QUALITY COSTS

Activity-based cost management provides agencies with an opportunity to measure quality and quantify the cost of quality (Exhibit 9–3). "Measuring quality costs can provide a useful stimulus to the process of quality improvement, serve as a method for determining refinements in the systems that drive quality, and identify specific opportunities for management attention. Moreover, monitoring quality control and improvement costs reinforces the value of a total quality philosophy."[8]

Measurement of quality is possible through the assignment of attributes to every activity tracked within the agency. Two types of costs have been associated with quality. The first cost is investment in quality. This is composed of activities that are designed to prevent customers from having problems with the quality of the services that they receive. Prevention of activities builds quality into the ser-

Exhibit 9–3 Cost Measurement Using Quality Dimensions

	Investments in quality		Costs due to nonconformance	
Dimension:	*Prevention*	*Appraisal*	*Internal*	*External*
	Prevention of failures from occurring or building quality into the process	Activities that detect failures	Internal process failure discovered before service delivery	Failure that directly affects the customer and is discovered by the customer

Source: Adapted from Waress, B.J., Pasternak, D.P., and Smith, H.L., Determining Costs Associated with Quality in Health Care Delivery, *Health Care Management Review*, Vol. 19, No. 3, p. 55, Aspen Publishers, Inc., © 1994.

vice delivery process by making it proactive instead of part of an after-the-fact quality assurance process. This is accomplished by recruiting qualified staff, training all staff on the requirements of the customer population that is being served, and giving them the tools and the ability to be accountable for high-quality service delivery. "Prevention costs are not actual costs, but investments in quality, for they prevent failures from occurring. Spending dollars early in a service delivery process prevents costly mistakes from being made later in the process."[9]

The second type of activity within the investment in quality category is appraisal cost. This is the detection of possible quality problems before the customer would become aware of a deficiency. This typically has been one of the roles of quality assurance. Appraisal activities focus on reviewing operations, contracts, programs, and administrative operations to determine whether there is a current or potential problem with the quality of services being provided.

The second cost associated with quality is the cost of nonconformance. Nonconformance cost is differentiated between internal and external failures. Internal failures are costs associated with problems before the customer is aware that there is a problem. Typically, this is the cost of rework, wasted activities, overtime not related to fluctuations in volume, nonproductive time, reinspection, excess inventories, and wasted supplies.

> Any nonachievement that impacts an internal customer eventually impacts the ultimate customer—the patient—in higher cost for service, longer wait, inefficiency, and other dysfunctional ways. A failure discovered by a customer or patient has at its root cause an internal system breakdown. The distinction between internal and external nonachievement is not a distinction based on causality, but upon geography. An internal nonachievement is a failure found before the customer receives the service or is an inefficiency in the service delivery process.[10]

The external cost of nonconformance is the cost of quality deficiencies that the customer has discovered. These types of costs could create ill will between the agency and its customers, potentially cause contracts to be lost, or create costly litigation. "This category reflects a failure that has been discovered by the customers and that impacts them directly. The intangible component of these costs is quite substantial, for it incorporates the ideas of trust, reputation, and customer loyalty. Thus, the dollar amount of external nonachievement may be less than the amount of internal nonachievement, yet the overall impact of external nonachievement is more severe because external nonachievement directly undermines marketing efforts, erodes the customer base, and diminishes professional reputation."[11]

Exhibit 9–4 is a list of costs associated with quality.[12] These activities do not reflect the cost of labor for normal service delivery. They do, however, reflect administrative activities that are attributable to the cost of quality.

> The cost of quality is typically 15 to 25% of revenues, though the appropriate range for most companies is from 5 to 8%. Even if it is higher, the amount itself is not as important as how management uses the information gained from calculating the cost of quality. Cost of quality analysis can be useful for three reasons. First, cost of quality analysis identifies the cost of not meeting customer needs and highlights opportunities for cost reduction. Secondly, the cost of quality analysis quantifies progress made as a result of adopting a total quality management program, and finally, the cost of quality analysis identifies ways to improve processes and activities continuously.[13]

COST MANAGEMENT

Cost management is a philosophy that should be pervasive in any home health agency that is interested in surviving in the highly competitive managed care environment. Cost management is the responsibility of everyone within the organization. An ABC system will identify the processes that consume resources; however, it is up to the employees of the agency to use these data to become more efficient. When cost data are linked to measures about quality, there is a wonderful opportunity to shape organizations to thrive in a highly competitive environment.

Prior to managed care, home health business was driven by the rules and regulations of Medicare. Providers learned how to play within the Medicare rules and, consequently, developed elaborate administrative structures. These structures work fine in a cost-reimbursed environment. However, in a highly competitive environment that is characterized by the ratcheting downward of revenue streams, this strategy will place providers at a major disadvantage.

Exhibit 9–4 Costs Associated with Quality

Prevention Costs
- Research on managed care utilization requirements by population
- Education of the patient or caregiver about medications, treatments, exercises, etc.
- Community outreach programs
- Case management
- Continuous quality improvement training/education
- Continuing education for all classes of employees—paid by the agency
- Employee education regarding agency policy and procedures, contract requirements, and care protocols
- Preventive maintenance on home medical equipment, infusion pumps
- Credentialing of personnel, review programs, and updates
- Development of operating standards
- Development of critical pathways
- Development of supplier standards for quality, education, and core competencies

Appraisal Costs
- Patient problems/nursing intensity level
- Insurance verification/service limitations/current enrollment
- Review of discharge information/lab results/initial assessment
- Review of clinical pathways variances
- Staff recruitment and development/quarterly goal setting and reviews
- Clinical and administrative team review
- Organizational utilization review/by team/by payor/by referral source
- Joint Commission on Accreditation of Healthcare Organizations accreditation
- Contract review: supplies, MCOs, payors, staff, or community health accreditation program

Internal Failure
- Nonbillable charges
- Amount of time from discharge until the admission visit was performed
- Amount of time to wait for follow-up services (physical therapist)
- Ability to contact proper agency personnel via telephone
- Rework
- Premium paid to external staffing agencies or independent contractors
- Risk management activities
- Workers' compensation claims
- Working capital tied up in excess supplies/accounts receivable
- Inability to collect accounts receivable on a timely basis
- Infusion or home medical equipment failure

External Failure
- Emergency visits
- Improper matching of staff to patient
- Inability to meet customer expectations/PT/MCO/referral source
- Customer complaint resolution
- Disallowed services
- Provision of excessive services
- Loss of contract
- Malpractice/insurance premiums

Strategies that will make sense are those that adopt a low overhead philosophy and manage costs from a prudent buyer perspective. This approach views resources as scarce and seeks to make sure that employees and processes are as efficient as possible. Complexity of service delivery is dropped for simplicity.

> No company can be successful over time if inflation-adjusted total costs do not follow a steadily declining pattern. Management must place unrelenting pressure on the entire organization for measurable cost reductions and productivity gains, year after year. The rate of improvement may vary annually but should never fall below inflation. Vigilance is critical because it is so difficult to regain cost competitiveness once it has been lost. Costs should not be allowed to get out of line in the first place. If your costs have become noncompetitive, then probably traditional expense reductions alone—cutting back here and there, reducing overhead, saving on travel—won't do the job. Even deep cuts along the way generally won't do. You need to think in a different way—eliminate big chunks of structured cost, to design cost out of the product and system, and to greatly improve efficiencies everywhere.[14]

NOTES

1. G. Cokins, et al. *An ABC Manager's Primer* (Montvale, NJ: Institute of Management Accountants, 1993), 30.

2. B.J. Brinker, *Handbook of Cost Management* (Boston: Warren, Gorham & Lamont, 1994), A1-23.

3. G. Cokins, *An ABC Manager's Primer*, 35.

4. L.J. Soloway, "Using Activity-Based Management Systems in Aerospace and Defense Companies," *Journal of Cost Management* (Winter 1993) 55–66.

5. B.J. Brinker, *Handbook of Cost Management*, A1-24.

6. L.J. Soloway, Using Activity-Based Management Systems, 55–66.

7. L.J. Soloway, Using Activity-Based Management Systems, 55–66.

8. B.J. Waress, et al., Determining Costs Associated with Quality in Health Care Delivery, *Health Care Management Review* 19, no. 3 (1994): 52–63.

9. *Ibid.*

10. *Ibid.*

11. *Ibid.*

12. *Ibid.*

13. B.J. Brinker, *Handbook of Cost Management*, A1-28.

14. C.B. Ames and J.D. Hlavacek, Vital Truths about Managing Your Costs, *Harvard Business Review* (January–February 1990): 140–47.

Part IV

Management Accounting

Chapter 10

Customers of the Financial Department

Home health is a service business. Successful home health agencies have a service orientation that is based on the needs of their customers. Customers can be external or internal to the organization. External customers are outside of the agency. They include patients and their caregivers and the organizations or people who control the referral of patients to the agency and/or have the power to change the referral stream. Internal customers are the employees of the agency and include all levels of staff, management, owners, and the board of directors. Customers, both external and internal, define service quality. It is up to the agency to determine whether it is meeting the needs of its customers. External and internal customers are listed below:

- External customers
    - Patients and their family/caregivers
    - Physicians
    - Referral sources
    - Case managers
    - Managed care organization (MCO)/payor/fiscal intermediary
- Internal customers
    - Employees
    - Departments
    - Management
    - Owners
    - Board of directors

Customer service is especially difficult because of how the health care system is structured. In almost every other industry, the customer pays the service provider directly, thus forming a direct relationship between the customer and the provider.

Only a few patients pay their home health providers directly. The rest pay premiums for insurance, and it is the insurance company that pays the home health provider. This creates two customers for every patient interaction. In fact, this is compounded because of the involvement of physicians, the patient's family or caregiver and, potentially, referral sources.

Customer service is the responsibility of everyone within the organization. Customer service is practicing what you preach and listening to the customer. Every interaction that an employee has with a customer will leave an impression regarding the organization that the employee represents. An impression can be positive, negative, or indifferent. The goal is to have everyone within the agency working toward a common goal: superior customer service.

Customer service is a strategy that will make a difference to the long-run viability of any organization. Home health agencies (HHAs) that adopt a customer service approach differentiate themselves from their competitors because everything that they do is oriented toward the customer. Customer service is experiential, demonstrable, and easily differentiated from mere lip service. Superior customer service can be severely affected if the external service delivery processes are out of sync or if internal processes are dysfunctional. This chapter will identify several elements of superior quality service that are necessary elements of the customer service strategy before transitioning into discussion of the customers of the financial department.

QUALITY SERVICE

Figure 10–1 identifies 14 elements of quality service.[1,2] The 14 elements are basic, down-to-earth concepts that apply to all forms of service delivery regardless of whether an internal or external customer is being served. The core of the service delivery strategy is represented by reliability, responsiveness, empathy, caring, and communication. Eight elements revolve around the core. These eight elements represent how service delivery and quality is approached by the HHA. The final element, listening, encompasses all of the preceding elements. Listening provides the filter between the customer and the HHA's approach to customer service. Active listening helps the evolutionary process of quality service delivery adapt to the changing needs of the customers who are served.

Listening

The act of listening is a continuous process on the quality service path. Listening provides a mechanism to hear customers' expectations, concerns, complaints, and desires. Listening provides a medium for translating customer expectations, concerns, complaints, and desires into a service delivery strategy that is customer

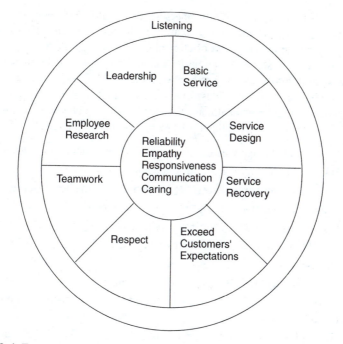

Figure 10–1 Fourteen Elements of Quality Service

focused instead of provider focused. This is especially important considering the diverse range of customers that an HHA has.

The concept of continuous evolution is also very important. The expectations of case managers, physicians, patients, MCOs, and payors change regularly. Expectations can be explicitly stated in a conversation, formally written into a contract, or implicitly stated. The last form of expectation presents a challenge for agency personnel and requires active listening to determine whether the provision of services is meeting or falling short of customer expectations. For instance, it may be very difficult for a sick individual to state in no uncertain terms what outcomes he or she expects from an interaction with the home health provider. This places the responsibility on the home health provider to help the patient and his or her family, or caregiver, to understand how the healing process works from a home health perspective. Listening to feedback and evaluating body language will provide clues to how well the message was received. Listening is an active research method, and it is ongoing.

Listening will also provide clues to changes in service delivery that the customer expects as part of the home health process and that the agency may need to implement. From a physician's perspective, this could be changes in follow-up practices regarding patient communication protocols. From an MCO's perspective, it may be the development of clinical pathways and outcome measurement practices. "A 1994 survey of home health-care patients revealed that the most important thing to the patient was how well the home health agency handled requests to change nurses or aides. The survey, which included responses from 7,000 patients of 25 home health agencies, was conducted by Press, Ganey Associates, Inc. The survey listed the top 10 patient satisfaction issues"[3]:

1. How well the agency handles requests to change nurses or aides.
2. Whether the family is kept informed about treatment.
3. How much the family is involved in planning home health services.
4. How much the nurse is concerned for patient comfort.
5. How much the aide is concerned for patient comfort.
6. Whether the nurse contacts the patient if he or she will be late or absent.
7. How well the nurse teaches patients to care for themselves.
8. How many technical skills the nurse demonstrates.
9. How well the initial plan for health care or treatment meets the patient's needs.
10. How helpful the person who made initial arrangements was toward the patient.

One of the key elements of listening is the ability to interpret correctly what is being communicated. Everyone has his or her own set of prior programming, terminology, and interpretations of the way things should be. It is very important that one of the elements of listening includes the development of a common understanding of what the customer's expectation really is. Once a common understanding is agreed upon, then the listener will need to act on the information that has been received.

Action is complex. Action is complex because of organizational dynamics and the level of employee accountability. Action could be handled immediately, if it is within the ability of the individual who has just received the customer's expectation or complaint, or action may require passing the information along to others so that the service delivery process can be completed. Action may require the modification of existing practices. In either situation, proper handling of the situation is critical from a customer service perspective.

Every employee within an agency is responsible for participating in quality service delivery. It does not matter whether the employee deals with external or internal customers. Listening provides a vehicle to understand when there are problems with meeting customer's expectations, regardless of what point in the service delivery process they occur. Listening is a form of customer research. "Customer research reveals strengths and weaknesses of a company's service from the perspective of those who have experienced it."[4]

The Core: Reliability, Responsiveness, Empathy, Caring, and Communication

> The importance and personal nature of health care encourage patients to seek the highest possible quality. Consumers and purchasers of health services are typically not capable of assessing the technical quality of care they receive. Because of this lack of ability to assess technical quality, consumers and purchasers utilize quality attributes associated with the delivery of health care. Results from this study suggest that patients define health care quality in terms of empathy, reliability, responsiveness, communication, and caring. These are human dimensions related to how the health care service was delivered, not the technical competence of the provider.[5]

Empathy is understanding the customer's feelings, situation, support system, needs, and expectations. It is the ability to relate to the customer, provide one-on-one care, and design a care plan specifically for the patient's problem. Empathy has always been part of the home health delivery process, and rightfully belongs in the core of quality service. Attempts can be made to enhance this element of customer service by evaluating practitioners' ability to interact with their customers. It may be that an individual has excellent technical skills but may need to work on interpersonal skills.

Reliability assures customers that service delivery is dependable and customer expectations will be met. It does not matter whether the expectation is that bills for the month will be submitted to a third party by the third day of the following month, all patients will be seen within 12 hours of acceptance of a referral, or the nurse will be at your house between 9 A.M. and noon.

> Reliability is the core of quality service. Little else matters to customers when a service is unreliable. When a firm makes frequent mistakes in delivery, when it doesn't keep its promises, customers lose confidence in the firm's ability to do what it promises dependably and accurately. Friendliness from the staff and sincere apologies do not compensate for unreliable service. Although most customers appreciate an apology, the apology does not erase the memory of that service. If a pattern of service failure develops, customers conclude the firm cannot be counted on, friendly and apologetic, or not.[6]

Responsiveness is an individual's, department's, or organization's sensitivity to the needs of the customers that it serves. This is the ability to react to changing expectations and, if necessary, to find alternative approaches to customer needs. This is also the ability to be flexible. Flexibility is measured by how quickly patients can be discharged from a hospital to the HHA, whether the agency can handle complex patient needs over the weekend or on a holiday, and how willing the agency is to go the extra mile.

From an internal customer perspective, this is the ability to produce a report or some other form of output when requested. It does not matter whether the request is preprogrammed or an adhoc request. What matters is the willingness to produce results when requested and the attitude with which it is approached. A 10-year study of more than 1,900 customers of 5 large, well-known U.S. corporations identified that reliability and responsiveness are the elements of service quality that customers value most.[7]

Caring is the ability to provide care and to care about the patient. Caring is another integral element of the home health delivery process. Caring is taking an interest in the well-being of the patient who is being served, waking up in the middle of the night wondering if he or she is all right, or worrying whether a different medication may have been more effective.

The service delivery dimensions of empathy and caring pertain to both the external and internal customer. Internal customers have feelings and need to be recognized for their efforts as part of a contributory process to accomplish the larger organizational objectives. Lack of consideration for internal customer needs contributes to dysfunctional organizations. This can be averted through actions that acknowledge and respect everyone's contribution and can be as simple as doing employee evaluations on a timely basis.

"Communication means keeping customers informed in language they can understand and listening to them. It may mean that the company has to adjust its language for different consumers, increasing the level of sophistication with a well-educated customer and speaking simply and plainly with a novice."[8] A home health practitioner will help patients to understand the home health process by teaching them about medications, side effects, transferring techniques, and changes in physical condition to monitor. Nurses will communicate with case managers if there is a need for additional services. Internal customers will outline specific projects, timelines, and project requirements, and then explain the bigger picture to staff of how a specific project will be used.

Communication that is not clear will cause problems from an outcome perspective as well as negatively cloud customer perceptions of quality. Communication is most effective when there is some form of verification that the initial message or communication is understood. This can be accomplished by soliciting feedback, summarizing to make sure that the message is understood, or including written instructions.

Not only is communication a means to becoming clear about an outcome, but also a method of completing the listening loop. The outer membrane of the quality service circle is listening. Listening makes providers aware of what the customer is saying. Listening requires a secondary step. That secondary step is some form of response. The response could be an acknowledgment that there is a problem, an immediate action that will correct a problem, or a communication to other members within the organization. *Communication* is a vehicle to provide background, resolve problems, and enhance the service delivery process.

> Consistent monitoring of these dimensions should allow administrators to learn of current quality perceptions and identify specific problem areas. Technical competence will always provide the baseline standard of quality, but it is important to recognize the patient's and the purchaser's perspective. Strict attention to the provision of technical quality will result in consumer complaints of tardy, unresponsive, and uncaring service. The result will be a decline in volume and difficulty in attracting new patient groups. Providers who satisfy consumer quality perceptions will secure an important competitive advantage.[9]

Performance measures can be established for the five core elements to be included as part of the activity-based management concepts discussed in the preceding chapter. Performance measures can be identified as part of customer (MCO, patient, and employee) surveys for specific periods of time and then matched to the activity cost. Trending of this information over time will identify whether there is a positive correlation between high-quality services and low cost.

Contributing Elements of Quality Service

Contributing elements of quality service are a reflection of agency efforts to build upon the core elements of quality service delivery. The contributing elements identify the who, what, why, and how of service delivery. Service delivery becomes the responsibility of everyone within the organization. Excellence in service delivery "requires the building of an organizational culture in which people are challenged to perform to their potential and are recognized and rewarded when they do."[10]

Basic Service

Basic service from an external customer's perspective is providing technically sound patient care services. The amount of services provided to patients as basic service is changing. This is due to the effect that managed care has had on the home health industry. It has created a paradigm shift from "more visits are better" to "more services for less cost." Beyond utilization, the other ingredients to basic service include breadth of services and clinical and administrative capabilities.

Breadth of service includes the range of services offered by the HHA. Services could be limited to nursing; physical, speech, and occupational therapies; social services; and home health aides for the provision of skilled intermittent services. The agency may have expanded services to include private duty, homemaker services, meals on wheels, home medical equipment, infusion therapies, respiratory therapies, and so forth. Other agencies may have developed specialized programs for pediatrics, oncology, patients with human immunodeficiency virus (HIV), and patients with mental health requirements.

Regardless of what services are being provided, the HHA must have the necessary technical competence to provide the service, the service must be reliable, and it must be responsive to the needs of the customer. Service provision must be available to the population being served. This may include providing home health services in dangerous environments, 7-days-a-week admissions, round-the-clock services, initial visits performed within 12 hours of referral acceptance, patient calls returned within 15 minutes of the initial call, physician follow-up, and communications on patient status with a case manager.

Basic service from an internal customer's perspective would be determined by what his or her role was within the agency. Each employee and department would be responsible for different processes within the agency. Each process would have inputs and outputs related to it. Basic service requirements would be understanding how process outputs were used in each subsequent step in the overall process. Service requirements can be enhanced through a cross-functional analysis of the entire process from beginning to end.

An important element in basic service design is not to overstate the capabilities of the organization. This will raise customers' expectations. In the event that the agency is unable to live up to the overstatement, there is the potential for creating customer problems.

Service Design

Service design includes all the processes within an agency from patient intake through discharge. If all of the elements are working in sync, then service delivery is smooth. If there are scheduling problems, coordination of delivery problems, or difficulties in collecting paperwork, then the agency has service delivery problems. Some of the service delivery problems will be visible to the customer; others will not. The prior chapter identified internal and external nonconformance as two types of problems that would affect quality.

Service delivery is the life blood of any service organization. If service delivery is inefficient, then the customer will eventually become unhappy. "Delivering the basic service customers expect depends in part on how well various elements function together in a service system. These elements include the people who perform the specific services in the service chain, the equipment that supports these performances, and the physical environment in which services are performed. Design flaws in any part of a service system can reduce quality. It is tempting to blame poor quality on the people delivering service but frequently the real culprit is poor service system design."[11]

From the customer's perspective, poor service delivery may be not knowing when someone is coming to visit. This could be exacerbated by an agency scheduling problem that caused the home health aide to arrive in the morning to give the patient a bath and, as soon as he or she was dressed and back in bed, the physical therapist arrived. Now the patient has to get up, go through the exercise regimen, perspire, and, before long, the benefits of the home health aide's visit are negligible.

Inefficient service delivery is also more expensive than efficient service delivery. Inefficient elements of the service delivery process include not getting sufficient information on the patient at time of intake, provision of services that will not be paid for, lack of inventory, insufficient or improperly trained personnel, improper coordination of services, and others. Efficiency of service delivery could be as simple as providing directions to patients' homes so that providers do not get lost or spend more time than necessary in transit. Salaried personnel who spend a lot of time in transit increase the agency's total cost because this is nonproductive time. Nonproductive transit time could be due to inefficient scheduling, lack of agency personnel, customer discharge patterns, geographic area, or myriad other factors. The goal is to identify service delivery problem points and work toward streamlining the entire process.

Nonproductive time is not limited to transit time. Nonproductive time could be attributable to scheduling of services so that every field employee has a full caseload or delivery of supplies or equipment prior to the nurse's arrival so that he or she does not have to wait for deliveries, or down time could be administrative in nature. Service delivery encompasses all aspects of an agency. This includes administrative processes and functions. Meetings, computer down time, rework, rebilling because of incomplete or inaccurate information, and many other nonvalue-added activities contribute to inefficient service delivery.

"Delivering quality service is in part a design challenge. The lesson of service design involves developing a holistic view of the service while managing the details of the service. Both perspectives deepen managers' understanding of the service, making it easier to fit it to the customer's expectations."[12] Adopting a holistic approach incorporates agency processes, employees, and customers into the service chain. The end result will be customer satisfaction, contract renewal, and financial viability.

Analysis of internal processes will help to identify how an agency is currently providing services. Once the internal processes have been identified, management can begin to question whether there is a better way of providing services. The goal of service delivery enhancement "is to redesign the service system to be simpler, more reliable, more efficient, more responsive, or improved in some other way. Customer input is critical."[13] Customer input will determine the performance measurement indicators that provide the base or initial benchmarks from which to measure organizational improvement efforts. Once redesign has taken place, it is important to review whether the new design is meeting customer expectations. Service enhancement can be the result of advances in information technology, development of service protocols and procedures, clinical pathways, efficient use of subcontracted services, incentive alignment, elimination of repetitive tasks, efficient resource utilization similar to New York City's Cluster Care program, or removal of tasks that do not add value to the customer.[14]

The more complex the organization, the more challenges will be faced in developing efficient service delivery. Control of the elements of the delivery process so that the entire behind-the-scenes process is blind to the customer will transition service delivery to "seamlessness." Service delivery is also the result of senior management's interactions with the customer. "Top level managers need to spend a day in the life of key customers in their distribution (or service) chains. There is no substitute for managers' instincts, imagination, and personal knowledge of the market. It should be the essence of corporate strategy. Only in that context can analytical devices like customer-satisfaction indices, market-share data, and, benchmarking results become servants rather than masters. And only with market-focused leadership can companies continuously and quickly reinvent themselves to meet new market needs."[15]

Service Recovery

Another element of the service delivery process is service recovery. Service recovery is a term used to describe how employees handle service delivery problems that have been raised by their customers. Customer complaint resolution will depend on the type of complaint. At a patient level, is the complaint something that can be resolved immediately, or was the complaint discovered as a result of a postdischarge satisfaction survey?

If the result was discovered after the fact, it should be identified by provider, classified, trended, and dealt with as part of an ongoing quality improvement process. Feedback should also be provided to the customer. If the customer complaint was a symptom of a larger problem, then effort should be expended immediately to correct the source of the problem before any additional problems happen. "Three possibilities arise when a customer experiences a service problem: the customer complains and is satisfied with the company's response, the customer complains and is not satisfied with the company's response, or the customer does not complain to the company and remains dissatisfied. Companies that do not respond effectively to customer complaints compound the service failure; they fail the customer twice."[16]

Addressing process flow removes individual blame and judgment and moves the analysis to a level that is consistent with higher purpose organizational objectives. Service recovery also speaks about organizational values. Organizational values flow down from the top, and it is the behavior at the top that is modeled by all members of the organization. Senior management needs to provide all employees with the tools of problem and conflict resolution, continuing education, and a reward system that makes customer satisfaction everyone's responsibility, and should interact visibly at the customer level.

Management should also make the resources available to enhance communicative abilities between the agency and its customers. This may require investment in information systems that enhance the service delivery process, new phone systems, an additional receptionist, or designated staff to handle customer complaints in a timely fashion. Communication is critical, and to allow customers to get lost in an agency's voice mail system is unacceptable.

Exceed Customers' Expectations

Companies are supposed to be reliable; they are supposed to provide the service they promise to provide. Thus, it is difficult for firms to exceed customers' expectations by being reliable. The process dimensions of service, however, provide the opportunity to surprise customers with uncommon swiftness, grace, courtesy, competence, commitment, or, understanding. The opportunity is present to go beyond what is expected. In effect, exceeding customer's expectations requires the element of surprise, and, the best opportunity for surprising customers is when service providers and customers interact. Companies must seek excellence on both the outcome and process dimensions of a service to develop a reputation for truly outstanding service. Excellent service reliability allows a company to compete. The addition of excellent process service creates a reputation for superior service quality. This is the "wow" element of service delivery.[17]

This is the ability to understand how the customers think and to answer their questions or address their problems before they have been able to put their thoughts into words. From an internal customer perspective, it is going beyond the request to provide additional value beyond merely providing output (a report, a response, an element of a process). If the customer is a case manager, the "wow" may be finding a solution to a difficult patient problem. Keep track of the large successes. They can be used advantageously at some other point in time.

Respect

Efficient service delivery requires respecting all elements of the service delivery chain. Customers need to be respected along each step of the process, employees need to be respected, vendors need to respected, and organizational objectives need to be respected. Customers have expectations regarding reliability, responsiveness, and basic service. They do not expect that inferior services, supplies, or procedures will be substituted.

Service providers expect that they will be paid for services that have been rendered. Employees expect that they will be treated fairly, that they will be rewarded for working toward organizational goals, and that their job and benefits will be secure. The common theme is that every link within the service chain expects to be treated fairly, honestly, and consistently. "Customers expect service companies to treat them fairly and become resentful and mistrustful when they perceive otherwise. Fairness underlies all the customers expectations. Customers expect service companies to keep their promises, to offer honest communication materials, to provide prompt service, to be competent and courteous, and to provide caring personalized attention. Fairness is not a separate dimension of service, but, rather touches the very essence of what customers expect."[18]

The transition from a Medicare to a managed care paradigm initially will create a challenge for providers of home health services. This is because the old paradigm focused on providing a greater amount of services to help meet the needs of the population that was being served. The managed care philosophy wants to provide only necessary and appropriate services. Until the new philosophy is totally integrated, there will be a feeling of shortchanging the patient.

Teamwork

Teamwork from a service delivery perspective is no different from watching or participating in sports. It is very obvious when a group of individuals is working as a team and when a group is not. Whether it is handing a baton to the next link in the chain or whether it is timing the delivery of a pass so that a team member can achieve the outcome of a completed pass, the concept is the same. Efficient service delivery requires that everyone within the organization function in a team-like fashion. This includes rooting from the sideline when team members have exceeded customer expectations or helping them when they encounter customer problems.

Services coordinated through teams become more efficient because the combined effort of the group is focused on achieving a specific outcome. This concept, when applied to the provision of patient care, combines multidisciplinary expertise in determining the best mix of services to meet the needs of the customer. This approach moves away from discipline-oriented outcomes to patient-oriented outcomes. Additionally, through developing trust with team members and a commitment to a common cause, everyone becomes accountable for achieving outcomes, thereby making the achievement of the group greater than the individual achievements. "It is common for employees to be stressed by the service role that they become less caring, less sensitive, less eager to please. The presence of service "teammates" is an important dynamic in sustaining servers' motivation to serve. Coworkers who support each other and achieve together can be an antidote to service burnout. Team involvement can be rejuvenating, inspirational, and, fun. Our research shows convincingly that service performance shortfalls are highly correlated with the absence of teamwork."[19]

Teamwork crosses functional boundaries. Efficient service provision requires the support of the internal agency staff. Staff members must understand what the processes and activities within an agency are and how they affect each element of the process. By understanding what each subsequent department's expectations are, it is possible to support the overall processes within an agency. Development of common goals, performance objectives, and performance rewards that are linked to service delivery reinforces that service delivery is everyone's responsibility.

Employee Research

Employee research is as important to service improvement as customer research, for three reasons. First, employees are themselves customers of internal service, and thus are the only people who can assess internal service quality. Because internal service quality affects external service quality, measuring internal service quality is essential. Second, employees can offer insight into conditions that reduce service quality in the organization. Employees experience the company's service delivery system day after day. They see more than customers see and they see it from a different angle. Employee research helps reveal why service problems occur, and what companies might do to solve these problems. Third, employee research serves as an early warning system. Because of employees' more intensive exposure to the service delivery system, they often see the system breaking down before customers do.[20]

Organizations that take advantage of their employees' research and observations are accomplishing two things at one time. First, they are addressing internal nonconformance problems before they become external nonconformance problems. Second, if action is taken on employee recommendations, this encourages employees to seek to improve themselves and the efforts of their organization continually. Encouraging employees to be proactive and demonstrating that management responds favorably to suggestions and will take appropriate action help to expand the employees' range of influence. (See Figure 10–2.)

Every employee interacts within his or her peer groups, within families, within communities, at business meetings, at professional seminars, with local vendors, and with politicians. Every employee should be viewed as a potential source of information and as an agency ambassador of good will. The last thing that any organization needs is for a disgruntled employee to bad-mouth his or her employer, coworkers, or the services that are provided. This type of communication is remembered and difficult to correct.

Leadership

Leaders

understand that in the new economics of service, front-line workers and customers need to be the center of management concern. Successful

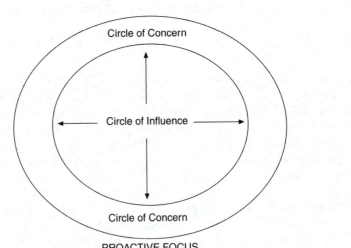

PROACTIVE FOCUS

Positive energy enlarges the circle of influence.

Figure 10–2 Circle of Influence. Source: Reprinted from *The Seven Habits of Highly Effective People* by S. Covey, p. 83. Copyright © 1989 by Stephen R. Covey. Reprinted by permission of Simon & Schuster, Inc.

service managers pay attention to the factors that drive profitability in this new service paradigm: investment in people, technology that supports front-line workers, revamped recruiting and training practices, and compensation linked to performance for employees at every level. And they express a vision of leadership in terms rarely heard in corporate America: an organization's "patina of spirituality," the "importance of the mundane."[21]

These leaders realize that customers want value from the services that they purchase. They recognize that their employees are the key to efficient and effective customer service, and they "believe in the capacity of people to achieve, view their own role as setting a direction and a standard of excellence, and giving people the tools and freedom to perform. Because these leaders believe in their people, they invest much of their personal energy into coaching and teaching them, challenging them, inspiring them, and of course, listening to them."[22]

The transition that will occur is that members of every level of management will begin to recognize that they need to focus on the customer, regardless of whether the customer resides within or outside the agency. This change is being stimulated by the changing health care delivery system. The winners in this new era of health care delivery will be the providers who can meet customers' expectations; provide cost-effective, outcome-oriented care; and remain financially viable.

Leaders are being challenged with this new paradigm. One of the answers lies in how they choose to respond to the changing environment. Adopting the 14 elements of quality service, enlisting the support of their employees, adopting efficient cost-management approaches, and striving to improve process continuously are strategies that will make a difference.

THE ROLE OF THE FINANCIAL DEPARTMENT IN SERVICE DELIVERY

The finance department has an opportunity to play a key role in helping its organization enhance the service delivery process. Service delivery is a team effort. Representatives from the accounting or financial departments can provide insights into the costs of different activities, process flow, and external customer requirements. In fact, by participating as members of multidisciplinary task forces, work groups, or teams, finance will help to achieve balance between operational priorities and financial realities.

One of the key roles that finance can play in the service delivery process is to work with its internal customers to develop reports (this assumes that information systems and finance are synonymous). Report development will depend on the customer. If finance is working with operations, then maybe the focus will be on extracting daily, weekly, and monthly information out of the information system regarding patient outcomes, utilization by referral source, utilization in relation to internally developed clinical pathways, staff productivity, scheduling efficiency, and cost of service by clinical pathway. If finance is working with the chief executive officer (CEO), then the focus would encompass all aspects of the agency. Topics might include operational forecasts for the balance of the year, cashflow requirements for the next month, costs of quality, performance indicators, or results of operations in comparison to forecasts.

Once reports have been produced, they should be analyzed, and, if necessary, corrective action should be taken. Review of a utilization by referral source may indicate that patients are being referred to the agency with a patient diagnosis that was excluded from a managed care contract. Identification of this fact will enable the agency to address its concerns with the MCO on a timely basis. Quick identification may correct potential problems before they occur. In this example, a specific patient diagnosis had been carved out from the managed care contract. Alerting the MCO to this issue should prevent any problems from occurring when billing the MCO on a per visit basis instead of including care under its capitated payment.

Inclusion of the finance department in operational analysis will expand both parties' perspectives. Finance can contribute an understanding of how costs fluctuate with service provision and what specific services and supplies have cost historically, and help to forecast what costs will be based on estimated utilization. Operations has an understanding of the dynamics of providing services, changes in service utilization, and utilization requirements by patient population. Combining the expertise of the two departments will provide a perspective that is larger than each department working in a vacuum. Collaborative efforts between operations and finance should be the rule rather than the exception.

Collaborative efforts are especially important as home health transitions into a prospectively paid service environment where payors are shifting risk to providers. Financial viability will be the responsibility of everyone within the organization. Financial viability will be the result of teamwork between all teams and functional departments, but it will especially require cooperation between operations and finance.

Entering into a service contract with an MCO is an element of basic service. It will require determining what services to offer; defining the service parameters that the agency will be accountable for; and estimating utilization, type of patient problems, anticipated cost of service, and agency profit. Successful negotiations will not be done unilaterally but, instead, draw on the strengths of the multidisciplinary team, of which finance should be a member.

One of the ways to approach managed care negotiations is to sit down with all members of the multidisciplinary team and begin to identify things that are critical to the success of the agency, what the agency's strengths are from a service delivery perspective, what the agency's weaknesses are, what type of services the agency wants to offer, what type of safety factors need to be included in the contract, and what type of information it wants to obtain from the MCO. Inherent in this process is determining the levels of organizational accountability. Organizational accountability in a managed care environment requires a cost-conscious mindset that focuses on appropriate utilization and maximization of employee efforts. Identification of who will be responsible for monitoring utilization; determination of accurate cost figures; daily, weekly, and monthly reporting; and the elimination of activities that do not add value to the customer will be some of the first steps toward organizational accountability.

Once information is obtained from the MCO, then finance and operations can work together to determine estimated patient population utilization requirements. The team would then attach costs to different types of patient problems, adjusting for service utilization ranges based on patient problem intensity, and develop a "what if" model to look at agency risk for fluctuations in patient utilization. Depending on the results of the analysis, the agency may decide that there is more risk than it is prepared to assume at this point in time, or it may want to explore identifying service exclusions to help lower the risk of the contract.

Service exclusion could be limited to equipment, supplies, infusion therapies, or specific patient problems and diagnoses. Service exclusion could also put caps on the dollar amount or number of services that an agency will provide. Codetermination of "safety nets" between finance and operations will help the agency to be financially viable. Assuming that all exclusions have been accepted by the MCO, exclusions have been entered into the contract, the contract executed, and the referring of patients has begun. This is where the real teamwork needs to begin.

Efforts should be made to develop reports and tools to evaluate utilization, cost, and quality on a daily basis. Monitoring of daily operations will enable management to determine how it is doing in relationship to contractual obligations, exclusion, and risk corridors. Beyond monitoring daily operations, the combined efforts of the finance and operations departments can focus on building economies into the service delivery system. It will be through the combined efforts that efficiencies and economies will develop. Activities aimed at building efficiencies into the delivery system will affect the bottom line positively in a prospective payment environment. Activity identification will be for both direct and support services.

There is no doubt that initially there will be finger-pointing regarding which department has the most amount of overhead. An approach that focuses on the mission and objectives of the organization will move this process to a higher level instead of getting stuck in a "we" and "they" battle. The answer is in approaching organizational efficiency from a process improvement perspective. Process improvement looks at the process and not the players. It incorporates customer expectations, employees, suppliers, performance measures, actual costs, and the organizational mission into continually improving the service delivery process. (See Figure 10–3.)

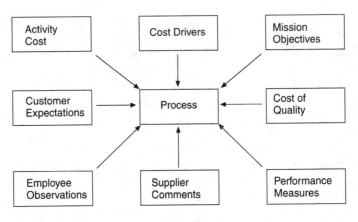

Figure 10–3 Processes Affect Every Element of the Agency

Finance can take a leadership or a participatory role in identification of process improvement opportunities. Regardless of the role, the important thing to remember is that efficient services translate to satisfied customers and profits. The obtainment of both objectives will allow agencies to continue to provide services, employ personnel, and invest in the future. Therefore, the balancing act between customer satisfaction, appropriate services, and financial viability becomes the responsibility of everyone within the agency. As a side note, agencies that have elected a not-for-profit status may object to the concept of profitability and service efficiency. In their case, service efficiency enables contributions, United Way grants, and other monies to be stretched across a larger population. Therefore, these principles are nothing more than prudent business acumen.

THE FINANCIAL DEPARTMENT AS EDUCATOR

The financial department has an obligation to its internal customers. This obligation is to make them informed consumers. Informed customers/consumers require that everyone in the company understand how the upstream and downstream processes affect their operations, how reimbursement is changing the way business is performed, and operational results. Sharing of operational results is a way to make everyone aware of how the business is doing, but, more importantly, it helps everyone to understand that there is more to work than their little world. This approach is a departure from the traditional role of finance, which previously has been characterized as having green eye shades, being concerned about beans (beancounters), and using financial information as a club in order to say, "I got you" or, "You exceeded your budget."

An open book approach to financial management within the agency accomplishes several things. First, by getting everyone involved in the numbers, it helps them understand the bigger picture. Understanding the bigger picture means supporting changing practice protocols and having the opportunity to participate in something that is bigger than yourself. Participation in something bigger than yourself means that now your circle of influence has increased, thereby making individual employee contributions more important than ever.

Second, the open-book approach helps develop common terminology and an appreciation of organizational goals and helps employees gain a basic understanding of organizational processes and informational requirements. Inherent in the education process are explanations regarding the effects of external influences like fluctuating payor mixes, changing reimbursement mechanisms, inflation, changes in case mix, statutory requirements, and operational overhead requirements on the agency. Providing internal customers with the results of operations only provides a snapshot of what is. True understanding will come from analyzing the influences, processes, and activities that are the cause of the symptoms.

Information sharing can begin with sharing the results of operations. An approach is to define common terms for the group that is presented with the results of operation. If the group is primarily clinical, then attempt to use their terminology, and build the presentation using their terms. Often nonfinancial employees will hear how much the agency charges for a nursing visit or a private-duty hour and think that the agency is making tons of money. However, they forget or are not aware of all the costs that are incurred to run an agency.

One of the challenges before the financial educators is helping employees with the new paradigm. This will require reprogramming employees who were educated in the more is better world. This world could have been part of their nursing education, administrative mandates, a cost-reimbursed mentality, or a personal presumption that more will ensure quality outcomes. The new view is appropriate care, by appropriate personnel, and without layers of administrative overhead. The opportunity is to create a unified work team that includes all employees, develop a common mission that is customer-/patient-centered, and build an organization that will be financially viable.

The Great Game of Business offers a practical approach to employee involvement. The basic premise is that employees will stop acting like employees if they adopt an ownership mentality. Adoption of an ownership mentality allows everyone to share in the profits and shift responsibility from owners and management to everyone. In addition, *The Great Game of Business* maintains that there are only two important things: (1) profit and (2) positive cash flow. Without either one, there will not be jobs.[23]

Linking rewards and incentives to continuous quality improvement (CQI), increased productivity, reduction of outstanding receivables, and profitability completes the loop. Now everyone has a stake in the financial viability of the agency beyond short-term salaries and benefits. One of the goals of employee involvement is to tie goals and objectives into quarterly and annual evaluations. Goals and objectives would link reductions in expense, quality improvement efforts, special projects, and normal job requirements to employees' reviews.

Another benefit is to have everyone participate in the budgeting process. Finance's role as an educator is to help departments and their chosen representatives through this process. The process would identify activity levels, variable and fixed expenses related to the activity levels, and quarterly and annual objectives. Finance would compile all the results, obtain executive approval, and begin the measurement process. Actual results would then be compared against the budget to determine how well the agency was doing against plan and prior activity. Variances in plan would be explained based on changes in volume, rate differentials, CQI efforts, quality indicators, and changes in activity cost.

EXTERNAL CUSTOMERS OF THE FINANCIAL DEPARTMENT

The fiscal intermediary (FI) was identified as an external customer of the agency. Finance's role with this customer is to make sure that quarterly periodic interim payment (PIP) reports and annual cost reports are completed correctly and accurately. Completion of quarterly and annual reports requires reconciling financial and operational results and reporting them in the required format. Cost reporting is part of the basic requirements of being a Medicare-certified agency.

From an FI's perspective, it relies on the work of the finance department to provide accurate information. In addition, developing a good work relationship with the FI will always be to the benefit of the provider. The service relationship can be enhanced by listening to suggestions that the auditors and their managers may make. Undoubtedly, the suggestions will be recorded in their workpapers for follow-up during their next encounter. Respect is another service element that may help to develop a good relationship with the FI. The FI is doing its job, albeit the FI can be difficult; however, increasing the agency's understanding of Medicare rules and regulations and doing research about how other agencies handle similar problems can prevent a lot of potential problems. This can be enhanced by providing prompt responses to inquires, maintaining good accounting records and accounting systems, reconciling visits to provider statistical and reimbursement (PS&R) reports, and developing a collegial relationship instead of an adversarial relationship. This is possible even though the FI's job is to disallow or allow costs, and finance's job is to maximize reimbursement.

The finance department is also responsible for the production of reports to third parties as required by MCOs, sundry payors, and regulatory agencies. In addition, finance is responsible for the application of correct charges against customers' escrow payments.

INTERNAL CUSTOMERS OF THE FINANCIAL DEPARTMENT

The financial operation of an HHA is a support function for basic operations. The majority of the internal customers were addressed above except for the board of directors. As a customer of the financial department, the board of directors expects timely and accurate financial statements; reports on operational variances, cashflow forecasts, and capital expenditure plans; and budgets for review.

The board's expectation is responsiveness to their informational requests, reliability in the facts and figures that are being provided, and timely communication. In return, the board helps to provide direction to the agency, secure credit, and generate funds.

OTHER CUSTOMERS OF THE FINANCIAL DEPARTMENT

In addition to the external customers identified in the beginning of the chapter, finance has a subset of customers that depend on the work of the finance department. These customers include the bank, vendors, financial auditors, and the Internal Revenue Service (IRS). The credit function is a very important role in any business. The banking relationship depends on accurate information, favorable business results, and the development of a working relationship.

Vendors need to be paid for the services and supplies that they provide the agency. When cash is tight, vendors will not be paid. If there is not a good relationship with vendors they may cut the agency off from ordering more supplies until their bills are paid. A good relationship with vendors may help to buy some time for the agency.

Financial auditors rely on the financial controls that have been established by the finance department. Reliance on the financial controls helps to reduce audit cost. The IRS relies on the data that are filed by the finance department. Of all the customers, the IRS has the biggest club, so accuracy and responsiveness are keys to dealing with this customer.

ALIGNING THE FINANCIAL DEPARTMENT'S MISSION WITH DEMING'S 14 POINTS FOR QUALITY IMPROVEMENT

Adoption of W. Edwards Deming's 14 points for quality improvement will provide a common framework for all members of the finance department. One of the goals of any support operation is to develop a customer orientation, continually strive to improve processes, and deliver high-quality products. Deming's 14 points offer a tool to focus the department on its role in service delivery.

Point 1: Create Constancy of Purpose

Constancy of purpose speaks to the need to recognize that the finance department has customers. Customers are both internal and external to the organization. It may require development of an internal mission statement that recognizes the need to attempt continually to improve one's abilities, to improve the services that are provided, and to be willing to change. Included in this mission statement is the department's approach to dealing with its customers.

Constancy of purpose is a long-term view that goes beyond the moment or the task at hand. It seeks to educate all team members about what their individual roles are and how their respective activities fit into larger processes. It is an understanding that everyone within the organization has a set of similar goals.

Point 2: Adopt the New Philosophy

The new philosophy is one of quality, cost management, and service delivery. These are the responsibilities of everyone within the agency and are strategies that require everyone's assistance. Quality, cost management, and service delivery are all bottom-line strategies that focus on the customer, value-added services, and long-run financial viability. The goals are to eliminate unnecessary steps, rework, and waste.

Adoption of the new paradigm requires that employees and their managers get out of the blame game. No longer will it be acceptable to point fingers; the new philosophy requires raising consciousness to the next level. The next level looks at the organizational mission, process objectives, and activity inputs and outputs in relation to the customer. Without continual emphasis on the goals of the collective, there is the ever-present possibility to slide back into old patterning.

The new philosophy requires understanding every customer's expectations. It requires understanding how each customer within the process stream prepares inputs to the finance department (upstream) and how each customer utilizes the outputs of the finance department (downstream). Once processes are understood, the new philosophy requires that the processes be benchmarked, improved, and made more efficient. The new philosophy requires a willingness to make a difference, to be accountable, and to help educate fellow employees.

The new philosophy will require a new paradigm for every employee. The new paradigm will necessitate flatter organizations, increased productivity, and a personal investment in improving the processes of the agency.

Point 3: Cease Dependence on Inspection

Inspection is a costly proposition. After-the-fact inspection implies that there are defects in the process, the output will require rework, and the system produces waste. Adoption of an attitude of pride in one's work, ownership, and accountability is one of the first steps in reducing the need for inspection. A secondary step is to invest in information technology that employs validation processes. This will eliminate the need for manual processes on the back end.

Point 3 identifies the need to identify process outcomes. Process outcomes should be internally identified. They are a statement of expectations in relationship to the customer base that is being served. This establishes the rules by which everyone needs to play, regardless of whether you are a manager, a supplier, or another team member. Establishing clear expectations assists in transitioning from an industry that has been characterized by retrospective review to one that is outcome-oriented. Furthermore, inspection can then be replaced with inspections based on random sampling.

Deming developed an alternative to inspection known as the *kp rule*. The following is an example of the kp rule as applied to a billing error.[24]

- $k_1/k_2 > p$, then no inspection
- $k_1/k_2 < p$, then 100 percent inspection
- $k_1/k_2 = p$, then 0 percent or 100 percent inspection based on historical experience
- p = average proportion of efforts or mistakes produced by a service process (a billing error)
- k_1 = the cost to inspect one service process unit (one bill)
- k_2 = the cost to rework the error or mistake (such as audit and inspection, data entry, customer service, mailing and collection fees)
- k_1/k_2 = break-even quality

Example: A $20,000/year billing supervisor is employed to audit (inspect) 20 bills per day for critical documentation errors. On average, one critical documentation error is found per day.

- $p = 1/20 = 0.05$
- k_1 = Cost to inspect one bill = $4.00

- k_2 = Cost to rework bill = $20
Therefore:

- $k_1/k_2 = 4/20 = 0.20$
- $0.20 > 0.05$ = no inspection

It is uneconomical to spend $20,000 on the billing supervisor's salary and another $5,200 on annual rework costs. The supervisor's time and the money should be invested in more productive work. This will yield a first-year savings of

$25,200. Continuous quality process improvement adds value to service. Workers should spend their time preventing problems instead of inspecting for them.

Point 4: End the Practice of Awarding Business on Price Tag Alone

Deming has identified that the low-cost supplier, service bureau, lawyer, accounting firm, or employee may cost the agency more money in the long run. His belief is that supplier identification should be based on whether the supplier will meet the needs of the agency. Need definition identifies the service levels that are expected by the agency, identifies what efforts are being made by the supplier as part of its quality improvement efforts, and develops a common mission.

Furthermore, Deming states that "striking deals with the cheapest supplier is the accepted American way of doing business. Certainly thrift is an admirable quality, and costs are important. But if low cost guarantees low quality anywhere in the supply chain, then the final product, though it may be cheap, will also be of low quality. Indeed, often low quality of the final product can be traced back to problems with incoming materials."[25]

The new paradigm will require all suppliers, both external and internal, to be reliable, responsive, and dependable. Their approach to service delivery must be consistent with agency processes, and coordinated efforts need to be made to enhance service delivery efforts continually.

Point 5: Improve Constantly and Forever the System of Production and Service

Process improvement crosses every functional boundary. It is the difference between efficient and inefficient service delivery. Process improvement identifies ways of enhancing the payables process; improving vendor relations; and eliminating payroll efforts, bad check runs, and restatement of financial statements. Process improvement requires identification of the process as it exists now, identification of better practices, and continuous attempts to improve the quality of the services provided. An example would be reduction of the days of outstanding accounts receivable from 105 to 90 days within a 3-month period.

Process improvement requires that employees understand their jobs and how they relate to every element of the process. Sufficient investments in continuing employee education are a critical element of process improvement, as is involvement with other teams and departments. Additionally, small successes will help to build employees' confidences (expand their circle of influence) to address other problem areas.

The Shewhart Cycle illustrates the concept of process improvement (Figure 10–4). First, one begins by identifying the process; second, processes are identified from an input and output perspective across cross-functional boundaries. Next, representatives are brought together from the various departments that con-

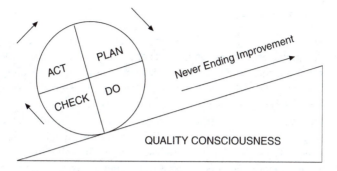

Figure 10–4 Shewart Cycle of Process Improvement. Source: Reprinted from *The Deming Guide to Quality and Competitive Position* by H.S. Gitlow and S.J. Gitlow, p. 79, with permission of Prentice Hall, © 1987.

tribute to the process. Activities are dissected, and consensus is reached about what the needs are of every customer within the process, what factors (cost drivers) influence the activities, and what goals (performance measures) need to be established. Results are monitored and shared with cross-functional participants. Further adjustments are made as necessary.

Point 6: Institute Training and Retraining

Employees are an asset that is not reflected on the balance sheet. Employees need to be trained in all aspects of the department's activities. Common terminology needs to be developed, as does an understanding of who the finance department's customers are, what their expectations are, and what individual roles are in achieving those objectives. Additionally, employees need to be cross-trained.

One of the first steps is hiring appropriate employees. Employees must have similar values to the organization. Without similar values, the concepts of teamwork, process improvement, and service delivery will always be at odds. The second step is to educate employees as to the policies, procedures, and practices of their new employer. Clear identification of expectation needs to be addressed, and quarterly review dates need to be established to monitor the new employees' progress. Finally, an investment needs to be made in the continuing education of all employees. Training can include problem-solving techniques, conflict resolution techniques, software training, college course work, use of statistical methods, management training, and supervisory training. Coestablishment of applications within the department is essential, and informational sharing with the entire staff helps everyone to benefit. Furthermore, improperly trained employees are inconsistent with the new paradigm of quality, efficient service delivery, and cost management.

Point 7: Institute Leadership

Management has a responsibility in the new paradigm to be accountable. This requires that managers become proponents of customer-oriented service delivery. If managers adopt an attitude that cost management is for everyone else, customer service exists only when they are interested, or any approach that is contrary to the objectives of the new philosophy, the process will be sabotaged.

Managers must begin by setting an example, encouraging two-way communication, being willing to experiment, promoting cross-functional relationships, and educating their staffs. Without actively participating, listening to the concerns of their staff, and taking a genuine interest in making a difference, employees will recognize a lack of commitment and label efforts as another management fad. Furthermore, performance evaluations need to be an integral component of all staff members' reviews.

Establishing management survey tools helps the agency evaluate the effectiveness of its managerial staff. If managers receive poor grades from their staff, this should be investigated and attempts made to correct management styles or behavior. No one is exempt in the new paradigm.

Point 8: Drive Out Fear

According to Walton,

> People are afraid to point out problems for fear they will start an argument, or worse, be blamed for the problem. Moreover, so seldom is anything done to correct problems that there is no incentive to expose them. And more often than not there is no mechanism for problem solving. Suggesting new ideas is too risky. People are afraid of losing their raises or promotions, or worse, their jobs. They fear punitive assignments or other forms of discrimination and harassment. They are afraid that superiors will feel threatened and retaliate in some fashion if they are too assertive or ask too many questions. They fear for the future of their company and the security of their jobs. They are afraid to admit they made a mistake, so the mistake is never rectified. In the perception of most employees, preserving the status quo is the only safe course.[26]

This is unacceptable.

Point 9: Break Down Barriers between Staff Areas

Elimination of a "we" versus "they" attitude is necessary for process improvement to occur. Normally, this attitude develops because of problems caused by one department or another not having an appreciation for the other's work requirements. This can be remedied through education, identification of cross-functional processes, and the development of common objectives and incentives. The following are several reasons for barriers[27]:

- *Poor Communication or Lack of Communication*—Poor communication could occur between departments, within departments, between bosses and subordinates, or within the extended process. It creates barriers because people feel excluded, confused, scared, or demeaned.

- *Ignorance of the Organization's Overall Mission and Goals*—Ignorance leads to the pursuit of individual departmental goals as opposed to working for the overall good.

- *Competition between Departments, Shifts, or Areas*—Competition is often encouraged by management as a way to motivate employees. Actually, it results in underachievement overall.

- *Too Many Levels of Management that Filter Information*—Individuals filter information. The more times that information is passed between individuals, the more the original meaning changes.

- *Differences between Departments*—Accountants, nurses, and marketers speak different languages and have different work cultures. There are different norms of behavior among these groups, which make it difficult for them to communicate.

- *Decisions and Resource Allocation without Regard to Social Memory*—A group can give up something for the common good as long as it is remembered, and the group is eventually rewarded for it. A sense of community and civic-mindedness will exist in this type of environment. An example would be when a department voluntarily gives up an opportunity to have its offices redecorated because another department needs the money. If this department is not remembered for this act and eventually rewarded for it, resentment will occur and will create barriers.

Point 10: Eliminate Slogans, Exhortations, and Targets for the Workforce

Goals have to have meaning and be measurable, and everyone must know the required steps, actions, and timeframes necessary to achieve the stated goals. Slogans that sound good but do not provide clear steps, actions, timeframes for accomplishment, and means to achieve are meaningless rhetoric. Examples include the following: decrease costs by 12 percent next year, decrease days outstanding to 50 days, and do it right the first time.

Point 11: Eliminate Numerical Quotas

Quotas lead to a short-term perspective. Quality, service delivery, and cost management require long-term perspectives. Management should develop an outcome orientation that links internal performance measures to customer expectations. Adoption of a horizontal perspective allows management to evaluate whether the processes within the department or agency are consistent with a customer-oriented philosophy.

Point 12: Remove Barriers to Pride of Workmanship

"Workers complain that they do not know from one day to the next what is expected of them. Standards change frequently. Supervisors are arbitrary. They are seldom given feedback on their work until there are performance ratings or raises, and then it is too late."[28] Some of the challenges for management are to be clear in establishing objectives, to reduce emergencies and "fires," and to help streamline processes. Processes that are repetitive, require cleaning up a problem, or are inconsistent with organizational objectives will create disharmony and lead to dysfunctional service delivery.

Pride in workmanship is possible by allowing employees to have ownership in the process, giving credit when and where credit is due, and providing feedback to the employees of how their work is used downstream from their actual site. Providing employees with the proper tools to do their job will also help to increase the pride that they take in their jobs.

Point 13: Institute a Vigorous Program of Education and Retraining

"Training and retraining should develop employees for changes in their current jobs, in respect to procedures, materials, machines, techniques, quality characteristics, and operational definitions. Everyone's job will be changing to incorporate statistical methods, from management to hourly workers. Education must be provided so that the transformation process can occur smoothly. The purpose of education and training should be to fit people to jobs and to responsibilities for which they are well suited."[29]

"Management has to look toward the future, develop new products and services, and put resources into research, training, and education. As products and services are continually improved, the organization must look for new and innovative ways to meet customers' needs. Appropriate job retraining will have to be instituted to qualify employees for the new job opportunities created. Retraining involves teaching employees new skills so that they can keep up with technological advances."[30]

"Education and training can prevent employee burnout because employees are exposed to new information and are provided with a forum to discuss problems. This can be very valuable because it stimulates interest in the job and encourages involvement in problem solving. Training in new jobs and methods can also rekindle the desire to participate on the part of employees who have written off their jobs as a source of fulfillment."[31]

Point 14: Take Action To Accomplish the Transformation

Quality, efficient service delivery, cost management, and process improvement are number one organizational priorities for those finance departments that are going to be leaders in the new paradigm. It requires walking the talk and being willing to change. It also requires the adoption of system thinking. System thinking looks at process inputs and outputs and recognizes the dynamic nature of a service business with multiple customers and changing requirements.

Point 14 is also about honoring the workers and the process, because without the workers and processes there is nothing.

CONCLUSION

The concepts of customer service transcend all elements of a service organization. Regardless of whether an employee is *front line* or *back of the office*, all employees must participate in exceeding customer needs. Furthermore, whether one subscribes to the principles of Juran instead of Deming, the important point is to practice quality, integrate CQI activities into daily operations, and use these principles to further staff members and the agency in realizing the agency's mission and vision.

NOTES

1. L.L. Berry, et al., Improving Service Quality in America: Lessons Learned, *Academy of Management Executives* 8, no. 2 (1994): 32–44.
2. M.R. Bowers, et al., What Attributes Determine Quality and Satisfaction with Health Care Delivery? *Health Care Management Review* 19, no. 4 (1994): 49–55.
3. Making Patients Part of the Evaluation Process, *Quality Progress* 28, no. 4 (April 1995): 14–17.
4. L.L. Berry, Improving Service Quality, 32–44.
5. M.R. Bowers, What Attributes, 49–55.
6. L.L. Berry, Improving Service Quality, 32–44.
7. *Ibid.*
8. M.R. Bowers, What Attributes, 49–55.
9. *Ibid.*

10. L.L. Berry, et al., Improving Service Quality, 32–44.

11. *Ibid.*

12. *Ibid.*

13. L.L. Berry, et al., Improving Service Quality, 32–44.

14. W. Balinsky and J.F. LaPolla, The New York City Shared Aid Program (Cluster Care): A Model for the Future, *Home Health Care Services Quarterly* 14, no. 1 (1993): 41–54.

15. F.J. Gouillart and F.D. Studivant, Spend a Day in the Life of Your Customers, *Harvard Business Review* (January-February 1994): 116–25.

16. L.L. Berry, Improving Service Quality, 32–44.

17. *Ibid.*

18. *Ibid.*

19. *Ibid.*

20. *Ibid.*

21. J.L. Heskett, Putting the Service-Profit Chain to Work, *Harvard Business Review* 8, no. 2 (1994): 32–44.

22. L.L. Berry, Improving Service Quality, 32–44.

23. J. Stack, *The Great Game of Business* (New York: Bantam Doubleday, 1992).

24. D.M. Sloan, *How To Lower Health Care Costs by Improving Health Care Quality* (Milwaukee, WI: ASQC Quality Press, 1994), 19.

25. M. Walton, *The Deming Management Method* (New York: Putnam Publishing Group, 1986), 63.

26. M. Walton, *The Deming Management Method*, 72.

27. H.S. Gitlow and S.J. Gitlow, *The Deming Guide to Quality and Competitive Position* (Englewood Cliffs, NJ: Prentice Hall, 1987), 142.

28. M. Walton, *The Deming Management Method*, 81.

29. H.S. Gitlow and S.J. Gitlow, *The Deming Guide*, 182.

30. *Ibid.*

31. *Ibid.*, 183.

Chapter 11

Teams

The concept of teams has gained a great deal of recognition in the past several years. Teams are a way to bring people together for a common purpose. Teams can be formed for specific or for ongoing projects. Projects could include the development of clinical pathways, study of quality indicators such as patient and employee satisfaction, or formation of a risk management group to identify safety precautions. Regardless of the task, teams are a way of assembling personnel for purposes of achieving desired outcomes. This chapter begins with the elements of effective teams, identifies necessary ingredients for developing teams, and specifies types of teams. The chapter concludes with a discussion of using teams for continuous process improvement and radical process improvement or re-engineering.

WORK GROUPS VERSUS TEAMS

It is important to begin by differentiating between teams and work groups. (See Exhibit 11–1.) Often, the term *team* is applied to both work groups and teams. The difference is that work groups are a group of individuals that comes together to perform a common task. Often a work group is characterized by a department or a function within an organization. The members of the work group do their job and help members in the group but are evaluated based on their individual contributions. There is very little concern for the other elements within the department; however, as a whole, the work group achieves a level of output that is used by the organization. The individual elements of the work group are held together by a supervisor or manager who directs the daily activities, organizes the pieces, and delegates activities to achieve the work group's objectives.

Teams have a common mission that is known by all and takes precedence over individual missions. There is a common understanding of what needs to be done, there is a common ownership of the process, and individuals are evaluated on their efforts as well as the efforts of the collective. Individual performance goals mesh with team goals and organizational goals. "Teamwork represents a set of values that encourages listening and responding constructively to views expressed by others, giving others the benefit of the doubt, providing support, and recognizing the interests and achievements of others."[1]

"Teams differ fundamentally from working groups because they require both individual and mutual accountability. Teams rely on more than group discussion, debate, and decision: on more than sharing information and best practice performance standards. Teams produce discrete work-products through the joint contributions of their members. This is what makes possible performance levels greater than the sum of all the individual bests of team members. Simply stated, a team is more than the sum of its parts."[2]

A team can be greater than the sum of its parts because each of the parts works toward accomplishing a goal that is larger than any one of the individual parts. The objective or mission of the team transcends individual priorities, thus creating a collective. A collective is a group of individuals that comes together for a specific purpose and works together toward a common goal. Team members within an organization are typically cross-trained, understand what is required of them individually as well as collectively, and build on each team member's individual strengths. Their common goal can be either internally or externally developed. However, the path toward accomplishing the objective is usually determined by team members.

Exhibit 11–1 Comparison of the Characteristics of Teams versus Work Groups

Work groups
- Strong, clearly focused leader
- Individual accountability
- The group's purpose is the same as the broader organizational mission
- Individual work-products
- Runs efficient meetings
- Measures its effectiveness indirectly by its influence on others
- Discusses, decides, and delegates

Teams
- Shared leadership roles
- Individual and mutual accountability
- Specific team purpose that the team itself delivers
- Collective work-products
- Encourages open-ended discussion and active problem solving meetings
- Measures performance directly by assessing collective work-products
- Discusses, decides, and does real work together

Source: Reprinted with permission from Jon R. Katzenbach and Douglas K. Smith, "The Discipline of Teams," *Harvard Business Review*, March/April 1993.

DEPARTMENTAL TEAMS

Departmental teams can be very powerful within their own domain. Individual departments become highly specialized because of dealing with one aspect of the business process. Departmental teams run the risk of getting into an "us versus them" syndrome with other teams. This may be because of the department's leadership, lack of cooperation from the other departments, or lack of understanding of how all the pieces within the organization fit together.

Departments can even become adversarial. "When this occurs, tribes (departments) are missing the basic point of why organizations are created in the first place. To accomplish complicated tasks in the most efficient ways, 'organizations' combine various groups under one roof to accomplish two things: first, division of labor, and second, shared resources and interdependence. When the collision between tribes occurs, the value of the first step, division of labor, is being emphasized, but no attention is being paid to the equally important second step, shared resources and interdependence."[3]

A remedy to this syndrome is to help each department within the agency understand what departments are its suppliers and what departments are the customers of its outputs. Identification of departmental inputs, outputs, and objectives is the first step in this process. This helps to define measurement criteria, but, of equal importance, the process identifies what is needed, why it is needed, and when it is needed. Inputs are identified from both the supplier department's perspective and the customer department's perspective. The customer department identifies what and how it wants information (inputs) to look. It also identifies when it wants its inputs, what supporting information is required, and so forth. This process can be performed for each department to develop an understanding of how each department uses inputs and outputs from other teams. Additionally, it will help to develop a common understanding between teams of what is expected of them. The development of a common reward system, unification of leadership, and the development of a leadership structure that does not support conflict will foster professionalism and enhance the obtainment of organizational goals.

Management has a role in this process. It needs to

> provide employees with the necessary training and support so that they are both willing and able to provide excellent service to internal and external customers; seek constant feedback on internal customer satisfaction with performance, and use it to improve the quality of service provided; in addition, top management should structure internal service functions and processes so that different departments can work together to support one another. Senior management needs to operate on the realization that internal customer satisfaction and external customer satisfaction are inextricably related.[4]

TEAM CHARACTERISTICS

Teams can be departmental or cross-functional or designed for special purposes. Teams, regardless of their charter, will exhibit similar characteristics. One of the first characteristics of effective teams is the range of experiences, expertise, and functional or technical abilities and skills that each team member brings to the team. Teams are assembled to achieve a specific objective. If the team is very specific in its charter, such as a finance department, then the range of skills, experience, and expertise will be structured for the finance function. Depending on the scope of the finance function, expertise may require in-depth understanding of accounting, payroll, taxes, cost reporting, auditing, banking, cash management, and financial reporting. Every member of the team will have varying degrees of expertise depending on their specific function or assignments. If the team is cross-functional in nature, it will draw from departmental resources across the entire organization.

It needs to be noted that, for a department truly to be a team, there is no longer a subordinate relationship within the department. Teams offer equal status to every team member. There is no differentiation between clerks, assistants, supervisors, managers, and senior managers. Decisions are democratic and not autocratic and are based on the team's ability rather than a team member's ability. Recognition and rewards are shared with the entire group and not taken by the supervisor.

Team selection should be made based on ability instead of personality. It is extremely important to have a harmonious and synergetic team; however, the primary goal is to achieve the objective for which the team has been assembled. Therefore, to choose someone for a team because he or she is a friend, the person gets along with another team member, or a reason not related to the primary purpose or objective of the team will ultimately hold the team back. "No team succeeds without all the skills needed to meet its purpose and performance goals. Yet most teams figure out the skills they need after they are formed. The wise manager will choose people both for their existing skills and their potential to improve existing skills and learn new ones."[5]

Successful teams draw members who have various skills. One of the required skill sets is "Problem solving and decision making skills. Teams must be able to identify the problems and opportunities that they face, evaluate the options they have for moving forward, and then make necessary trade offs and decisions about how to proceed. Most teams need some members with these skills to begin with, although many will develop them best on the job."[6] Problem solving requires the ability to recognize when there is a problem. Problems may be the result of an error in the service delivery process and brought to the employee's attention by a customer, part of an internal problem that will affect an internal department, or a potential problem caused by changes in regulatory structure.

Problem recognition requires that employees cannot function with blinders. They need to be cognizant of their piece of the process as well as the larger process or system. Problem recognition requires that team members be clear about what their objectives are, the objectives of other teams, and organizational goals. This requires the ability to think systemically. Systemic thinking is linear, in that one process affects the next process and so on. Problem recognition can also be based on intuition. "Intuition in management has recently received increased attention and acceptance, after many decades of being officially ignored. Now numerous studies show that experienced managers and leaders rely heavily on intuition— that they do not figure out complex problems entirely rationally. They rely on hunches, recognize patterns, and draw intuitive analogies and parallels to other seemingly disparate situations."[7]

Problem resolution requires that team members determine whether problems are an isolated occurrence or part of a larger system problem, whether problems are a one-time event or recurring, or the scope of the problem. Problem resolution also requires that team members be accountable for resolving problems and have the ability to resolve problems. This may require creativity or innovation when resolving problems, the assistance of other team members, or the assistance of other teams within the organization. In any situation, if team participants are not provided the latitude to resolve problems and work with their team members at problem resolution, then teams will never have the ability to achieve their maximum potentials.

Team members must have good interpersonal skills. "Common understanding and purpose cannot arise without effective communication and constructive conflict, which in turn depend on interpersonal skills. These include risk taking, helpful criticism, objectivity, active listening, giving the benefit of the doubt, and recognizing the interests and achievements of others."[8] Not only are team members required to have good interpersonal skills, but also there should be a forum for resolution of team problems. Resolution may require the use of an outside intermediary, a facilitator, or simply the willingness to move problems to a higher level instead of shutting down or becoming defensive.

Interpersonal problems could occur because of cultural differences between team members. These differences could be due to training, personal biases, departmental or cultural jargon, or myriad other factors. They are complicated because each individual has a set of values, departments have their own values, and team members have their own values. Therefore, it is imperative that teams develop an ability to communicate with one another and resolve conflict among themselves and with other team members. This can be accomplished by recognizing that everyone approaches problems in different fashions; they have different thinking patterns and have different orientations, thus requiring an approach that honors individual differences but recognizes the need for prompt resolution in order to move the process to a higher level.

Problem resolution also requires the ability to see things from different perspectives. This is analogous to saying that there are 360 different ways of looking at a particular perspective. By rotating 1° to the right of a stationary object, the viewer is able to obtain a slightly different perspective as his or her orientation changes. This is out-of-the-box thinking, a willingness to look at things from different perspectives and not opt for old solutions to new problems. It is moving away from the blame game and the easy answers of, "It is accounting's problem," or "due to the personnel department." The new paradigm requires a leap in faith and a willingness to accept the possibility that the old way may not be the best way.

Other team characteristics include a willingness of all team members to be accountable for the team's outcome. This is mutual accountability; it enables the team to become larger than the sum of its pieces. Accountability can occur when the objectives of the team are clear and known by all members of the team. They know what is expected of them on an individual and collective basis, that workload is fairly distributed, and that a common approach has been developed to achieve a specific outcome:

> All effective teams develop rules of conduct at the outset to help them achieve their purpose and performance goals. The most critical initial rules pertain to attendance (for example, "no interruptions to take phone calls"), discussion ("no sacred cows"), confidentiality ("the only things to leave this room are what we agree on"), analytic approach ("facts are friendly"), end-product orientation ("everyone gets assignments and does them"), constructive confrontation ("no finger pointing"), and, often the most important, contributions ("everyone does real work").[9]

THE CHANGING ORGANIZATIONAL STRUCTURE

Originally, HHAs followed the traditional business design of American business. This design was a top-down approach. It is the typical hierarchical organization that had layers of supervisors and management. Senior management negotiated with customers, understood their needs, and communicated its interpretations to the next lower layer of staff. This structure was employed because members of senior management felt that they were the only ones who could correctly interpret the needs of the customer (this also presumes that the customer's needs and expectations were being acknowledged). "Layers of middle management were positioned to make sure the organization functioned according to plan. The military structure of low risk and high control dominated. Managers and employees were good soldiers."[10]

This model had several limitations and was inverted to reflect an emphasis on the needs of the customer and the employee. Organizations began to focus their service delivery needs on the customer. Efforts were made to make the organization more responsive to the customer. Employees were expected to be accountable for customer service, customer expectations were to be funneled to senior management, and senior management was to determine whether these expectations were consistent with their values. This was a bottom-up approach to quality management. (See Figure 11–1.)

This approach helped to make significant strides toward honoring the customer; however, it did not make any advances toward aligning the agendas of the three employee groups in relationship to the customers who were being served, reducing cost, increasing efficiency, and honoring the customer and the employee. This required the organization to make another transformation.

This new organizational structure recognized the importance of customer-focused teams. Customer-oriented teams would then revolve around the customer,

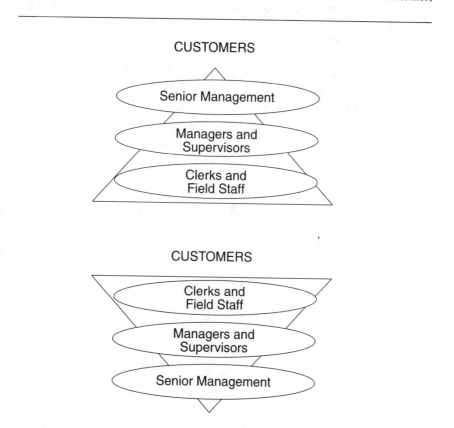

Figure 11–1 Changing of Approaches to Customer Service

listening to its needs and expectations and then integrating these needs and expectations into the agency's basic service delivery plan. This approach recognized that all elements of the agency team had to be linked to the service delivery program. Figure 11–2 identifies the interrelated needs of the external and internal customer.

MULTIDISCIPLINARY TEAMS

One of the first steps toward this new model was the development of multidisciplinary teams. Multidisciplinary care teams were developed that had representation from all elements of the care process. Nursing, the therapies (speech, occupational, respiratory, and physical), home health aides, and case managers came together to begin to build comprehensive care plans to serve their clients better. By combining the efforts of all of the care disciplines, it became possible to eliminate duplication of activity, to isolate approaches that did not work or only produced modest returns, and to develop joint accountability for achieving patient outcomes.

This process encouraged team participants to identify where they could improve their clinical approaches to focus on the care processes as a whole, instead of as one element of a larger process. This shift in perspective helped to eliminate

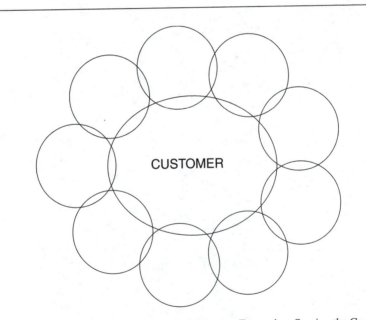

Figure 11–2 An Evolving Organizational Structure Focused on Serving the Customer

agendas by discipline in favor of a care plan that honors the patient and the combined efforts of all participating team members.

Multidisciplinary teams have been used in clinical pathway development. The development of clinical pathways provides a benchmarking system that focuses on patient outcomes. Clinical pathways identify how each member of the multidisciplinary team interfaces with the patient, what interventions are to be performed, and the timing of interventions, and establish individual patient milestones as well as expected patient outcomes. Once the entire process was laid out, it became possible for the individual team members to identify how their efforts contributed to the larger picture.

Beyond clinical pathways, teams can be used for joint case management. Clinical pathways provide a beginning measurement for home health care. There are numerous variables that affect patient problems and, depending on the severity of patient problems, the clinical pathways would need to be altered to conform to specific patient needs. The alteration process can be accomplished through the input of the multidisciplinary team. Furthermore, as the team becomes well versed in working together, it has the ability to perform case management activities, thus eliminating a supervisory layer within the agency.

INTRODUCTION OF INTERDISCIPLINARY TEAMS

Expanding the ranks of the multidisciplinary teams to include a representative from finance, information systems, and senior management and possibly the managed care liaison would create an interdisciplinary team. The addition of these representatives would increase the power of the multidisciplinary team. For instance, clinical pathways can now have costs attached to the care delivery process. This would enable team members to monitor the cost of a clinical pathway or an episode of care according to a customized clinical pathway, and calculate a variance. Inclusion of costs allows team members to evaluate financially quality of care, identify savings that could accrue from altering the care delivery process in relationship to outcomes, and identify their contribution toward organizational viability.

The information systems representative will ensure that the multidisciplinary teams can obtain results of operation to evaluate their efforts. This may require the development of specialized reports identifying key success factors that can be included as performance measures, thus enhancing a team's ability to collect information on its clients. This could be as simple as acquiring lap-top computers or as complex as developing a specialized clinical documentation system that incorporates clinical pathways and clinical pathway customization on a patient-specific basis. Regardless of the approach, the information systems representative would begin to understand the complexities of the clinical operation. This understanding would enable the building of an interdisciplinary bridge that allows higher organizational outcomes to be achieved.

Blending the talents and the expertise of finance and information systems together will allow the multidisciplinary team members to analyze the results of operation from a cost perspective: cost in relationship to units of service, quality, or outcomes. The bridging of disciplines will enable the respective team members to appreciate everyone's contribution to the current process, but, more importantly, the bridging will provide a vehicle for continuously refining the care process, the costing process, and the data collection and reporting process. Results and learnings can then be shared with other team members.

EVALUATION OF TEAM RESULTS

Results can be captured and disseminated as part of an ongoing continuous quality improvement process. This process will help to identify where teams are working well together and where individual team members may need additional training. Results analysis could group together actual results by team, patient problem, diagnosis-related group (DRG), age group, clinical pathway, or myriad other indicators. Evaluation of results will help the agency to determine where there is room for improvement. A variance from plan may identify the need for additional clinical pathways or pathway redesign. Redesign may be attributable to one team having measurable success by increasing the frequency of home health aide visits on the front end, thus reducing the patient's overall amount of time on service.

Results evaluation should include agency results in relationship to team contributions. Decreasing revenue streams, episodic payments, and capitated payments will all have different ramifications on agency viability. It is important that teams understand their contribution as well as other agency costs. Several benefits should appear as a result of information sharing. First, teams should be able to improve continually on their results by learning what works and what does not work in relationship to other team results. Utilization statistics regarding the number of patients per team, severity of patient problems, and team member volume will help to stimulate an understanding of what needs to be accomplished from the patient and organizational perspective.

TEAM SPECIALIZATION

Interdisciplinary teams can become highly specialized by product line. Product-line specialization may include separating teams based on expertise. Expertise could be defined by patient age groups (e.g., pediatrics, young adults, older adults, and geriatrics). Expertise could also be defined by service specialty (e.g., hospice, traditional intermittent visits, private duty, respiratory therapy, or community-based family support services). Within service specialty, there is an opportunity for further differentiation. Specialization could occur based on program character-istics (e.g., cardiac, wound care, obstetrics, high-risk mothers and infants, reha-bilitation, and an assortment of other programs).

Specialization allows teams to concentrate on their specialty. Specialization leads to process refinement and enhancement of the service delivery process. This is especially beneficial when teams are assigned to physicians who have specialty practices. Assigned teams can work with the physician to develop clinical path-ways that are tailored to the needs of the patient. This also develops a close work-ing relationship between teams and referral sources. The added benefit of this type of relationship is that it honors two sets of customers: (1) the patient and (2) the physician. Team members have the ability to coordinate services, provide follow-up to the physician, and suggest new and innovative approaches to the provision of home health services. A good working relationship will lead to the development of a collegial relationship between a potential managed care gatekeeper and the HHA. This relationship will be of long-term benefit to the agency as physicians band together to control the patient population.

Specialization can also be of interest if the agency is interested in working closely with specialty hospitals. Identification of specialty needs will provide the agency with a vehicle to work closely with the hospital, its physicians, and staff to develop comprehensive clinical pathways. This relationship has the potential to become a win–win for both the agency and the hospital in the managed care envi-ronment.

SUPPORT DEPARTMENTS

The development of multidisciplinary and interdisciplinary teams will advance service delivery to the external customer. Figure 11–2 illustrates this concept. Un-fortunately, service delivery from an internal customer perspective may still be stuck in Figure 11–1. Patient care is the primary purpose for an agency's exist-ence. All other departments and activities should be designed to support this proc-ess.

Departmental specialization has created little hierarchies that have not transitioned into teams, but, more importantly, these departments have not ac-knowledged the new paradigm in service delivery. Service delivery requires ev-eryone to be as efficient as possible. The new paradigm requires support depart-ments to justify the costs of their support activities to the primary service teams.

No longer can the following be accepted: "inferior quality of many internally produced products and services; lack of cooperation between divisions and departments; constantly rising headcounts in many support departments; ever-increasing overhead costs; frequent conflicts over transfer prices; and widespread apathy and complacency among affiliated divisions and departments."[11]

> Every "support" function must be assessed in terms of its value-added contribution. To ensure equity, the assessment must be accomplished by the contingent already found to add value to the organization—the customers of the support departments. It is imperative that the review not be performed by such traditional decision-making groups as management, human resources, or any other support function. This will surely lead to rationalization and perpetuation of the status quo. It would be like asking the fox if he should be in the chicken coop. Internal customer evaluation would certainly have a tremendous residual effect on the groups responsible for providing the service. Wow, would this increase communication and service to our internal customers.[12]

Support departments must transition into a team mentality whose sole mission is to exceed its internal customers' needs. This transition will require understanding what is needed by the internal customers, developing protocols to meet those needs, and eliminating all activities that do not provide value to their customer base. This transition will be difficult for departments such as personnel and finance, which historically have viewed themselves as the organizational gatekeepers.

Building on the merits of quality improvement, support departments can transition from back-end gatekeepers by developing quality audit programs. Quality audit programs will identify the special needs of teams. Needs can vary depending on product line, specialty program, referral source, type of service, organizational structure, or any number of reasons. Transitioning into a prospectively oriented process, support teams begin to anticipate the needs of the internal customer departments that they serve. Linking a quality audit program to service provision will enable teams to identify areas to improve processes currently and prospectively.

INTRADISCIPLINARY TEAMS

Alignment of organizational objectives can occur by developing intradisciplinary teams. Intradisciplinary teams would reflect each of the organization's processes within its team structure. This cross-representation will require that teams bear their respective cost of providing care and administrative costs. Administrative costs will represent support processes that enable teams to provide services. Representatives will begin to understand how each of the processes under their control contributes to each team and to the whole. Intradisciplinary team cost reflects all costs related to the activities of the team.

The goal of developing intradisciplinary teams would be to eliminate all activities and costs that do not support the team. Intradisciplinary team representatives would be challenged to make their individual elements as efficient as possible. Costs that are out of line would be negotiated, targeted for reduction by finding alternate practices, or eliminated. An example of a cost that could be targeted for reduction would be the cost of monthly financial statements. Team members may find that they can manage their operations with flash reports that show daily utilization in contrast to pro-rated capitation payments. By applying a previous quarter's standard overhead rate, they are able to determine operational profitability, and financial statements can be moved to a quarterly basis.

Intradisciplinary teams can be used to develop scorecards that honor the entire organization. The development of scorecards that honor the entire organization can then be linked to the performance measures that were addressed in Chapter 9. Balanced scorecards will be addressed in Chapter 17.

CROSS-FUNCTIONAL TEAMS

Cross-functional teams are another way of describing inter- and intradisciplinary teams. These teams have representation from various departments within the agency. Team membership will depend on the purpose of the team. Teams can be ongoing in the case of multi-, inter-, and intradisciplinary teams, or they can be brought together for a specific purpose.

The concept behind cross-functional teams is that diversity builds on the strength of the team. They accomplish this by using the same team format, except by obtaining cross-departmental or functional representation, all elements of the organization can be represented. "The diversity of team members supports collaborative and creative work efforts. The central advantage of a cross-function team is that it brings together information, knowledge, and skills that might not otherwise be readily available. By design, the information, knowledge, and skills the cross-function team can draw on are crucial for the effective resolution of complex problems involving technology and the coordinated development of product and service."[13]

Team members bring an understanding of each of the functions that they represent. This enables all elements of the organization to have a fair representation and input into cross-functional team activities. For instance, if the objective of the cross-functional team were to identify all of the processes within the organization, it would be able to accomplish this task because every function would be represented on the team. The team would begin by asking one person to identify tasks in his or her area of expertise. This process would also spark or stimulate other team members to identify additional processes in their departments or realize that they have a piece of the same process. Once all team members had identified all the different processes within their areas, the list would be combined and consolidated to identify all the processes within the agency. Processes would then be identified in the order of occurrence, linkage points identified between suppliers and customers, and then expectations identified for each customer within the process.

Figure 11–3 identifies 13 activities that take place within an agency. The two primary processes are the provision of patient care and billing. Included in billing is the subprocess of data entry, submission, and collection-type activities. The cross-functional team would identify all activities from intake through discharge and all support activities that include billing, practitioner payment, and collection activities.

Process improvement activities would begin by tracing how information collected at different parts of the process could be enhanced. For instance, problems with third-party responses, rebilling, and collection activities may be due to problems in the intake process. The symptoms or problems appear at the end of the process list; however, the root cause was at the top of the process.

Other areas for consolidation or improvement can also be identified. Intake, case management, and coordination of services could be consolidated into the responsibilities of the team. Rotation of teams to handle intake on a daily basis, coordination of incoming services, and case management activities could be

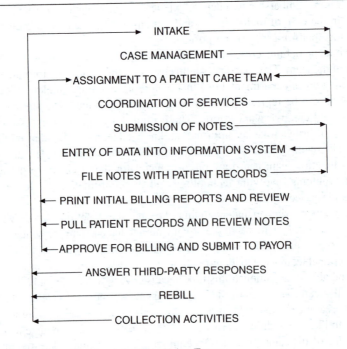

Figure 11–3 Cross-functional Analysis Using Teams

handled by the designated team. New referrals could be assigned to the appropriate team based on patient need, specialized service requirements, or team census. Process identification enables the organization to rethink the way it wants to provide care.

Advances in information technology would enable an agency to combine submission of notes, data entry, and records management into one process. Teams would enter data directly into lap-top computers, and data would be transmitted from the field to the agency's system, eliminating the need for note transcription and data entry by someone not familiar with patient specifics. Streamlining this process improves the quality of patient documentation and has the opportunity for transitioning records management into an electronic process. Notes would be retained within the system as an electronic chart printed on an as-needed basis for submission, and any documents that were not directly entered could be scanned into the system to complete chart documentation.

Printing initial billing reports for review, pulling patient records, and approving for submission could be enhanced through information technology, team review prior to submission, and changing perspectives from quality assurance to quality improvement. Building quality improvement into the front end of this process would require educating all team members on what customers expect for patient documentation, developing the information system to prompt practitioners for care specifics, and employing random spot checks to identify problems. Problems can be eliminated by including the quality improvement audit as part of the multidisciplinary team format.

Identification of process time and cost enables teams to identify alternative approaches to service delivery, to establish benchmarks to measure process improvement outcomes, and to target areas for improvement (Table 11–1). For instance, a review of the above processes could financially justify the acquisition of new computer technology or lap-top computers to enhance the documentation and billing process.

An estimated reduction in staff time was used to arrive at the potential savings that could accrue from converting to a documentation system that was entered directly by field staff into their lap-top computers and transmitted into the agency's main system (Table 11–2). The estimated savings of $23,579 could then be used to justify the expenditure for lap-tops and training. It is important that this is not a one-time analysis but that it is reviewed to determine whether actual savings were close to what had been forecasted.

USE OF INPUT AND OUTPUT INDICATORS FOR VARIANCE ANALYSIS

Tracing processes through the organization, establishing supplier outputs, customer expectations, and timeframes, is one of the first steps to defining internal

Table 11-1 Example of Activity, Time, and Cost

Activity	Time (hours)	Cost ($)
Intake	500	10,763
Case management	1,600	44,280
Assignment to a patient care team	3,000	77,490
Coordination of services	1,800	25,461
Submission of notes	650	14,391
Entry of data into information system	3,500	45,203
Filing of notes with patient records	1,100	8,118
Printing of initial billing reports and records	100	1,722
Pulling of patient records and reviewing of notes	500	4,613
Approval for billing and submission to payor	300	6,458
Answers to third-party responses	600	11,070
Rebilling	100	1,538
Collection activities	400	7,380

benchmarks and standards. Internal benchmarks help to identify the person(s) responsible for a process, the quantities that can be expected, and the quality of output. Variances from these standards will help to isolate improvements, problems, and fluctuations due to volume.

Workflow may be rather simple, calling for little search for information and infrequent problem solving. The greater the complexity in a workflow, the higher the need for teamwork, since no one team member is likely to have as much expertise as is needed for dealing with a specific work problem. High variability causes increased difficulties in planning and a greater need for flexibility. All of this calls for greater coordination than does the low-variability setting, for which a few standard sets of rules and procedures may provide adequate coordination across units.[14]

Table 11-2 Quantification of Quality Improvement Objectives Using the Performance Measures of Time and Cost

	Time (hours)	Cost ($)	Reduced Time (%)	Reduced Cost ($)
Submission of notes	650	14,391	10	1,439
Entry of data into information system	3,500	45,203	40	18,081
Filing of notes with patient records	1,100	8,118	50	4,059
Total savings				23,579

Identification of key benchmarks will help to monitor the process. Identification of many benchmarks will make monitoring expensive and time consuming. An inexpensive approach to tracking variances would be to begin by coming to agreement with the supplying department on exactly what the customer department's needs are. List the needs on a publicly visible document. Record results at the appropriate intervals and then continually work to improve those results, increase expectations, enlist the help of all members of the organization, and never settle for only adequate results.

ANALYSIS OF SUPPLIERS

Identification of supplier expectations does not need to be limited to the internal organization. External suppliers can become part of the team organizational structure. W. Edwards Deming identified the need to reduce the number of suppliers an organization had. His philosophy was that it was better to develop a long-term strategic relationship with a single supplier than to have relationships with multiple suppliers and constantly have them compete against one another for purposes of obtaining the lowest possible bid. This philosophy recognized that a long-term relationship would enable the agency and its suppliers to work toward the agency's objectives.

This requires that suppliers be treated as team members. Participation within the organizational structure enables suppliers to understand the challenges of service delivery within the agency and to work toward developing a much more efficient service delivery process. Potential suppliers to include as team members would be suppliers of medical supplies, home medical equipment, or infusion therapies. Team objectives might identify the need to reduce the amount of time between patient discharge and the delivery of supplies or infusion therapies, confusing billing practices, service delivery problems, stock outages, discourteous drivers, or any number of other factors.

Suppliers would then have an opportunity to work with the agency to correct problems in the service delivery process. Suppliers that are not willing to work with the agency, that have different agendas, or that have different perceptions of quality need to be replaced with suppliers who have the same quality orientation as the agency. The concept of suppliers can be expanded to include nurses, therapists, aides, or any other caregiver that contracts or is subcontracted to the agency.

Subcontracted or supplemental staff should follow the same strict guidelines the agency has developed for its own internal staff. This should include certification, evidence of continuing education, and inclusion in team results. The ultimate goal is to make the service delivery process as efficient as possible. This requires that all elements of the service delivery process participate in the never-ending quality improvement process.

CHASING THE ANTS WHILE THE ELEPHANTS RUN WILD

It is very easy to point fingers or attribute organizational problems to a person, department, or the point where the process is exploding. The difficult work is to trace through the process, identifying symptoms but not resting until the root cause is found. All too often, a decision is made to opt for the easy answer.

Ultimately, the goal is to develop an organization that is focused on customer service, efficient service delivery, measurable quality, low costs, and high perceived value. This new organization transcends personal egos. "We can no longer merely pass the cost on to the customer (or Medicare). So we must make tough decisions on what is the most beneficial approach. Do we retain the service residency or do we outsource? If the service is retained only the direct users should be burdened with the cost. Only then will we find out who actually needs the service support."[15]

MANAGED CARE IS CREATING COMPETITION

The health care delivery system is in the process of consolidating to compete effectively in a managed care environment. Providers are recognizing that the fragmented delivery system can become more efficient by aligning all aspects of the delivery process. This is creating the need for individual providers to demonstrate value, prove cost-efficiency, accept risk, and demonstrate outcomes. In a sense, this is not dissimilar from a global economy where providers and MCOs compete for patients.

Patients will choose providers based on individual and systemwide scorecards. Therefore, to succeed will require the integration of new values. One set of values is demonstrated by Exhibit 11–2. Exhibit 11–2 looks at the organization holistically. It identifies 19 customer-oriented principles that apply to all aspects of the evolving organization.

The 19 customer-oriented principles provide an outline of 8 areas that will help HHAs to survive in a managed care environment. The first area, "General," speaks about the need to know the customer, both internal and external. Efforts need to be made to understand upstream and downstream processes from the customer's perspective. Regardless of whether an agency is part of an organized delivery system or remains free-standing, efforts must be made to improve service delivery, increase response time, eliminate duplicative testing, and monitor outcomes. This requires staying on top of advances in technology, working with everyone in the entire delivery chain, and no longer being content with, "This is the way we always did it."

Improvements in organizational design will lead to cost reduction, improved efficiency, and increased customer satisfaction. Organizational improvement may require a leap in trust for a new model that is not complicated; fosters trust and

Exhibit 11–2 Principles of World-Class, Customer-Driven Performance

General

1. Get to know the next and final customer.
2. Get to know the competition.
3. Dedicate yourself to continuous, rapid improvement in quality, cost, response time, and flexibility.

Design and organization

4. Cut the number of components or operations and number of suppliers to a few good ones.
5. Cut the number of flow paths (where work goes next).
6. Organize product- or customer-focused linkages of resources.

Operations

7. Cut flow time, flow distance, inventory, and space along the chain of customers.
8. Cut set-up, changeover, get-ready, and start-up time.
9. Operate at the customer's rate of use (or a smoothed representation of it).

Human resource development

10. Develop human resources through cross training (for mastery), continual education, job switching, and multiyear, cross-career reassignments.
11. Develop operator/team-owners of products, processes, and outcomes.

Quality and problem solving

12. Make it easier to produce or provide the product without error (total quality).
13. Record and retain quality, process, and problem data at the work place.
14. Ensure that line people get first crack at problem solving before staff experts.

Accounting and control

15. Cut transactions and reporting; control causes not costs.

Capacity

16. Maintain and improve present resources and human work before thinking about new equipment and automation.
17. Automate incrementally when process variability cannot otherwise be reduced.
18. Seek to have plural instead of singular work stations, machines, and cells of flow lines for each product or customer family.

Marketing

19. Market and sell your organization's capability and competence.

Source: Reprinted with the permission of The Free Press, a Division of Simon & Schuster Inc., from *Building a Chain of Customers: Linking Business Functions To Create the World-Class Company* by Richard J. Schonberger. Copyright © 1990 by Richard J. Schonberger.

growth among managers, suppliers, and employees; encourages personal growth; and defines success as a balance between the needs of the customer, clinical operations, financial viability, and employee needs.

The elimination of nonvalue-added activities, waste, and delivery times will increase organizational efficiency. Organizational efficiency is a necessary ingredient of financial viability. It requires eliminating those steps and activities that do not provide value to customers. Activities that need to be eliminated occur because of poor communication, repeated data entry of the same information, not fully understanding customers' expectations, and holding on to the status quo.

Traditional views toward human resources will need to change radically as agencies adopt the principles of a world-class organization. The human resources department historically has been a gatekeeping department that recruited personnel, offered preliminary training and orientation into company policies, and determined job classifications and pay increases. The new paradigm will require human resources to justify its existence to the teams that it supports and focus on outcome-oriented activities.

Outcome-oriented activities will include developing training programs to meet the specific needs of the teams that it supports. This could include educating team members on conflict management, effective presentations, statistical analysis, or effective transfer techniques. Policy creation will need to be flexible and provide guidance, but no longer will be a tool for back-end control.

Quality and problem solving go hand in hand. Employees need to be able to understand quality, measure their own processes, and determine how they can improve. Team members provide resources to help other individual team members get up to speed. Additional growth will come from team learning and the assistance of training departments and outside consultants.

Accounting and finance is a support department that will need to change its orientation. No longer can the accounting department's existence be for the sole purpose of producing financial statements. "Over the last decade, the organizations that made the most progress in changing performance measurement systems to support improvement initiatives were the ones in which Accounting adopted the perspective of being a service provider rather than the producer of financial reports."[16]

The new paradigm will see accounting and finance become strategic partners to teams. This new relationship will have a training element, a reporting element, and a common focus. The common focus will be on developing the tools that enable teams to accomplish their missions. A common focus will enable teams to measure their performance by criteria that honor the entire organization instead of one element of the entire process (e.g., clinical operations or financial operations). Performance measures will include customer satisfaction indices, financial viability indicators, employee satisfaction, and other indicators of process efficiency.

The constricting of revenue streams will bring capacity issues to the forefront of customer service. Excess capacity is a form of inefficiency. Capacity issues include personnel, office space, and information systems. Employee capacity addresses productivity, process efficiency, and employee psychology toward additional projects. Office space should be maximized and evaluated for workflow efficiency. Information systems provide an opportunity for everyone in the organization to enhance their individual processes. Enhancements come from moving from single machines to networks, use of a centralized database, and a system that only requires entry of data once.

APPROACHES TO PROCESS IMPROVEMENT

Process improvement begins with first understanding the processes that take place within an organization. Once processes are known, improvement begins by identifying ways to improve the process. One approach is to work at process improvement in a gradual fashion. This approach is commonly referred to as *continuous quality improvement* (CQI). For this process to work, processes must be identified, be measurable, be linked to outcomes, and be measurable from the customer's perspective. The goal is to work at process simplification, eliminating activities that are not required by the customer, and recognizing that processes move across the agency in a horizontal fashion, not functionally or departmentally.

Some of the core concepts within CQI are the following:

- Customer service is about exceeding customer expectations.
- Customer expectations must be known in order to be met and exceeded.
- Clinical pathways are a method of standardizing care to measure outcomes.
- Cost-efficiency includes appropriate use of agency personnel, supplies, and space.
- Management needs to support the process.
- Everyone needs to be accountable.
- Quality is measurable.
- Performance measures honor the entire organization.
- The process is never ending.

Identification of cross-functional processes will highlight those processes that no longer serve the organization. Process elimination will free up organizational resources to focus on activities that have value. Elimination of processes could lead to workforce reduction. Indiscriminate reduction of the workforce can lead to fear and disincent employees. Therefore, efforts need to be made to assist with redeploying human assets to areas where the organization will benefit. Efforts need to be made to work with the remaining employees to educate them and help them with the transition.

The changing reimbursement environment, managed care, and the changing health care delivery system are forcing providers to become as efficient as possible. Some advocate more aggressive approaches than CQI efforts. These strategies have been called *delayering, downsizing, rightsizing, reengineering,* and *restructuring*. The net effect is that they change the way the organization appears and functions.

> Restructuring is concerned with moving, shrinking, or eliminating organizational units ("boxes"), reengineering has to do with changing the way work is carried out. The argument for reengineering, at its most basic, goes as follows. Too many corporations (and other organizations) historically have been organized vertically, by functions—research and development (R&D), manufacturing, marketing, finance, and so on. As a consequence, employees' mindsets have become defined by their particular function—or "silo" or "chimney" or "stovepipe," as some have put it.[17]

Restructuring and reengineering are two methods that eliminate processes, activities, and people. Their goals are bottom-line oriented; their approaches are harsh; and their victims are the organizations' internal processes, suppliers, and customers.

> Customers could care less, however, about internal organizational design. All that matters to them is composite output—in terms of quality, cost, and time. The challenge, therefore, is to improve on current competitiveness by reorganizing into work processes that make the most sense from the customer's point of view. This change is typically described as moving to a horizontal flow of tasks that cuts across the various functions. The new arrangement, ideally, is a work system comprised of a set of business processes—each with a definable beginning and ending—such as new product development, customer acquisition, and order fulfillment.[18]

Therefore, agencies that adopt a management structure that supports continuous quality improvement, cross-functional teams, and innovative process improvement will have the ability to determine what their customers need. The major difference between CQI and restructuring or reengineering is approach. CQI tends to be oriented tactically and incremental, while restructuring and reengineering tend to be oriented strategically and radical. CQI is a bottom-up approach, and restructuring and reengineering are bottom-down approaches.[19] "The key is to create an organizational culture that encourages innovation, through participative work practices, at all levels of the organization. For many employees this will translate into small-scale improvement activities; for others located in strategic positions, this will result in a large-scale redesign. Management's job is to provide appropriate resources to employees to further these outcomes."[20]

Ultimately, the goal of any approach is to link organizational processes to the strategic objectives of the organization. CQI is a method to improve the ongoing process, restructuring is a method of shedding excess baggage, and reengineering is a vehicle to change the way work is performed. Once restructuring or reengineering has been completed, CQI efforts can resume.

A long term perspective that encompasses CQI, restructuring, and, reengineering should explicitly build a concern for human development. For today's employees will almost certainly play a crucial role in determining the corporate tomorrow. Firms should strive to use reengineering not to eliminate jobs, but to increase the desirability of their products and services in the marketplace. This is the only way to employ the reengineering concept and preserve employee morale and loyalty, and to successfully enlist employee ideas for better processes. A humanistic orientation is instrumentally sensible from the corporation's standpoint. Strategic advantage clearly depends on capable, committed, empowered employees in all areas, at all levels.[21]

NOTES

1. F.R. Katzenbach and D.K. Smith, The Discipline of Teams, *Harvard Business Review* (March-April 1993): 111–20.
2. *Ibid.*
3. P.C. Neuhauser, *Tribal Warfare in Organizations* (New York: Harper Business, 1988), 18.
4. T.R.V. Davis, Satisfying Internal Customers: The Link to External Customer Satisfaction, *Planning Review* (January-February 1992): 34–40.
5. F.R. Katzenbach and D.K. Smith, The Discipline of Teams, 111–20.
6. *Ibid.*
7. P.M. Senge, *The Fifth Discipline* (New York: Bantam Doubleday, 1990), 168.
8. F.R. Katzenbach and D.K. Smith, The Discipline of Teams, 111–20.
9. *Ibid.*
10. J.L. Escover, Focus: Value, *Business Horizons* (July-August 1994): 47–50.
11. J. Magidson and A.E. Polcha, Part II: Creating Market Economies within Organizations: A Conference on Internal Markets, *Planning Review* (January-February 1992): 34–40.
12. J.L. Escover, Focus: Value, 47–50.
13. M. Sashkin and M.G. Sashkin, *The New Teamwork: Developing and Using Cross-Function Teams* (New York: AMA Publications, 1994), 10.
14. *Ibid.*, 59–60.
15. J.L. Escover, Focus: Value, 47–50.
16. J.R. Dixon, et al., Business Process Reengineering: Improving in New Strategic Directions, *California Management Review* (Summer 1994): 93–108.

17. R.W. Keidel, Rethinking Organizational Design, *Academy of Management Executives* 8, no. 4 (1994): 12–27.
18. *Ibid.*
19. J.R. Dixon, Business Process Reengineering, 93–108.
20. R.E. Cole, Reengineering the Corporation: A Review Essay, *Quality Management Journal* 1, no. 4 (1994): 77–85.
21. R.W. Keidel, Rethinking Organizational Design, 12–27.

Chapter 12

Management Accounting

This chapter focuses on management accounting issues as they relate to the home health agency (HHA). The beginning of the chapter concentrates on the development and use of the budget as a management tool. Once the budget has been developed, it can be used in conjunction with financial statements for purposes of variance and financial analysis. The chapter concludes with a description of a financial model.

BUDGETS

Budgets, when used properly, provide management with a tool to assess what the financial position of the agency will probably look like given the current set of assumptions. Budgets are a snapshot of the future based on the best guesses of the individuals who contribute to the budgeting process. Budgets can either be used as a tool by management or thrown in a drawer to collect dust until the next budgeting period. Those HHAs that throw their budgets in a drawer have wasted a great deal of effort. A budget is a management tool that, if used properly, will provide an early warning system to respond proactively to opportunities or threats instead of reacting and forcing a transition to survival mode.

The metamorphosis that causes budgets to change from a worthless piece of paper to a tool is management's approach to the budgeting process. It is a philosophical difference in the way an organization is managed. If the organization is proactive, requires staff and management accountability, and takes pride in doing what it says it is going to do, then the budget will become a tool. This does not mean that the agency needs to be rigid and highly structured to use budgets. What it means is that the agency has developed an internal benchmarking system that it uses to measure its financial performance and create organizationwide ownership of agency results.

To become a tool, budgets must be compared against actual results. Comparison of actual results against budget will create a variance. Variances from plan can be either favorable or unfavorable. It is the job of team members and management to evaluate variances from plan and to determine whether a problem exists and corrective action needs to be taken. Budgets need to be created in sufficient detail to allow management to evaluate how well the agency is doing. Additionally, budgets will become increasingly important as the cost reimbursement safety net slips away.

Of equal importance, the budget is a tool that is relied on by bankers, creditors, the board, and other external customers. Therefore, the budget is a statement of management credibility. Bankers are responsible for the loans that they make. An HHA that presents a budget that is unobtainable will create friction between the HHA and the credit facility. Therefore, budgets should be presented that are realistic and achievable. Unfortunately, if funds are made available and the agency is not able to achieve budgeted results, funds are used and variances cannot be explained in a reasonable fashion, possibly jeopardizing future credit availability.

THE TRADITIONAL APPROACH TO BUDGETING

The budgeting process can be approached from a top-down or a bottom-up orientation. A top-down process is dictated by senior management, and no input is solicited from other members within the agency. Although this process is typically more expedient, it does not foster ownership of the budgeting process. Lack of ownership leads to a mindset that ignores the budget because it is "theirs" and not "mine."

A bottom-up approach requires that department managers and supervisors contribute to the process. This process is more labor-intensive and usually requires more time, but it helps to build accountability for achieving organizational results. Accountability is also enhanced if employee evaluations are linked to operational results in respect to the budget. However, it is important to note that rewards and the evaluation of results need to be consistent across the entire operation; otherwise, inequalities will disincent employees.

A bottom-up approach can follow the traditional organizational chart where every department develops its own budgets in response to volume estimates, history, or departmental goals. Departments are asked to forecast budgeted expenses for the upcoming year. Budgets are developed by calculating departmental salary costs, employee benefits, operating expenses, and facility overhead expenses. Costs are based on history and inflated for employee increases and rising supplier costs. Operating and facility expenses are based on history and adjusted for new programs or changes in the operational infrastructure. Costs are then accumulated across the entire agency.

Departmental managers who have been through the budgeting process attempt to build "fat" or extra costs into their budgets. The reason for this is twofold. The first is that it allows for departmental inefficiencies. The belief is that as long as the entire department is under budget, then unfavorable variances will be ignored. Therefore, by incorporating a cushion into the annual departmental cost, the likelihood of being scrutinized for operational excess is minimized. The second reason is that the budgeting process usually consists of two or three passes. The first pass produces an inflated version of the budget, requiring a second pass be made at the budgeting process. The second pass will usually incorporate mandatory reductions of expenses. Those managers who had not built fat into their budget would then be in a bind when it came time to trim the excess. If the budgeting process goes to the third phase, then managers would need to become very serious about cost reduction.

Unfortunately, this process has the potential of being detrimental to an organization's health, especially when managers are requested to reduce operating budgets based on total outlay of expenses. This is because total expenses do not provide managers with an understanding of the actual processes and activities that will take place within an agency for those costs to be consumed. Without this knowledge, costs are eliminated regardless of whether or not they provide value to the customer. Costs that have been eliminated during the budgeting process but are integral to the primary and support processes within an agency will be incurred regardless of whether the cost was budgeted for, thus reducing some of the value that could have been gained from the budgeting process.

AN ACTIVITY-BASED APPROACH TO BUDGETING

Activity-based budgeting is an approach that links primary and support processes for purposes of developing the budget. This differs from the traditional approach to budgeting. The traditional approach looks at what resources will be consumed instead of what caused resources to be consumed. Process identification looks at the flow of data within the organization from suppliers through eventual output to the customer. Activities are related to cost drivers. Cost drivers could be volume-oriented, such as the number of visits an agency is anticipating performing during the upcoming year or the number of patients (by patient problem) that it will have on service.

Figure 12–1 illustrates the flow of data through an agency. Employees, contractors, supply vendors, and other suppliers provide the resources that will be used by the processes within the agency in providing patient care to the customer. Processes will also address other customers of the agency. As discussed in Chapters 8 and 9, there are multiple processes and activities that take place within an agency. Figure 12–1 simplifies these processes into two major categories: (1) primary customer-oriented activities and (2) support activities. Understanding the cost of activities provides management with a tool to manage the process; therefore, budgeting by activities and processes provides an internal benchmarking system that is consistent with how costs are recorded.

This process is more holistic than the traditional financial approaches to financial reporting and budgeting. It honors the entire organization by developing performance measures that look at overall agency performance from four different perspectives simultaneously. These four indicators were developed by Robert Kaplan of Harvard University. They include measures that evaluate (1) financial performance, (2) customer satisfaction, (3) internal operations, and (4) innovation and improvement.

The budget is then built based on the anticipated activities and processes that will take place within the agency. Activity cost is accumulated within major processes and assigned to the operational units that consume the resources. Utilization of this approach provides several benefits for the management of an HHA.[1] First, costs are assigned based on who benefited by their consumption not because of an arbitrary allocation. This simple benefit has the impact of reducing the potential for organizational friction, which is typically part of the budgeting process.

Budgeting by activities provides managers with a tool that is more comprehensive than traditional budgeting methods, improves the quality of management in-

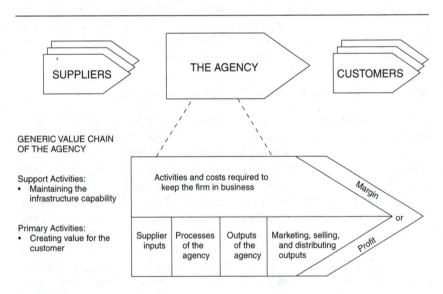

Figure 12–1 Interrelatedness between Support and Primary Activities in the Value Chain. Source: Reprinted with permission from *Emerging Practices in Cost Management: Activity-Based Management* by B.J. Brinker, p. D6-4, © 1994, Warren, Gorham & Lamont, 31 St. James Avenue, Boston, MA 02116. All rights reserved.

formation, and provides managers with a methodology for managing process improvement in an activity-based costing environment. The assignment of costs to internal customers is then based on their needs, thus forcing support departments to become as efficient as possible. Additionally, activities can then be linked to internal and external performance measures. Identification of performance measures allows managers to structure the processes within an agency for the purposes of achieving maximum customer value, improving organizational performance, and achieving organizational objectives.

The difference in traditional budgeting versus activity-based budgeting is illustrated by Figure 12–2. Figure 12–2 is an activity-based budgeting system that provides a closed loop. The closed loop looks at how resources are used by agency processes, identifies whether those processes achieved their output objectives or performance targets, and then evaluates how the process can be improved. Conversely, the traditional budget process identifies how much money was spent in relation to how much was budgeted to be spent. Therefore, management's ability to control outcomes and processes is enhanced with the implementation of activity-based costing and budgeting processes.

THE TRADITIONAL BUDGETING PROCESS

The budgeting process usually starts several months before the end of the fiscal year. Usually, a budget timeline is established and published to all budget participants. The timeline could look like the following:

1. Hold budget kick-off meeting.	October 15
2. Develop key objectives in relationship to the strategic plan.	October 22
3. Develop capital budget.	October 29
4. Develop revenue forecast.	November 5
5. Develop expense forecast.	November 12
6. Integrate capital, revenue, and expense budgets.	November 19
7. Develop cash forecast and evaluate in relationship to cost limits.	November 26
8. Review results and adjust.	December 10
9. Package final presentation including assumptions.	December 17
10. Obtain final approval and present to the board.	December 24
11. Incorporate into financial reporting.	

Budgeting processes can be long and drawn out. The process begins with an introductory budgeting meeting. It is during this meeting that organizational goals and

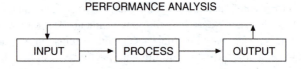

Figure 12–2 Understanding Process Flow Is the Key to Performance Analysis

objectives are identified and shared with all budget participants. This process may include creative techniques like brainstorming, visualization, and dream sharing. On the other hand, it could be coupled with a more traditional process such as SWOT (strengths, weaknesses, opportunities, and threats) analysis. Once the initial budget guidelines have been disseminated, participants are asked to follow the timeline for submission of information. Generally, the chief financial officer (CFO) and the chief operating officer (COO) have the majority of the work in the budgeting process.

The second meeting will identify departmental and operational objectives and strategies with respect to the mission and objectives identified in the first meeting. This is where anticipated volumes are estimated, fundraising activities identified, employee productivity and increases defined, departmental spending limitations reviewed, estimates for inflation identified, and departmental objectives outlined. This information is then used for departments to develop capital, revenue, and expense budgets. Budgets are then forwarded to the finance department, which integrates all of the raw data, develops a cash budget and balance sheet, and evaluates cost in relationship to the Medicare limits. Results are then reviewed and adjusted until management has a budget that it is willing to present to the chief executive officer (CEO), the board, or any other interested party.

Often, this process results in forcing the budget to approximate a bottom line. To arrive at an arbitrarily determined bottom line, managers will increase revenue streams or decrease costs. Often seasoned managers will backload revenue increases to provide time to achieve their estimates. Incentives often are based on performance measures that only consider one part of the entire operation. For example, incentives that are based solely on increases in revenue could ignore whether the new revenue stream is profitable to the agency. This is another reason activity-based budgeting makes sense.

The Capital Budget

The capital budget is a forecast of the agency's anticipated expenditures for assets that have a life greater than a year. Typically, capital budget items fall into the following categories: furniture, office equipment, building improvements, vehicles, land, buildings, and other. Purchases of assets are due to renovations, new program development, enhancement of the agency infrastructure, or equipment that has worn out and needs to be replaced.

Capital budgeting is important from a financial management perspective. Knowing when asset acquisitions are anticipated allows finance to determine the appropriate vehicle for acquiring the capital asset. Acquisition could be made by cash from operating funds, special purpose funds, or restricted funds. Assets could be acquired by a bank loan, leasing, or installment payments. The financing vehicle will depend on the type of asset being purchased, financing alternatives available from the vendor, and the agency's cash and financial position.

The capital budget will identify who has placed the request, a description of the asset to be acquired, justification, anticipated acquisition date, purchase cost, and any other relevant information. Additional justification could be performed by working with the finance team. Justification could be based on cost savings, additional revenue flows, opportunity cost, safety, or enhanced efficiency. Finance can then rank acquisitions based on organizational benefit. Acquisitions may need to be approved by the board of directors.

The Revenue Budget

The revenue budget is the anticipated annual revenue for the HHA. It is the aggregate of all service or product lines that are housed within the company. Typically, the revenue budget is built on a series of assumptions regarding the number of admissions, admissions by payor source, utilization, mix of visits, and supply cost. Obviously, the starting point is estimating the amount of referrals that the HHA will obtain from various referral sources. Referrals can be based on history, adjusted to reflect current trends, or increased for anticipated marketing efforts. For example, if the referral source is a hospital, and the hospital is closing down a wing or discontinuing a specialty, this may have a material impact on the number of referrals that the agency will receive. Other factors to consider regarding referral sources are when physicians take vacations, seasonal fluctuations for operations, seasonal fluctuations due to geographic considerations, holidays, and the development or discontinuance of existing programs.

Admission estimates will also be influenced by the type of strategies that an agency is pursuing. Volume estimates will need to be made for anticipated contracts that the agency may enter into with an MCO, large employer, or other third party. It will be necessary to know the timing, composition of patients, and patient requirements for completion of the budgeting process.

Estimating admissions is a two-step process. The first step is to identify the number of admissions by referral source taking into consideration some of the factors discussed above. The second step is to categorize referrals by payor source. Identification of admissions by payor source will provide management with a tool to evaluate profitability by payor source in relation to the budget, allow the budgeting process to incorporate changes that are taking place at the referral sources that will affect the composition of the HHA's payor sources, and enable the budget to calculate revenue by payor source.

Once admissions are known, it is possible to estimate an anticipated visit mix for each payor. Visit mix could be based on prior history, payor peculiarities, or changes in the HHA's approach to service provision. Visit mix can also be based on the composition of the patients received from a referral source, patient problems, and patient demographics. For example, a referral source that discharges patients with psychiatric needs will require more social services, whereas admissions for rehabilitation patients will require more physical therapy. Visit estimates may be constrained because of the inability to obtain physical therapists or transportation difficulties in inclement weather.

Visit estimates and admissions allow the agency to track its anticipated patient census for the entire year and utilization by payor mix. Patient census, admissions, and discharges are the drivers for other agency support costs. Estimating utilization helps to quantify that visit estimates are consistent with the patient admission estimates. If the agency is adopting a policy of service delivery efficiency, then the utilization statistic by payor should exhibit a downward trend. From a capitated contract perspective, it is beneficial to track the number of covered lives on a monthly basis, estimated admission utilization percentage, admissions, and service utilization once admitted.

Total visit volume by payor provides the base for determining gross revenues, contractual allowances, discounts, and net reimbursement. The above process is completed for each service line within the agency. Other service lines could include hospice, infusion therapies, resale supplies, and private duty. Each service line develops a patient referral base and specialized indicators such as number of days on service, type of supply, type of infusion therapy, or hours of private duty by discipline or type. Once the patient base has been developed by service line, it is possible to develop volume estimates, massage the data to reflect prior trends or new developments, and summarize by payor. These data will then provide the base for identification of the revenue budget, cost of service, and many of the support functions. It is important to quantify assumptions so that estimates have meaning.

The development of a payor table provides a vehicle to convert volume estimates into revenue forecasts. A payor table identifies gross and net payments by type of service and depend on payor specifics. Gross revenue is calculated by extending total visit volume by the HHA's charges on a discipline basis. Gross revenue is the aggregate of the total discipline cost. Calculation of net revenue, discounts, and contractual allowances depends on the payor. It depends on payor payment policies and contractual relationships.

Some payors will pay on a per visit basis, some will discount charges, some will pay based on an episode of care or a per member per month arrangement, and others will be cost-reimbursed. The construction of the payor table depends on how the agency will be paid for services. Cost-reimbursed payors like Medicare do not require identification of a net rate by discipline. Instead, one rate could be used based on aggregate costs. This rate would be calculated once all costs and volume are known. The balance of the payors would have specified rates. Rates could be specific by discipline or based on an episode of care. Episodic rates would need to be identified and linked back to patient admission estimates. Identification of gross charges in relationship to episodic payments identifies how much the agency is discounting its services. Capitated payments are an extension of the negotiated per member per month rate by the number of covered lives. Identification of gross charges for capitated contracts identifies how much the agency is discounting its services. Contractual allowances are the difference between gross charges and net revenue.

The agency may offer discounts to payors based on visit volume. If this is the case, then discounts will need to be included in the formula. Discount calculation could be based on the number of referrals, the volume of services, or aggregate charges. The difference between the negotiated rate without a discount and the discounted rate is the amount of discount. This is summarized to identify the total amount of discounts by payor for the budgeting period.

Expense Budget

Once volume estimates have been established, it is possible to build the expense budget. The expense budget is composed of direct patient care or cost of service, support costs and activities, and facility costs. Some expenses are directly identifiable on a patient-specific basis and will fluctuate with volume. Other costs associated with patient care will fluctuate indirectly with volume. There will be many different cost drivers associated with these costs.

Development of direct cost of services begins with the estimated volume statistics. It requires understanding how the agency is choosing to provide services. An agency may choose to provide all services through employees. Another agency may choose to supplement its service provision through the use of subcontractors and staffing agencies. The mix of service provision is important because it can help to explain changes in cost of service. Cost of service can fluctuate because employees are not being used as productively as possible. This could be due to scheduling problems, geographic area, an abundance of meetings, or visit requirements. Any of these factors will cause more subcontracted services to be used, thus increasing cost of services.

The distinction is important for two reasons. First, the cost may be significantly different between employees and subcontracted staff. Employees have a lot of incremental costs associated with them. In addition to payroll taxes, health benefits, life insurance, and workers' compensation, there is professional liability insurance, continuing education, and paid holidays. The other reason is reimbursement for travel expenses. Employees are typically paid for travel costs, whereas subcontractors include it in their rates. Other costs that are identifiable at this level are the cost of escorts into high-risk areas and interpreters.

Cost of service identification begins by identifying cost on a discipline-by-discipline basis. Once aggregate cost of service has been calculated, use of the above payor mix ratios can be applied to the cost of service totals. This facilitates budgeting profitability by payor.

Cost of service for nursing would be the aggregate of employee costs and subcontract costs. The calculation of employee costs begins with identifying how many full- and part-time nurses are on staff. For ease of calculation, a full-time equivalent (FTE) is used. An FTE converts all part-time employees into full-time employees.

Table 12–1 identifies an estimated visit forecast. Nursing visits are estimated to be 35,000 annual visits, and the agency has 20 FTE nurses. The next step requires estimating the average number of visits that each FTE will be able to provide

---

Table 12–1 Cost of Service Calculation Based on Service Estimates

Visit projections	
Nursing	35,000
Physical therapy	12,000
Occupational therapy	3,000
Speech therapy	2,000
Medical social services	1,000
Home health aide	45,000
Total Visits	98,500
Estimated visits per RN FTE	1,200
Number of staff RN FTEs	20
Total staff visits	24,000
Budget calculation	
Projected nursing visits	35,000
Staff visits	24,000
Subcontract visits	11,000

during the course of the year. A productivity factor of 5 was used to arrive at 1,200 annual visits. This was calculated at 5 visits a day for 48 productive weeks. Extending this sum by the number of FTEs indicated that 11,000 visits would need to be subcontracted.

Total nursing cost can now be determined. The subcontracted portion would be 11,000 visits multiplied by a contractually determined rate. The employee cost would be salary plus benefits and other employee costs. Salary cost would either be a function of individual salaries, hourly rates, or per diem rates. If incentives or overtime are used as a method of increasing productivity and decreasing the amount of subcontracted work, then this needs to be factored into the equation. The cost of incentives and overtime will need to be included in the budget.

Benefit cost, payroll taxes, and workers' compensation can be determined once salaries are calculated. Benefit costs will depend on what the agency includes as benefits, what types of benefits are available to full- versus part-time staff, and any anticipated increases in benefit cost. Employer-related costs such as payroll taxes, unemployment insurance, and workers' compensation depend on the amount of gross payroll cost.

The above analysis would be calculated on a monthly basis to reflect cost of service correctly in relation to fluctuations in volume. Payroll taxes would be reflected when paid versus when the liability was incurred. The above analysis could be used to determine anticipated staffing levels and be linked to advertising expenditures, training costs, and replacement costs.

The above process would be completed for each discipline and service line. In addition to labor, supply cost would need to be estimated. Soft supply cost will depend on agency usage patterns. It could be calculated based on discipline visit volume by extending the number of visits by some historic factor. Analysis of supply cost may yield agency efficiencies.

Once labor and supplies have been calculated, it is time to address the balance of the costs associated with the direct provision of care. Travel expense has two types of cost associated with it. The first is travel time. Travel time is unproductive time from the agency's perspective, and the more travel time between visits, the less visits the employee will be able to perform. The second element is travel expense. Travel expense could be reimbursement for mileage, purchase of bus or train passes, taxi fares, or the cost of agency-owned automobiles. Travel cost will depend on the geographic area that is covered and how the agency chooses to address travel issues. Other issues related to travel are safety, automobile insurance, and flexibility.

In activity-based costing terms, the above section identified unit costs. Unit costs are identifiable for each unit of patient activity. The next element of the budgeting process is the identification of batch costs. These are support costs that are incurred from admission through discharge. These costs include intake, nursing supervision, case management, records management, quality improvement, scheduling, data entry, and billing.

Support costs would be aggregated on a departmental basis in the traditional budgeting process. Departmental operating cost and facility cost would also be included. Activity-based budgeting would then assign departmental resource cost to activities. Activities would then be assigned using activity drivers to cost objects. Cost objects could be teams, product lines, programs, or payors.

Budgeting of support department expenses would be based on activities and the needs of the customers who use their services, such as teams (Figure 12–3). During the development of the revenue budget, visit activity was identified by referral source. It is conceivable that each referral source has been assigned to a specific team. Therefore, volumes are associated with each team, revenues, and unit costs. Batch-level support costs can then be assigned to each team. Resource drivers (the mechanism that assigns resource cost to activities—time, admissions, patient census, etc.) are assigned to the activities that support each team's efforts. Activities can then be assigned to teams based on how many resources each team consumes. Exhibit 12–1 identifies possible activity cost that could be assigned to the teams.

Assignment of business-level cost would be made to the product line or program that benefits by its cost. This could be the cost of marketing, specialized recruitment, or interest. These costs should be identifiable based on the type of service provided, for example, marketing based on new contracts or referral sources, the number of new hires, or outstanding receivables by product line. Facility or enterprise cost would be assigned to each department prior to assignment at the team level.

Estimating expenses for the upcoming year is fairly straightforward. Budget estimates need to incorporate assumptions for pay increases, inflation, volume changes, strategic plans, and departmental and organizational objectives. Em-

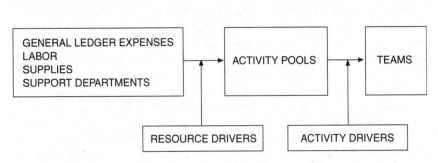
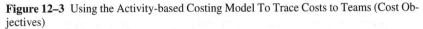

Figure 12–3 Using the Activity-based Costing Model To Trace Costs to Teams (Cost Objectives)

Exhibit 12–1 Possible Activity Pools

Hands-on patient care	Travel	Case management
Documentation	Case conferencing	Logistics coordination
Benefit verification	Insurance verification	Record filing
Record retrieval	Chart review	Billing
Collections	Claim investigation	Personnel recruitment
Employee training	Policies and procedures	Photocopying
Phone reception	development	Mail distribution
Order placement	Customer service	Vendor payment
Special projects	Financial reporting	Cash and credit management
Cost reporting	Customer surveys	Report creation
Field staff payroll	Customer meetings	Manual payroll
Tax reporting	Administrative staff payroll	Audits—fiscal intermediary
Audits—financial	Staff meetings	Facility management
Contract management	Budgeting	Training
	Disciplinary action	

ployee cost will need to be evaluated in relationship to anticipated volumes to determine whether support personnel requirements need to be increased. Other costs will fluctuate with volume or other factors, such as seasonality, anticipated changes to the organization's infrastructure, investment in new assets, organizational expansion or contraction, and special projects.

Linking resource cost to activities and then combining activities into major processes enables managers to evaluate whether these processes are of value to the HHA. Some refer to this process as *priority-based budgeting*.

> Priority based budgeting is a planning and budgeting tool which can constrain or reduce levels of budgeted expenditures quite dramatically and effectively, and in most cases with the full support of management. This is because they clearly see how equitable the process actually is. Its use is typically triggered by the recognition that there has been some unchecked "cost creep" in some of the more "traditional overhead" areas. It is particularly potent in challenging and prioritizing all the activities and costs which are claimed to be necessary for keeping the firm in business and maintaining the infrastructure and capability of the firm to carry out its work. The degree of challenge is most effectively encouraged by linking internal activities to the internal customers who are driving the need for the activities to be performed at a particular level of quality, timeliness and cost. When used together, activity based budgeting and priority based budgeting produce a cogent combination to ad-

dress the issue of what is the optimum level of resources the business needs to allocate to achieve its chosen business objectives.[2]

The Balance Sheet and Cashflow Budget

The balance sheet and the cashflow budget should be produced simultaneously. This ensures that the balance sheet, cashflow budget, and income statement are all in balance. It also helps to verify that assumptions are realistic. Basically, the cashflow budget is a summary of cash inflows and outflows, the income statement is a summary of revenue and expenses, and the capital budget identifies acquisitions and starting points for depreciation expense. When revenues and expenses are added to the ending balance sheet, the new balance sheet is extremely distorted. This is because revenue streams and payments have not been taken into consideration. Inclusions of cash inflows and outflows will determine proper ending balances for the balance sheet.

Cash inflows from revenue-producing activities such as the provision of patient services will depend on the payor. Some payors pay in 30 days, others in 120. This will affect cash inflows. Cash outflows will depend on the agency policy for payment of employees, vendors, and acquisition of assets. Creditors such as banks, leasing companies, and vendors who have the ability to charge high interest rates dictate when payments will be made. The net difference between cash inflows and outflows identifies the agency's working capital requirements. Interest cost can be calculated based on outstanding loan balances plus or minus working capital draws.

Calculation of Cost Reimbursement Rates

Once the expense budget has been updated for interest, depreciation, amortization, and local taxes, the cost-reimbursed rate can be calculated and added to the revenue budget. Unlike prospective payors, cost-reimbursed payors require that all expenses be known and adjusted for costs that are nonallowable. Nonallowable costs would include advertising for the purposes of patient solicitation, the difference between accelerated depreciation and straight-line depreciation, and interest expense due to the owner.

Costs would be pumped through a cost report model to arrive at an interim rate. The interim rate would then be used for purposes of the annual rate to be used for the upcoming year. Quarterly PIP reports should also be calculated if the agency is a PIP provider. This is necessary to determine the effect changes in volume will have on cash flow. Increases in visit volume will cause the agency to experience cash shortages, thus causing a lump-sum adjustment in the subsequent quarter.

Decreases in visit volume will cause the agency to be overpaid, thus creating an overpayment liability. In either case, the agency needs to plan accordingly.

Adjustments, Approval, and Integration into Financial Reporting

Once the initial budget has been developed, it is time to circulate and review the budget in relationship to the organizational objectives that were determined at the beginning of the process. This may be accomplished by circulating the initial budget to the contributing members of the agency, for the review of senior management only, or by conducting other analysis. Other analysis could include comparing the initial budget to current year operations, historical trends, or some other indicator. Once changes have been integrated, and the budget has been approved, it is time to circulate the budget. The budget package will include a breakdown of all assumptions, summary statements, and detailed monthly statements. Everyone who has accountability for results or contributed to the process should receive a copy.

Monthly operations can then be compared to plan. Explanation of variance is everyone's responsibility and can be accomplished through several different methods. Ideally, this process should be completed before financial statements are submitted to senior management. Variance analysis can be formalized as part of a monthly presentation or done in a report format.

Regardless of what approach is used, variance analysis should identify favorable and unfavorable variances. Variances are typically composed of a volume and an efficiency element. Table 12–2 illustrates several variances for the current month's operations. Variances would be explained for both the current and year-to-date periods.

Tables 12–2 and 12–3 are two different statement formats that can be used as part of the financial statement evaluation process. Table 12–3 displays actual and budget results in a current period and year-to-date format. Table 12–2 includes percentages. Percentages numerically quantify the amount of the budget variance. The percentage change is calculated by taking the variance and dividing it by the budgeted amount. Income variances are calculated by subtracting plan from actual. Expense variances are calculated by subtracting actual from plan. The reason for changing the sequence is to have positive variances and negative variances. A positive revenue variance would be an increase of revenue over plan. A positive expense variance would be to have less expense than originally anticipated.

Financial statement presentation depends on who will be receiving the financial statements. Generally, board members, bankers, and executives like to see summarized statements. Others like to see very detailed statements. Very detailed statements would identify patient service revenue by discipline and segregate costs by payor. Support services would also include much more detail. This can be

Table 12–2 Comparative Statement of Revenue and Expenses: Format A

Sample Home Health Agency
Statements of Revenue and Expenses and Changes in Fund Balance
As of April 30, 1995

	April	Plan	Current month		Year to date	
			Variance	% Change	Variance	% Change
Net patient service revenue	$552,320	$540,000	$12,320	2.28	$ 25,235	1.18
Other revenue	1,000	3,000	(2,000)	-66.67	(1,000)	-8.33
Total revenue	553,320	543,000	10,320	1.90	24,235	1.13
Expenses						
Professional care of patients	370,150	366,375	(3,775)	-1.03	(19,525)	-1.36
General and administrative	142,000	140,625	(1,375)	-0.98	(7,351)	-1.35
Occupancy	12,100	12,150	50	0.41	(300)	-0.62
Provision for bad debts	6,350	6,210	(140)	-2.25	(1,500)	-6.52
Depreciation	2,835	2,835		0.00	0.00	0.00
Interest	2,300	2,160	(140)	-6.48	(125)	-1.39
Total expenses	535,735	530,355	(5,380)	-1.01	(28,801)	-1.39
Income from operations	17,585	12,645	4,940	39.07	(4,566)	-6.15
Nonoperating gains						
Contributions						
Investment income	300	450	(150)	-33.33	(200)	-11.11
Total nonoperating gains	300	450	(150)	-33.33	(200)	-11.11
Revenue and gains in excess of expenses	17,885	13,095	4,790	36.58	(4,766)	-6.27
Fund balance—beginning	203,409	212,965	(9,556)	-4.49	(9,556)	-6.37
Fund balance—ending	$221,294	$226,060	$(4,766)	-2.11	$ (4,766)	-2.11

Table 12-3 Comparative Statement of Revenue and Expenses: Format B

Statements of Revenue and Expenses and Changes in Fund Balance
As of April 30, 1995

	April	Plan	Variance		April	Plan	Variance
Net patient service revenue	$552,320	$540,000	$12,320		$2,160,235	$2,135,000	$ 25,235
Other revenue	1,000	3,000	(2,000)		11,000	12,000	(1,000)
Total revenue	553,320	543,000	10,320		2,171,235	2,147,000	24,235
Expenses							
Professional care of patients	370,150	366,375	(3,775)		1,455,325	1,435,800	(19,525)
General and administrative	142,000	140,625	(1,375)		552,351	545,000	(7,351)
Occupancy	12,100	12,150	50		48,900	48,600	(300)
Provision for bad debts	6,350	6,210	(140)		24,500	23,000	(1,500)
Depreciation	2,835	2,835			11,340	11,340	
Interest	2,300	2,160	(140)		9,125	9,000	(125)
Total expenses	535,735	530,355	(5,380)		2,101,541	2,072,740	(28,801)
Income from operations	17,585	12,645	4,940		69,694	74,260	(4,566)
Nonoperating gains							
Contributions							
Investment income	300	450	(150)		1,600	1,800	(200)
Total nonoperating gains	300	450	(150)		1,600	1,800	(200)
Revenue and gains in excess of expenses	17,885	13,095	4,790		71,294	76,060	(4,766)
Fund balance—beginning	203,409	212,965	(9,556)		150,000	150,000	
Fund balance—ending	$221,294	$226,060	$(4,766)		$ 221,294	$ 226,060	$ (4,766)

accomplished using the statements shown in Tables 12–2 and 12–3 and providing supplemental schedules for those individuals who like to see more detail. However, supplemental schedules by themselves will require an explanation, thus requiring a variance analysis.

Variances should be explained from both a volume and efficiency perspective. Both statements indicate a $12,320 positive revenue variance. This is the result of increased volume and a deterioration of the average charge. This is illustrated by Table 12–2. Table 12–2 illustrates the calculation of both volume and rate variances. Volume is the difference in total visits for the period extended by the budgeted revenue. Visits grew by 205 for the current period, or 2.7 percent. Unfortunately, the growth in visits was to a payor group that skewed the average rate downward by $0.32. The decline would then be explained because of changes in payors, visit mix, or referral patterns. Table 12–4 is an example of a volume and efficiency analysis format for revenue.

The same technique could be used to explain differences in the cost of patient care. The increase of 205 visits should have caused a negative variance of $10,014. The actual variance was $6,241 less because of efficiencies in the average cost of service. The efficiency variance would need to be investigated and explained. Some of the causes may be a result of factors discovered in the revenue variance, such as a change in the visit mix. Other factors could be due to higher employee productivity, less travel expense, or an adjustment of some sort. All of these factors would be spelled out. Table 12–5 is an example of a volume and efficiency analysis for cost of service.

Ultimately, the purpose of variance analysis is to meet the needs of the consumers of the financial statements. Variance analysis is similar to the budgeting proc-

Table 12–4 Revenue Variance Analysis Using Volume and Efficiency Measures

	Volume	Rate ($)	Total ($)
Volume			
Actual	7,705	72.00	$554,760
Plan	7,500	72.00	540,000
Volume variance			14,760
	Actual rate ($)	Plan rate ($)	
Efficiency			
Actual volume			7,705
Rate	71.68	72.00	(0.32)
Efficiency variance			(2,466)
Revenue variance			$12,294

Table 12–5 Patient Care Variance Analysis Using Volume and Efficiency

	Volume	Rate ($)	Total
Volume			
Actual	7,705	48.85	$376,389
Plan	7,500	48.85	366,375
Volume variance			(10,014)

	Actual rate ($)	Plan rate ($)	
Efficiency			
Actual volume			7,705
Rate	48.04	48.85	0.81
Efficiency variance			6,241
Cost of service variance			$(3,773)

ess and the production of financial statements. They are time-consuming processes. Internal consumers must be clear that this is the process and format that yield the best return from a management and cost perspective.

OTHER TYPES OF ANALYTICAL PRESENTATIONS

Often, accountants use various supplemental schedules and statement formats to illustrate changes that are occurring. Table 12–6 is a trend analysis. A trend analysis displays the results of similar periods of time side by side. Similar periods are usually monthly or annual results. Trend analysis allows users to identify balances that are uncharacteristic with respect to previous results.

Table 12–7 is referred to as a *common size financial statement*. The common size financial statement begins with the assumption that net revenue is equal to a dollar. All costs are calculated in relationship to this base. Therefore, it provides the user with a vehicle to explain expenditures in relationship to a unit of measure that everyone understands, the dollar.

Table 12–8 is a per visit financial statement. This statement restates revenue and expenses on an average per visit basis. This statement has more value when per visit cost is separated by payor and product line.

The Rolling Budget

The rolling budget is an advanced budgeting tool. The rolling budget requires that every month the annual budget be updated for current changes. This process causes the budget to become a "living" document that currently reflects all known opportunities and challenges. The rolling budget enables management to be in-

Table 12–6 Trend Analysis

Statements of Revenue and Expenses and Changes in Fund Balance
As of April 30, 1995

	Jan	Feb	Mar	Apr	YTD
Net patient service revenue	526,329	541,097	540,489	552,320	2,160,235
Other revenue	3,000	3,000	4,000	1,000	11,000
Total revenue	529,329	544,097	544,489	553,320	2,171,235
Expenses					
Professional care of patients	350,924	367,876	366,375	370,150	1,455,325
General and administrative	135,826	133,702	140,823	142,000	552,351
Occupancy	12,150	12,500	12,150	12,100	48,900
Provision for bad debts	5,900	6,125	6,125	6,350	24,500
Depreciation	2,835	2,835	2,835	2,835	11,340
Interest	2,220	2,250	2,355	2,300	9,125
Total expenses	509,855	525,288	530,663	535,735	2,101,541
Income from operations	19,474	18,809	13,826	17,585	69,694
Nonoperating gains					
Contributions					
Investment income	450	400	450	300	1,600
Total nonoperating gains	450	400	450	300	1,600
Revenue and gains in excess of expenses	19,924	19,209	14,276	17,885	71,294
Fund balance—beginning	150,000	169,924	189,133	203,409	150,000
Fund balance—ending	169,924	189,133	203,409	221,294	221,294

formed constantly of how internal and external changes are influencing the agency's operational results. The other benefit is that the rolling budget forces managers to link strategies to operational budgets because now the variance analysis process includes revision of estimates for the next 12 months to be consistent with current results and future plans. This process is superior to revising the budget after 4 or 6 months of operations to reflect current results because it does not allow as much time to elapse before corrective action can be taken.

RATIO ANALYSIS

Ratio analysis adds another level of understanding to the results of operation. Ratios enable the user to draw conclusions about the financial results that would not be available by looking only at ending balances. "Financial ratios are not another attempt by financial specialists to confuse and confound decision makers. Financial ratios have been empirically tested to determine their value in predicting

Table 12–7 Common Size Statement

Statements of Revenue and Expenses and Changes in Fund Balance
As of April 30, 1995

	Jan	Feb	Mar	Apr	YTD
Net patient service revenue	0.994	0.994	0.993	0.998	0.995
Other revenue	0.006	0.006	0.007	0.002	0.005
Total revenue	1.000	1.000	1.000	1.000	1.000
Expenses					
Professional care of patients	0.663	0.676	0.674	0.669	0.670
General and administrative	0.257	0.246	0.259	0.257	0.254
Occupancy	0.023	0.023	0.022	0.022	0.023
Provision for bad debts	0.011	0.011	0.011	0.011	0.011
Depreciation	0.005	0.005	0.005	0.005	0.005
Interest	0.004	0.004	0.004	0.004	0.004
Total expenses	0.963	0.965	0.975	0.968	0.968
Income from operations	0.037	0.035	0.025	0.032	0.032
Nonoperating gains Contributions					
Investment income	0.001	0.001	0.001	0.001	0.001
Total nonoperating gains	0.001	0.001	0.001	0.001	0.001
Revenue and gains in excess of expenses	0.038	0.035	0.026	0.032	0.033
Fund balance—beginnning	—	—	—	—	—
Fund balance—ending	═	═	═	═	═

Table 12–8 Per Visit Trend Analysis by Profit and Loss Category

Statements of Revenue and Expenses and Changes in Fund Balance
As of April 30, 1995

	Jan	Feb	Mar	Apr	YTD
Net patient service revenue	$73.10	$72.63	$71.07	$71.68	$72.10
Other revenue					
Total revenue	73.10	72.63	71.07	71.68	72.10
Expenses					
Professional care of patients	48.74	49.38	48.17	48.04	48.58
General and administrative	18.86	17.95	18.52	18.43	18.44
Occupancy	1.69	1.68	1.60	1.57	1.63
Provision for bad debts	0.82	0.82	0.81	0.82	0.82
Depreciation	0.39	0.38	0.37	0.37	0.38
Interest	0.31	0.30	0.31	0.30	0.30
Total expenses	70.81	70.51	69.78	69.53	70.14
Income from operations	$ 2.29	$ 2.12	$ 1.29	$ 2.15	$ 1.96
Visits	7,200	7,450	7,605	7,705	29,960

business failure. The results to date have been quite impressive: financial ratios can, in fact, discern potential problems in financial condition even five years in advance of their emergence."[3]

Ratio analysis is enhanced when results are reported consistently and ratios can be compared against an industry standard. Consistent reporting can be controlled internally. Industry standards are nonexistent. This is because of several factors that include the lack of uniform reporting, no central collection agency for proprietary results, and inconsistencies caused by cost reporting.

Financial ratios can be classified into four major categories: (1) liquidity, (2) activity, (3) profitability, and (4) capital structure. *Liquidity* is a term that is used to measure the agency's ability to meet its short-term obligations (payroll, vendors, and creditors). Liquidity is cash or how quickly assets can be converted into cash. Receivables that are collected provide the agency with a source of cash; those that are not collected use cash because now the agency has to find alternate sources to pay vendors, employees, and creditors. The following ratio calculations are based on Tables 12–10 and 12–11.

Liquidity Ratios

There are several ratios that can be used to monitor liquidity. The current ratio assesses the HHA's working capital requirements. Working capital is current assets less current liabilities. The current asset ratio is an indicator of the agency's ability to meet its short-term obligations. Typically, a ratio of 2.00 is considered a standard for most businesses. The calculation of the current ratio is shown below. The *current ratio* is showing that there has been an improvement in liquidity over the previous year:

	1995		1994	
Current assets	965,000		641,000	
	———	1.49	———	1.33
Current liabilities	647,000		483,000	

The *acid test ratio* eliminates prepaid expenses, inventory, and other receivables from the calculation. The concept is that prepaid expenses and inventory will take longer to convert to cash than accounts receivable and marketable securities; therefore, it is a better indicator than the current ratio. In this example, there has been improvement over the previous year. Additionally, the acid test indicates a weaker liquidity position than the current ratio:

	1995		1994	
Cash + investments + accts receivable	938,000		619,000	
	———	1.45	———	1.28
Current liabilities	647,000		483,000	

The *days in patient accounts receivable* is a ratio that evaluates one element of the working capital ratio, accounts receivable. Accounts receivable makes up the largest portion of an HHA's current assets; therefore, it becomes an excellent indicator of potential liquidity problems. The ratio shown below indicates that the days in accounts receivable have grown. This could be due to a change in payor mix, billing problems, or poor collection efforts. The increase in accounts receivable of 3.25 days over the previous year aging accounts for almost $36,000 in additional working capital requirements. This is demonstrated by the efficiency analysis illustrated in Table 12–9.

	1995		1994	
Net accounts receivable	752,000		476,000	
————————————	————	67.91	————	64.66
Net revenue/365	11,074		7,362	

The *average payment ratio* identifies on average how much is being paid out on a daily basis. Ratio results indicate that the average payment days have decreased. This indicates that there has been a change in payment policies, and the agency is using more cash than the previous year. The combination of decreasing payment days and increasing accounts receivable indicates that the HHA increased its cash requirements over the previous year. Since long-term borrowing went down, funds were available as a result of increased profits.

	1995		1994	
Current liabilities	647,000		483,000	
————————————————	————	60.43	————	66.96
(Operating expenses – depreciation)/365	10,707		7,214	

Table 12–9 Accounts Receivable Efficiency Analysis

	1995	1994	Variance
Net receivables	752,000	476,000	276,000
Net revenue/365	11,074	7,362	3,712
Days in patient accounts receivable			64.66
Variance due to volume			240,018
Days in patient accounts receivable	67.91	64.66	3.25
			11,074
Collection efficiency			35,991
Total variance			276,008

Activity Ratios

Activity ratios measure how well the agency manages its resources. These ratios are commonly referred to as *turnover ratios* because they provide an indicator of resource efficiency. The asset turnover ratio is exhibiting a positive trend. This ratio indicates that management utilized its assets more efficiently than in the previous year. "A high value for this ratio implies that the entity's total investment is being used efficiently; that is, a large number of services is being provided to the community from a limited resource base."[4]

	1995		*1994*	
Net patient revenue + other revenue + net nonoperating gains	4,106,000		2,746,000	
	———————	3.48	———————	3.22
Total assets	1,181,000		853,000	

The *fixed asset turnover ratio* is a subset of the asset turnover ratio. It measures how well management is using the agency's assets. The trend indicates a positive use of HHA assets:

	1995		*1994*	
Net patient revenue + other revenue + net nonoperating gains	4,106,000		2,746,000	
	———————	67.31	———————	52.81
Net fixed assets	61,000		52,000	

The *working capital turnover ratio* is another indicator of how well management is using HHA resources. Ratio results indicate a downward trend. This is consistent with the increase in the days in patient accounts receivable and the decrease in average payment days. Management could enhance its cash management techniques.

	1995		*1994*	
Net patient revenue	4,042,000		2,687,000	
	———————	12.71	———————	17.01
Working capital	318,000		158,000	

Profitability Ratios

Profitability ratios are indicators of the HHA's health and its ability to meet its financial obligations. These ratios help to identify trends that are caused by changing payor mixes, shifting funding sources, or run-away operating expenses. *Return on equity* indicates a positive trend between years.

"For health care firms without access to donor-restricted funds, government tax support, or other sources of new equity, asset growth will be limited to return on equity. This principle is referred to as 'sustainable growth.' The principle simply says that a firm cannot generate a growth rate in assets greater than its growth rate in equity for a prolonged period of time. If a firm can generate a return on equity of only 5 percent per year, its new growth in asset investment will be limited to 5 percent per year."[5]

	1995		1994	
Excess of revenues over expenses	177,000		98,000	
	———	0.41	———	0.39
Fund balance	429,000		252,000	

The *return on assets* is similar to the return on total asset ratio. It measures how well management is utilizing its resources.

	1995		1994	
Excess of revenues over expenses	177,000		98,000	
	———	0.15	———	0.11
Assets	1,181,000		853,000	

The *total margin ratio* is an indicator of what percentage of total revenues is being retained by the HHA. This ratio can be broken down into components to look at the portion that is attributable to operations versus nonoperating revenues.

	1995		1994	
Excess of revenues over expenses	177,000		98,000	
	———	0.04	———	0.04
Net patient revenue + other revenue + net nonoperating gains	4,106,000		2,746,000	

Capital Structure

These ratios are typically referred to as *leverage ratios*. They indicate how the agency has funded the growth in assets. The equity financing ratio indicates the portion of the assets that were purchased with equity. The long-term debt to equity ratio identifies the portion of debt used to purchase assets. Both ratios indicate a positive trend.

Higher values for the equity financing ratio and lower values of the long-term debt to equity ratio are indicators of positive financial health. "After all, if an entity had zero debt or a fund balance to total assets ratio of 1.0, there would not be any possible claimants on the entity's assets and thus no fear of bankruptcy or insolvency. The ratio indicates the percentage of total assets that has been financed with sources other than debt."[6]

Equity financing ratio

	1995		1994	
Fund balance	429,000		252,000	
	———	0.36	———	0.30
Total assets	1,181,000		853,000	

Long-term debt to equity ratio

	1995		1994	
Long-term debt	105,000		118,000	
———————	———	0.09	———	0.14
Total assets	1,181,000		853,000	

Times interest earned is an indicator of how well earnings are exceeding interest expense. A higher ratio indicates stronger ability to carry debt.

Even though a firm has a very low percentage of debt financing, it may not be able to carry additional debt because its profitability cannot meet the increased interest payment. Repayment of interest expense is a very important consideration in long-term financing. Failure to meet interest payment requirements on a timely basis could result in the entire principal value of the loan's becoming due. Meeting the fixed annual interest expense obligations is thus highly critical to solvency. The time interest earned ratio measures the extent to which earnings could slip and still not impair the entity's ability to repay its interest obligations. High values are obviously preferable.[7]

	1995		1994	
Excess of revenues over expenses + interest expense	193,000		117,000	
———————————————	———	12.06	———	6.16
Interest expense	16,000		19,000	

Debt service coverage expands on the previous ratio by including the principal portion of debt to determine how many times debt service can be covered by operating and nonoperating income. Depreciation is added back because it is a noncash outlay. "A standard minimum debt service coverage ratio value used by investment bankers in the hospital industry is 1.5."[8]

	1995		1994	
Excess of revenues over expenses + interest expense + depreciation	214,000		132,000	
———————————————	———	7.38	———	6.95
Principal payments + interest expense	29,000		19,000	

"The *cash flow to debt ratio* has been found to be an excellent predictor of financial failure, even as much as five years in advance of such failure. The numerator (cash flow) can be thought of as the firm's source of total funds, excluding financing. The denominator (total debt) provides a measure of a major need for future funds, namely, debt retirement. A low value for this ratio often indicates a potential problem in meeting future debt requirements."[9]

	1995		1994	
Excess of revenues over expenses + depreciation	198,000	0.26	113,000	0.19
Current liabilities + long-term debt	752,000		601,000	

Ratios, when used independently, can be confusing. Ratios used in conjunction with other ratios and consistently applied can provide management with a valuable tool to monitor home health operations.

MODELING

The budgeting process and any unique project analysis follow the general flow of input, calculations, and output. Every analysis requires defining a desired outcome. In the case of the budget, the outcome was a forecast of what the next year's operation will look like given the current operating environment and the assumptions that were built into the budgeting model. Unique analysis requires understanding what is the desired outcome of the modeling exercise. Outcomes could include determining whether to lease or buy an asset, purchase a building, bid on a managed care contract, start a new product line, or simply conduct a sensitivity analysis to determine current risks.

Figure 12–4 identifies inputs into the modeling process. The level of inputs will depend on the type of analysis, desired outcomes, and the level of modeling sophistication at the disposal of management. Factors that determine the level of input complexity will be the analysis timeframe (weekly, monthly, quarterly, or annually), the number of periods within each timeframe, the range of services offered by the agency, reimbursement structure (cost reimbursed, episodic, or capitated), the complexity of service delivery (bundled services), and the internal organizational structure (different pay rates, multiple programs, multiple companies, intercompany sales, and home office transactions).

Financial models should integrate investment, operating, and financing assumptions.[10] Investment assumptions include the rate of earnings on investments, amount and timing of capital expenditures (routine and projected), and depreciation calculations. Operating assumptions include inflation, changes in service utilization and volume, business risk, and intercompany transactions and transfer pricing. Financing assumptions identify the composition of debt (term notes, credit lines, bonds, and leases), timing of debt increases and decreases, equity funding, and working capital requirements and management practices (payment days and outstanding accounts receivable).

The calculation section will depend on whether the model is being constructed manually, on a PC spreadsheet like Lotus or Excel, or as part of a specialized

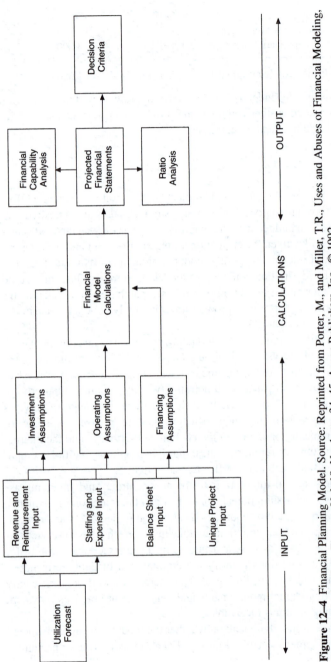

Figure 12–4 Financial Planning Model. Source: Reprinted from Porter, M., and Miller, T.R., Uses and Abuses of Financial Modeling, *Topics in Health Care Finance,* Vol. 19, No. 1, pp. 34–45, Aspen Publishers, Inc., © 1992.

Table 12–10 Comparative Balance Sheet

Sample Home Health Agency
Balance Sheets
December 31, 1995 and 1994

	1995	1994
Assets		
Current assets		
Cash and cash equivalents	$74,000	$41,000
Investments	112,000	102,000
Accounts receivable net		
of estimated uncollectibles of		
$61,000 in 1995 and $30,000 in 1994	752,000	476,000
Other receivables	27,000	22,000
Total current assets	965,000	641,000
Assets whose use is limited		
Cash	35,000	35,000
Bank certificates of deposit	100,000	100,000
	135,000	135,000
Equipment		
Medical & office equipment	56,000	39,000
Vehicles	50,000	37,000
	106,000	76,000
Less accumulated depreciation	(45,000)	(24,000)
Net equipment	61,000	52,000
Deferred finance charges,		
net of accumulated amortization of		
$15,000 in 1995 and $10,000 in 1994	20,000	25,000
	$1,181,000	$853,000
Liabilities and fund balances		
Current Liabilities		
Current maturities of long-term debt	$13,000	$13,000
Accounts payable	40,000	21,000
Accrued payroll and vacation costs	496,000	352,000
Estimated third-party payor settlements	28,000	31,000
Advances from third-party payors	70,000	66,000
Total current liabilities	647,000	483,000
Long-term debt less current maturities	105,000	118,000
Fund balance	429,000	252,000
	$1,181,000	$853,000

Table 12–11 Comparative Cash Flow

Sample Home Health Agency
Statements of Revenue and Expenses and Changes in Fund Balance
December 31, 1995 and 1994

	19X5	19X4
Net patient service revenue	4,042,000	2,687,000
Other revenue	27,000	32,000
Total revenue	4,069,000	2,719,000
Expenses		
Professional care of patients	2,714,000	1,835,000
General and administrative	1,042,000	675,000
Occupancy	90,000	83,000
Provision for bad debts	46,000	21,000
Depreciation	21,000	15,000
Interest	16,000	19,000
Total expenses	3,929,000	2,648,000
Income from operations	140,000	71,000
Nonoperating gains		
Contributions	19,000	15,000
Investment income	18,000	12,000
Total nonoperating gains	37,000	27,000
Revenue and gains in excess of expenses	177,000	98,000
Fund balance at beginning of year	252,000	154,000
Fund balance at end of year	429,000	252,000

modeling package. Data will need to be entered for purposes of the calculation or extracted from an existing database. Calculations are then based on parameters that are defined by the analyst. Calculations could use financial ratios, use relationships between fixed and variable expenses, or depend on prior events taking place.

Once the calculation is complete, the output should be in the form of pro-forma statements. Pro-forma statements allow the analyst to compare results and to fine-tune assumptions if necessary. "The process of constructing a financial model contributes significantly to a better understanding of how an organization functions. The interconnections of financial variables are particularly complex. If managers participate in the model development process, they will be forced to trace systematically through the various interrelated effects of their decisions. As a result managers should better comprehend the complex relationships that comprise their organization."[11]

CONCLUSION

The budget, variance analysis, performance measures, and ratios are tools that managers use to evaluate where the agency is in relationship to its stated goals and objectives. These tools provide a methodology to quantify results. Attempts should be made to integrate these tools prospectively into the management process; otherwise, if solely used in retrospective review processes, they tend to lose their power.

NOTES

1. B.J. Brinker, *Emerging Practices in Cost Management: Activity-Based Management* (Boston: Warren, Gorham & Lamont, 1994), D4-5.
2. *Ibid.*, D6-5.
3. W.O. Cleverly, *Essentials of Health Care Finance* (Gaithersburg, MD: Aspen Publishers, 1992), 134.
4. *Ibid.*, 146.
5. *Ibid.*, 153.
6. *Ibid.*, 142.
7. *Ibid.*, 144.
8. *Ibid.*, 145.
9. *Ibid.*, 145.
10. *Ibid.*
11. *Ibid.*

Part V

Financial Management Issues

Chapter 13

Human Resource Management

Individuals are the core element of a service business. Old models of personnel management subscribed to a belief that employees had to be supervised, tasks had to be reduced to the simplest possible task, and rigid policies and procedures had to be in place to keep employees in their place. Consequently, personnel management models developed layers of personnel, supervisors, managers, and executives. Whether this model was developed because it was a continuation of a military structure, "Theory X," or a bureaucratic structure that facilitated the building of fiefdoms is no longer important. What is important is the integration of a different philosophy into the management of human resources.

First, employees are a home health agency's (HHA's) assets. Human resources are not reflected on the traditional balance sheet but certainly contribute to the value of the organization. Without employees, a business does not exist. Employees bring value to an organization and, through their efforts, increase its value. Value is increased through individual growth, a willingness to work toward a collective goal, and a reward system that honors employees' contributions. Value can be measured by surveying customers, short- and long-term financial results, internal benchmarking and process improvement efforts, and the agency's willingness to learn and grow.

The new philosophy requires that employers make commitments to the employees they hire, and, in return, employees need to make commitments to their employers. This chapter looks at the development of an accounting department; discusses issues related to recruitment, training, and performance reviews; and concludes with issues related to human resource management.

THE ACCOUNTING AND FINANCE FUNCTION

The accounting and finance function is responsible for recording and reporting the results of operation; management of the processes related to cash, such as billing, collection of receivables, and payment of vendors and employees; and the credit function. Reporting functions include reporting to local, state, and federal taxing authorities, unions, fiscal intermediaries, benefit administrators, and others. In addition to the daily and monthly management of fiscal operations, the accounting and finance function interacts with internal customers in the development of forecasts, budgets, and special projects.

The members of the accounting department will have different levels of experience, training, accountability, and interaction with different customer groups. The accounting and finance department, hereafter referred to collectively as the accounting department, will consist of several primary positions. The number of positions will depend on the size of the agency, the amount of automation, and the complexity of the agency. Typically, the following positions exist and can be combined or expanded, can use different names, or can include other positions.

- Accounts payable
- Data entry or billing
- Bookkeeper or accountant
- Payroll
- Collections
- Controller or chief financial officer (CFO)

Each of these positions is responsible for different processes within the agency. Accounts payable is responsible for recording all agency liabilities; handling vendor inquiries and payment; and maintaining proper records of all payments, purchases, and adjustments. The volume of accounts payable activity will depend on the size of the agency, the amount of services being offered, organizational complexity, and the agency's approach to the utilization of temporary staffing agencies.

The payroll function is responsible for aggregating all time records, computing weekly or biweekly payrolls, and completing external payroll reporting requirements. The volume of payroll efforts will depend on the number of employees receiving checks, whether there are different payrolls for field staff versus administrative staff, data collection difficulties, and agency policies related to the issuance of manual checks. Payroll effort will also depend on who has responsibility for the tracking of paid time off, used and available health benefits, and other agency benefits.

The data entry or billing function is responsible for entry of activity into the agency's billing system. Activity data could be in the form of day sheets, tapes that need to be transcribed, or a combination of patient notes and other forms. The function is responsible for data entry, filing of support data, and the production and submission of bills to clients. Depending on the sophistication of the billing system, many tasks can be automated to enhance data retrieval and the billing process.

Collections personnel are responsible for responding to third-party inquiries, collecting delinquent accounts, and working with the billing personnel to reduce back-end collection problems. Other activities that may require additional personnel are the application of cash payments, credit verification, and reporting.

Accountants or bookkeepers have the responsibility of preparing financial statements, reconciling bank accounts, maintaining the general ledger, and preparing workpapers that support the financial statements. The volume of work will depend on the complexity of the agency, the degree of automation, and the other activities in which the accountant or bookkeeper may be involved. Smaller agencies may combine this position with an office management function, purchasing, or myriad other activities.

The controller or CFO has responsibility for the fiscal operations of the agency. This includes budgeting, financial and cost reporting, development of accounting policies and procedures, internal control functions, treasury functions, interaction with auditors or the board, and supervision of staff. The amount of effort required of this position will depend on the amount of support staff, the degree of automation, and how the chief executive officer (CEO) chooses to utilize this position. Some CEOs will create a position of CFO, but the position will basically be the head bookkeeper. Other CEOs will provide the space for the CFO to be part of the senior management team and a valuable contributor to the long-run success of the agency.

THE DEVELOPMENT OF AN ACCOUNTING TEAM

The development of a cohesive work group requires that every member of the accounting team understand his or her responsibilities in relationship to the efforts of the accounting department. This can be accomplished through meetings or having each employee document what his or her responsibilities are, what activities consume the day, and individual procedures. Concurrently, cross-training needs to occur.

Cross-training is an important vehicle for any department. Cross-training is having employees learn each other's jobs. This allows employees to take vacations and not come back to a desk full of work. More importantly, cross-training helps to educate department members on the responsibilities of the entire department. This way, if a problem needs to be handled, someone in the department will be able to handle it, and customer service is not impeded.

The development of a customer service orientation is another step in the development of a cohesive accounting department. Accounting is a support function and therefore supplies information to customers within and external to the agency.

The controller or CFO is responsible for educating staff on these concepts. Concepts that are critical are the identification of suppliers, customers, process input, processes, and process output.

One way to begin is by helping staff to identify internal and external customers. Each position will have a different subset of customers. Exhibit 13–1 identifies one of many potential internal and external customers by type of position as listed earlier. Customers' identification will lead to activity analysis. Activity analysis is composed of three parts: (1) input, (2) processes, and (3) output. The accounting department should attempt to identify individually, and as a group, how to evaluate and measure inputs, processes, and outputs.

Accounting activities historically have taken a back seat to operations. Therefore, to add more value to the accounting process, it will require tracing activities and processes upstream. As discussed in previous chapters, this will require help from other departments and teams. The development of teams that have cross-functional representation would enhance this process. An initial starting point, however, would be to ask other departments to sit in on accounting department meetings. These representatives could help with upstream activity identification and assist in beginning the process of activity streamlining.

Recruitment of Staff

Recruitment of qualified staff is a basic premise in the development of a strong accounting department. Recruitment efforts begin with determining what type of position is being recruited, what skills and education are required of that individual, and whether prior work experiences are essential for the successful candidate to succeed. Therefore, the recruiting process begins by defining what the job requirements consist of and what the ideal candidate will contribute and then determining whether the candidate's values are consistent with departmental and organizational values.

A recruitment process that hires from within will help to retain qualified staff and give employees an incentive to work at increasing their own contribution to the agency. Internal hiring practices are normally demonstrated by job postings that enable existing employees to be considered as potential applicants. If no internal applicant meets the posted job requirements, then an external job search can be initiated.

Recruitment efforts for someone to fill the accounts payable function will be much different from those to fill the CFO's position. Recruitment methods will also depend on where the agency is most likely to obtain qualified candidates. Recruitment for an accounts payable position could be accomplished by advertising in the local newspaper. Advertising in a local newspaper would produce responses from potential applicants who have a variety of experiences. Some of

Exhibit 13–1 Positions and Related Internal and External Customers

Position	Internal customer	External customer
Accounts payable	Nursing operations	Supply vendor
Payroll	Employee	Internal Revenue Service (IRS)
Data entry	Collections	Third-party payor
Collections	Controller	Factor
Accountant	Controller	Auditor
CFO	Accounting staff	Bank officer

these experiences may be transferable to the specific needs of the agency; others may not. If the agency is looking for someone with experience for a particular software package, then this should be stated in the advertisement to limit the amount of responses.

The search for a CFO would probably not use the local newspaper. This is because the skill set that an agency is looking for is of a specialized nature. Albeit, some of the skills are transferable from other industries; however, most CEOs want someone who will have prior home health experience, have very little transition time, and bring value to the operation. Recruitment for this type of position is usually through consultants, state or national home health associations, or advertisement in trade journals.

Advertisements soliciting responses should identify the type of position, experience and educational requirements, and a method for submitting resumes. Generally, enough information should be placed in the ad to enable potential candidates to determine whether they qualify for the position or whether the position appeals to them. Often the higher the position, the longer the job search will take. In some situations, the agency may choose to solicit the help of a recruitment agency to fill a position.

Recruitment agencies can help to expedite the hiring process by advertising, prescreening employees, and verifying references. This process is beneficial if time is of the essence or if qualified individuals are difficult to find. However, there is a cost associated with external recruiting firms. Fees are usually negotiable, partially refundable if the new hire does not live up to expectations, and dependent on the agency's relationship with the recruiter. Fees can range from 5 to 35 percent of the first-year salary and bonus.

Evaluation of Applicants

The first phase of the evaluative process is isolating prospective candidates from all of the responses. This can be accomplished by reviewing the submitted resumes. Resume review looks for several factors that will determine whether an interview should be arranged. The primary purpose is to determine whether applicants have applicable experience and training to meet job requirements. Candidates who have been in a highly specialized accounting function may not be able to make the transition to an accounting department that is composed of generalists. A person with a general accounting background in a different industry may be able to make the transition; however, there will be a learning curve due to terminology and the peculiarities of the home health care industry.

In addition to experience and training, stability is an important consideration when reviewing resumes. A person who changes jobs every couple of months may bring unwanted baggage to the accounting department or cause the recruitment process to be a never-ending process. Other considerations include prior salary history and responsibilities. A person who has been accustomed to supervising staff or earning more money than the position is paying may use the new position as a temporary assignment until he or she can find a job with a similar salary and responsibilities as previous positions.

The second phase of the evaluative process is to begin the interview process. The interview process should require the applicant to complete an employment application. Prospective applicants should complete information about themselves, educational experience if applicable to the job, and employment history. In addition to the employment application, the potential candidate should provide authorization to inquire about references. In addition to the employment application, the interviewer may want to develop questions related to the specific job. This technique enables the interviewer to obtain more information in advance, so that the interview can maximize the amount of information that is obtained. Additional questions could be developed regarding the handling of accounting transactions, the development of spreadsheet models using Lotus 1-2-3, or examples of how the candidate has handled certain situations in the past.

The interview process can be a two-stage process. The first stage would reduce the amount of potential applicants. The second stage would determine the applicant who has the desired experience, values consistent with the organization, and apparent best overall fit. Effective interviewers use open-ended questions and provide general information to encourage applicants to respond in detail to their questions. This can be accomplished by asking who, what, where, how, and why questions in response to statements, the applicants' resume, or their employment application. All interview results should be documented. Unsuccessful candidates should receive rejection letters. Successful candidates should receive acceptance letters.

Once hired, employees will need to become acclimated to their new position and company, complete appropriate paperwork like I-9s and W-4s, and familiarize themselves with company policies and benefits. The first several weeks will be spent learning existing processes and computer systems and meeting new people. Sometimes new employees are assigned a "buddy." The buddy will answer questions regarding how things work in the agency, offer assistance with organizational questions, and provide support with job-related questions. Selection of a buddy should be based on appropriateness and positive approach. The selection of buddies who have a negative approach or outlook could taint the new employees' views before they have had a chance to make their own assessment. Additionally, an informal accounting department luncheon is a way of introducing the new employees to their coworkers.

Training

Employees are recruited to the accounting department based on a set of skills and experiences that they have acquired preceding their employment at the agency. Their training and education needs to continue while they are employed at the agency. This is for several reasons. First, employers need to make a commitment to the employees they hire.

> Companies must shift from using and then harvesting employees to constantly renewing employees. Employees must feel valued, trusted, and respected members of the corporate community to be part of it. Both companies and employees are healthier if employees have multiple skills, if they can move easily across functional boundaries, if they are comfortable switching back and forth between regular duties and special projects. Additionally, all employees—not just bosses—must be much more aware that the purpose of the organization is to provide services that customers value, and that if the organization does not do that, nobody will have a job.[1]

Education and training are a way of providing employees value in addition to a timely paycheck and benefits. Education and training also provide a vehicle to keep employees challenged, motivated, and thinking about ways to improve agency processes. This last point is extremely critical in an environment that is measured by cost efficiency. The effects of managed care are forcing employees, departments, and agencies to become as efficient as possible. Efficiency is causing organizations and support departments to become flatter. At the same time, more employees may be asked for greater levels of output.

There are several ways that this can be accomplished, but a central theme still exists. That central theme is for all support departments, including accounting, to become as efficient as possible. So, by making a commitment to employee education, a win–win situation can occur. Employees increase their value through additional education, and the agency benefits by employees applying their new skills to their job. Additionally, "the processes employees use to think and the decisions they reach as a result of their thinking determine how they will proceed. If employees continually refine their thinking skills and hence sharpen their decision making capacity, the quality of what they do will be enhanced."[2]

Education and training are possible through external sources, such as colleges, technical schools, seminars, and workshops. Specialized accounting seminars can be obtained through state and national accounting associations. Training can also be brought in-house. This can be accomplished by purchasing videos that the entire department can watch, recruiting outside consultants, or sending one employee to a course or seminar and asking him or her to share the learning experience with the entire department.

Figure 13–1 demonstrates how this concept works. The employee or group of employees attends a workshop, seminar, or course. Prior to course approval, the employee and the manager codetermine course outcomes that they want to achieve. Outcomes could be to come back with specific skills, technical information, or some other benefit. Outcome identification would initially outline how the new information would be used in the employee's job or by the agency. This process would also identify how information would be disseminated. Initial benchmarks or evaluation points would also be determined.

Upon completion of the course, the employee follows the predetermined approach to disseminating information. If the workshop was payroll-related, the method of dissemination might be a memo attached to everyone's paycheck; if the course was related to collection techniques, then new approaches might be implemented. Courses would be evaluated for content in relation to desired outcome and benefit received. Depending on the type of course, it may require working with the material, returning to class, and then working with updated material. This approach would help employees gain maximum benefit from courses that are highly technical in nature.

An example would be software training. Software developers are creating very complex applications. Applications could be spreadsheet-oriented, like Lotus or Excel; database-oriented, like D-Base, Fox Pro, or Access; or the agency's unique information system. Often, when employees attend classes, they can only retain a limited amount of information before they get saturated. It is wise to have them implement their learning, integrate learning with the reading of manuals, share learning with coworkers, and then go back for additional training. The second training will build on an existing base, and more advanced information will be retained.

Training in appropriate uses of information technology will lead to improvement in processes. Process improvement requires that employees know what processes flow through the agency, who the suppliers and customers are of the process, and what service expectations are along the path. Employee training and education should not be limited to only technical accounting activities. One of the goals

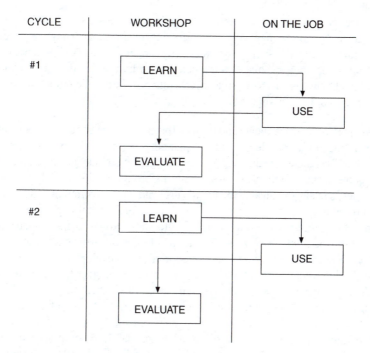

CYCLE	WORKSHOP	ON THE JOB

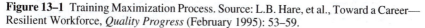

Figure 13–1 Training Maximization Process. Source: L.B. Hare, et al., Toward a Career—
Resilient Workforce, *Quality Progress* (February 1995): 53–59.

of employees' growth is to expand their horizons. Horizons can be expanded by
introducing employees to concepts of customer service, quality management, statistical thinking, changing management paradigms, and industry changes.

Employees' growth can also be accomplished by making it a mandatory part of
their personal performance measurement.

> One ingredient of a successful program is a system that helps employees
> regularly assess their skills, interests, values, and temperaments so that
> they can figure out the type of job for which they are best suited. An-
> other is a system that enables employees to benchmark their skills on a
> regular basis. These systems help employees understand both them-
> selves and the work to be done so well that, ideally, they routinely find
> their way into the right jobs and routinely update their skills. These sys-
> tems prod, awaken, and galvanize so that square pegs and round pegs
> find their way into right holes. Imagine how productivity would soar if
> most people had jobs that turned them on! By self-assessment, we mean
> a systematic process of taking stock of those attributes that influence

one's effectiveness, success, and happiness. Unless individuals understand the environments that let them shine, the interests that ignite them, and the skills that help them excel, how can they choose a company or a job where they can make their greatest contribution? Unless they understand how their personal style affects others, how can they function with maximum effectiveness?[3]

Another vehicle to educate and train staff is through the use of weekly meetings. Weekly meetings provide a forum for planning, review, training, and dissemination of information to team members. Meetings can include guests, who could be from other departments or teams or could be brought in specifically for training purposes, such as to enhance the team's oral and written communication skills.

Information dissemination can include "the larger picture," process improvement results, financial results, clinical outcomes, growth plans, legislative updates, book or article reviews, or the sharing of other departments' critical success factors. The controller or CFO has an opportunity to develop his or her associates, provide them with tools and a rationale for succeeding in the changing home health environment, and encourage staff to build on their successes. Thus, the controller or CFO begins to transition his or her role into that of a facilitator or coach.

Meetings are expensive. Therefore, meetings should be properly planned and have specific agendas. Meetings provide an excellent vehicle to reinforce team concepts, praise the collective team instead of a specific member of the team, and turn negative situations into learning experiences. Meetings can be used to develop team mission statements, to develop performance measurement criteria, and to address operational problems or issues.

> Many organizations tap the creativity well by using quality management, but the well goes dry after the initial reserves are drained. Relationship and ego boundaries around people and departments prevent the necessary awareness for more sustained improvement. But by looking directly to the human system and developing leaders who can go beyond their own emotional boundaries, organizations can tap deeper into the reserves to achieve significant change for quality improvement. Leaders who consciously cultivate the appropriate vision, create an environment conducive to learning, develop negative and positive feedback loops, and reward improved relationships will be the champions in this process. Because leadership is what one does and not what one says, these action-oriented leaders will seek greater understanding of their own psychological processes and habitual biases that inhibit their ability to listen, respond clearly, transform conflict, and maintain discipline toward a focused target.[4]

Performance Review

The annual merit increase (includes step and cost of living increases) is quickly becoming a concept of the past. Annual merit increases worked well in a cost-reimbursed environment; however, in a managed care environment, they are not consistent with cost efficiency and streamlined operations. Annual increases were probably developed as a mechanism to incent employees to work hard. However, some employees view the merit increase as a form of entitlement. Others have figured out ways to "game" the annual review process by increasing output immediately prior to their annual review and producing minimal output for the balance of the year. Additionally, annual increases tend to be short term in nature, to destroy teamwork, not to be process oriented, and to be subjective. Furthermore, "there is still a prevailing attitude among many managers that their role is to control, organize, direct, and evaluate employees' efforts. This conflicts with the TQM [total quality management] philosophy that proposes that employees must be empowered to directly affect their work. Many managers have yet to realize that their role, as Deming claims, must change from that of judge to coach."[5]

Bonuses fall into the same category. For example, a bonus that is based on increases in revenue can negatively affect an agency. By not considering all elements of the process, unscrupulous employees can increase revenue and sales to the detriment of the agency. Problems can occur because of contract administration, uncollectibility of receivables, high cost of service, or internal problems. Incenting managers on the end product ignores all of the personnel who were involved in making things happen. Additional problems could result because of cost reporting disallowances.

The review process should be designed to provide employees with feedback about how they are performing their jobs. Feedback should be designed to encompass all those areas that are critical to successful execution of job-related duties, to evaluate processes and process improvement, to incorporate customer feedback, and to provide a vehicle for employee growth and improvement. Annual reviews allow too much time to pass for purposes of providing feedback to employees; therefore, moving to a quarterly basis facilitates continuous quality improvement.

The new evaluative process incorporates the views of team members, internal and external customers, and managers. Managers are evaluated by their subordinates and employees are evaluated by peers. Performance criteria have a customer service orientation; are based on value added to the organization; are linked to personal, team, and organizational goals; and consist of monetary and non-monetary rewards.

Performance evaluation design should be consistent with the agency's orientation. If the agency is formed around teams, then evaluations should be designed and completed by team members. If the orientation is in transition from a functional to a process orientation, then a cross-functional or hybrid approach that combines the traditional employer–subordinate approach and the team's evaluation should be employed. Regardless of the current orientation, performance evaluations need to address the individual's role in the processes in which he or she is involved. This includes looking at inputs, the processes, the tools, and the outputs. The design of performance evaluations can complement activity-based costing and budgeting by determining value, frequency of events, cost drivers, resource drivers, and linkages to performance measures. Performance evaluations need to be dynamic to consider the evolving needs of both the employee and the agency.

Performance evaluations need to be tailored to the position and processes in which the employee is involved. A payroll clerk will be involved in different processes from an accounts payable clerk, and each will have different customers and different objectives. Individuals who handle the accounts payable and payroll functions will require specialized knowledge about their functions versus a controller, who will need general knowledge of all financial systems, third-party reimbursement, financial reporting, internal control, and other functions germane to that position. What will be common to all is their job knowledge, process indicators, interpersonal characteristics, customer service orientation, and growth plans. As responsibility increases, organizational and environmental considerations will come into play in evaluating team members. Exhibit 13–2 is an example of a performance measurement tool that could be used for a controller.

Evaluations can take each key area and attach a weight to it. For instance, the controller may have different weights attached to each of the evaluation centers. There is no rule as long as the total weighting is equal to one. Each of the evaluation centers would consist of a subset of evaluation points. For instance, job knowledge could consist of sections that address financial reporting, accounting systems, accounting theory, intercompany transactions, taxation, reimbursement, and internal controls. The customer service section would address factors that the accounting department had considered important to its service orientation, such as responsiveness, reliability, accessibility, timeliness, and accuracy. Process indicators could use an activity log that compares actual time spent versus budgeted time, actual improvements versus planned improvements, and actual metrics versus planned metrics.

This approach allows the evaluative processes to include customer feedback, employee feedback, and managerial or team member input. Furthermore, by expanding the customer service section to include the input of all customer bases, the evaluation considers the employees' contribution from the viewpoint of all who could be influenced by their efforts. Customers would include external customers, interdepartmental customers (operations, administration, etc.), and intradepartmental customers (team members, accounting staff, etc.).

Actual ratings could be jointly developed in the case of process indicators, for instance, days outstanding for accounts receivable personnel or the number of

Exhibit 13–2 Performance Measurement Tool

	Unsatisfactory	Satisfactory	Exceptional
Performance Measurement Tool			
Position: Controller			
Job knowledge			
Financial reporting			
• Accounting theory			
• Profit and loss statement	_____	_____	_____
• Balance sheet	_____	_____	_____
• Statement of cash flows	_____	_____	_____
• Footnotes	_____	_____	_____
• Consolidations	_____	_____	_____
Computer systems			
• Spreadsheets	_____	_____	_____
• Database systems	_____	_____	_____
• General ledger	_____	_____	_____
• Supporting systems	_____	_____	_____
Other			
• Statistics	_____	_____	_____
• Internal control	_____	_____	_____
• Third-party reimbursement	_____	_____	_____
• Outcome management	_____	_____	_____
• Budgeting	_____	_____	_____
• Strategic planning	_____	_____	_____
• Cash management	_____	_____	_____
• Taxation—local, state, & federal	_____	_____	_____
• Managed care contracting	_____	_____	_____

	Below standard	Standard	Above standard
Process indicators			
Financial			
• Bad-debt write-offs	_____	_____	_____
• Payroll errors	_____	_____	_____
• Vendor complaints	_____	_____	_____
• Cost-reporting adjustments	_____	_____	_____
• Billing errors	_____	_____	_____
Cycle time reductions			
• Monthly closings	_____	_____	_____
• Budgets	_____	_____	_____
• Age of outstanding accounts receivable	_____	_____	_____
Development of performance indicators			
• Staff	_____	_____	_____
• Self	_____	_____	_____
• Cross-functional indicators	_____	_____	_____
• Cost drivers	_____	_____	_____
• Resource drivers	_____	_____	_____

continues

Exhibit 13–2 continued

	Unsatisfactory	Satisfactory	Exceptional
Interpersonal characteristics			
Communication abilities			
• Oral	_____	_____	_____
• Written	_____	_____	_____
• Presentations	_____	_____	_____
Other			
• Ability to motivate staff	_____	_____	_____
• Assertiveness	_____	_____	_____
• Personal potential	_____	_____	_____
• Flexibility	_____	_____	_____
• Problem-solving skills	_____	_____	_____
• Vision	_____	_____	_____
• Analytical abilities	_____	_____	_____

	Below expectations	Meets expectations	Exceeds expectations
Customer service orientation			
External customers			
• Responsiveness	_____	_____	_____
• Reliability	_____	_____	_____
• Accuracy	_____	_____	_____
• Understands their needs	_____	_____	_____
Internal customers—Intradepartmental			
• Responsiveness	_____	_____	_____
• Reliability	_____	_____	_____
• Accuracy	_____	_____	_____
• Availability	_____	_____	_____
• Understands their needs	_____	_____	_____
Internal customers—Interdepartmental			
• Responsiveness	_____	_____	_____
• Reliability	_____	_____	_____
• Accuracy	_____	_____	_____
• Availability	_____	_____	_____
• Understands their needs	_____	_____	_____

	Below expectations	Meets expectations	Exceeds expectations
Personal growth plans			
• Continuing education	_____	_____	_____
• Team development	_____	_____	_____
• Application of learning to process improvement	_____	_____	_____
• Knowledge transfer to staff	_____	_____	_____
• Integration of professional & personal goals	_____	_____	_____

continues

Exhibit 13–2 continued

	Below expectations	*Meets expectations*	*Exceeds expectations*
Organizational and environmental			
• Educates other departments	_____	_____	_____
• Participates in professional organizations	_____	_____	_____
• Cross-functional development activities	_____	_____	_____
• Involvement in quality improvement	_____	_____	_____
• Ability to wear multiple organizational hats	_____	_____	_____

manual paychecks for the payroll personnel. Customer service ratings would be based on whether they did not meet, barely met, met, or exceeded customer expectations. Team member evaluations would be based on unsatisfactory, satisfactory, or exceptional levels of contribution. The mathematical sum of the evaluation points would be totaled by section, weighted, and combined with other sections. This would then determine the amount of increase to which an employee would be entitled.

When processes are linked to customer feedback, personal growth objectives, and team and organizational objectives, the evaluation becomes a tool for process improvement.

Today's superior organizations receive a broad range of contributions from their people. Employees own and continually improve their own processes and master multiple skills, as well as make products or provide services. Since they contribute in many ways, the rewards they receive should be of many kinds: a basket of rewards.[6]

Many of the basket's rewards are nonmonetary. One esteemed value is training. While yesterday's employees had job security on their minds, this era of endless downsizing has changed that. People today may be less concerned with job security than long-run work-life security. Training in and usage of multiple skills, including process improvement skills, provide more lines on a resume, should one be needed.[7]

Other nonmonetary rewards include being allowed to: work in teams, relate horizontally with customers at the next process, be a part of organizational and team goal-setting, go on trips to evaluate prospective new equipment, visit key suppliers or customers, use experience and mental acuity in improving processes, join professionals on projects, make presentations of proposed problem solutions, rate as well as be rated, and wear the same uniform and eat in the same company cafeteria as senior executives. Still others include being associated with whole processes, gaining satisfaction from self (team) recording of results, and being recognized in awards ceremonies or on walls of fame.[8]

Another class of rewards are no-cost or low-cost, such as best parking place, dinner at a fine restaurant, and ball-game tickets. Meaningful as well are team, site, and company celebrations (picnic, beer and pizza) for launching a product, completing a project, meeting a stringent quality target, achieving zero customer returns, and so on.[9]

On the monetary side—besides base pay—are bonuses, company stock or stock options, profit-sharing, gain-sharing, merit pay, pay for suggestions, and pay for knowledge. These payment options may be individual or group oriented.[10]

The old system—base pay and benefits—recognizes performance only in gross terms. The system must thus be supplemented. Some might say, however, that one or two supplementary rewards—not a whole basket—are sufficient. A profit-sharing advocate, for example, might argue that a share of profits provides adequate motivation and equity. But profit is time-biased. Last year's profits—before the organization began TQM and reengineering—may be owed to a booming economy. Next year, after improvement teams have raised quality and cut wastes by orders of magnitude, poor economic conditions may produce a loss. So no bonus. And the following year's high profit might be largely the work of key people no longer with the company. They did great work but got no bonus and left.[11]

Bonuses and gain-sharing involve another kind of bias. Everyone in the bonus group gets the same fixed or percentage share. Persons or teams that perform exceptionally feel poorly rewarded, and laggards over-rewarded. Pay for knowledge (or multiple skills) has still another, obvious kind of bias. It says nothing about past or current performance. Rewards are for potential or expected performance, which will not necessarily be obtained. Pay based on performance appraisal is so problematic that some in the quality movement (the late W. Edwards Deming for one) call for its complete elimination.[12]

When the content of the basket of rewards is meager, performance rating inequities loom large. However, when appraisal is just one of several avenues to reward and value, arguments against it begin to fade. Each of the rewards in the basket, when taken alone, is inadequate. Collectively, they provide enough kinds of rewards that most people will feel well treated. A member of a high performing team says, "We didn't get profit-sharing this period, but we got a bonus," or, "We didn't get profit-sharing or a bonus, but the company invested in us—80 hours of training in job skills and process improvement techniques." Those who garner new skills certificates may receive a pay increase—plus perceived improvements in work life security. And those who feel unfairly appraised may not stew over it long if other kinds of rewards are forthcoming.[13]

Exit Interviews

Exit interviews provide a form of closure for the employee and another data collection source for quality improvement. From a closure perspective, the exit interview allows employees to identify all of those things that they liked and disliked about their specific job, the people that they worked with, their supervisors and managers, company policies, and anything else on which they are willing to comment. From the department's or team's perspective, time should be allotted to acknowledge the departed person's contributions and determine whether anything can be learned from involvement with this individual. Possibly, the department or team will identify qualities to look for in new applicants and qualities to avoid and jointly develop a revised job description.

From a continuous quality improvement perspective, the exit interview is a vehicle to determine how things can be improved within the organization. It needs to be remembered that not all suggestions will be of value. This could be due to a mismatch between employee values and organizational values, systemwide changes, or interpersonal problems. However, if problems begin to repeat themselves (i.e., a specific manager or process), then complaints need to be investigated.

HUMAN RESOURCE COSTS

Human resource costs consist of base pay, incentives or bonuses, benefits, perquisites, and employer-related costs. Benefits typically consist of paid time off, health insurance, disability, and life insurance. Benefits packages can be increased to include deferred compensation, dependent health and life insurance, and tuition reimbursement. Benefits packages are usually designed to incent a worker to join a particular company and provide a safety net for the individual and the agency.

There is a substantial cost to benefits. Benefit costs are based on the range of benefits that are included in the benefits package, agency preferences, and the composition of the work group. Benefit costs will depend on the type of plan that is offered. For instance, a traditional indemnity plan may have a higher cost than a plan offered by the local health maintenance organization (HMO). This may be attributable to the indemnity plan having no out-of-pocket threshold or risk-sharing mechanism. Cost will also depend on the size of the agency, agency bargaining power, and whether health insurance can be purchased through a state organization or purchasing collective.

Over and above the actual premiums paid for health insurance is the cost of administration. Administrative cost has increased because of federal laws such as the Employee Retirement Income Security Act of 1974 (ERISA), the Age Discrimination Act (ADEA), the Americans with Disabilities Act (ADA), the Family and Medical Leave Act (FMLA), the Health Maintenance Organization Act, and the Equal Employment Opportunities (EEO) Act.

Health, disability, and life insurance represent tangible benefits to the employee. To the agency, they have a significant cost attached to their provision. As agencies strive to become more cost efficient, health, disability, and life insurance benefits will come under scrutiny. Benefit costs can be reduced by putting a ceiling on the amount that an employer will pay on behalf of its employees for coverage. Employers offer choices in health care coverage. If the choices available are between a traditional indemnity plan such as Blue Cross/Blue Shield and coverage from a local HMO, and a cost is identified for each, then the employee will be able to determine which plan he or she wants. The choice will be made with the knowledge that if the insurance plan costs more money than what the employer is willing to contribute, then it will come out of the employee's pocket. Benefit cost can also be reduced by adjusting the amount of the deductible, copayment, and range of services provided.

Some agencies prorate the amount of health insurance that they will pay on behalf of their part-time employees. This is typically accomplished by establishing a part-timer threshold. The threshold could be based on a minimum number of work hours, length of employment, number of visits, or a combination of factors.

One of the techniques for making the employer/employee cost-sharing mechanism more appealing is to introduce a cafeteria plan. A cafeteria plan allows employees to pay for their medical and life insurance benefits using pretax dollars. Cafeteria plans must meet specific conditions specified by the Internal Revenue Service Code. Cafeteria plans allow employers to structure a benefit menu to meet the needs of their employees. Other menu options could include dependent coverage, dental and vision coverage, flexible spending accounts for medical and dependent care, long-term disability, and 401(k) contributions.

> The Code specifies a number of requirements that a cafeteria plan must satisfy. Proposed regulations clarify the application of these requirements. According to the regulations, the cash element may be present in the form of employer contributions, employee salary reduction (pretax) contributions, or both. For example, in a full-menu cafeteria plan, an employer may offer:
>
> - Three medical options (e.g., insured low-option, insured high-option, and HMO)
> - Group-term life insurance at various multiples of annual salary

- Dependent care
- A cash or deferred plan under Section 401(k)

The employer might require employees to choose at least one of the medical options and at least the minimum level of group-term insurance. The employer would establish a budget (i.e., employer contributions), which the employees could allocate to the purchase of benefits as they saw fit. Employees who did not wish to spend the entire budget to purchase benefits could have the remainder paid to them in cash. On the other hand, employees who wanted to buy benefits that exceeded their budget could elect to have their salary reduced to pay for the excess benefits with pretax contributions.[14]

Payroll taxes represent a significant cost to the agency. Payroll taxes are at a federal and state level. Federal taxes are for social security (Federal Insurance Contributions Act; FICA) and unemployment. Social security is based on a percentage of gross wages up to a ceiling. The employer has responsibility for matching employee withholdings. Federal unemployment is also based on a percentage of gross wages up to a ceiling. State unemployment taxes vary by state.

It is the responsibility of the agency to withhold payroll taxes from all employees' payroll checks, remit tax withholdings on a timely basis, and complete quarterly and annual reports. Noncompliance will lead to fines, penalties, and possibly imprisonment. Payroll taxes are a cost of doing business. Payroll taxes can also be minimized by reducing turnover, use of cafeteria plans, and use of the common paymaster concept. For instance, the CEO is in charge of two agencies, one is a Medicare-certified HHA and the other provides unregulated private services. If the CEO were to draw a paycheck from both companies, and the combined total exceeded the social security ceiling, the consolidated effect would be an overpayment of social security tax for both the individual and the consolidated organization.

Therefore, if

> a group of corporations is considered a common paymaster group by meeting one of the following tests at any time during the calendar quarter: (1) they are members of a controlled group for federal income tax purposes as defined in section 1563 of the Internal Revenue Code except that "more than 50%" ownership is substituted for "at least 80%"; (2) 50 percent of one corporation's officers are officers of the other corporation; or (3) 30 percent or more of one corporation's employees are employees of the other corporation. While the savings can be substantial at the FICA level, the rules at the state and local levels vary widely. The controller should therefore check with all local taxing authorities to determine if similar savings are available.[15]

Attempts to minimize payroll tax liability have caused many agencies to explore the use of independent contractors. Independent contractors are responsible for their own taxes, benefits, and costs of providing services. However, from the agency's perspective, this may present a problem with control. Use of independent contractors should be consistent with the agency's legal counsel's opinions.

Documentation of employee dismissals is a vehicle to prevent increases in state unemployment costs. Employers have the ability to contest unemployment claims providing they can show cause for dismissal of the employee. Documentation is the key. Documentation should include policies and procedures that were violated, dates of warnings, acknowledgment of warnings by the employees, and actions taken. Claims that have been contested can be appealed and charges reversed if the employer is successful.

WORKERS' COMPENSATION

Workers' compensation is another cost related to human resources. Workers' compensation is an insurance policy that is paid for by employers on behalf of their employees. The insurance policy provides for the payment of medical expenses and a portion of lost income for those employees who are injured while conducting company business. Workers' compensation is calculated on gross wages, dependent on a rating scale developed by industry, the agency's claim experience, and state rules.

Although workers' compensation rules are different by state, most rates are established for the upcoming year, a deposit is made to the state fund or private placement agency, and a retroactive adjustment is made. The retroactive adjustment is based on whether gross wages changed from the original estimate. Therefore, calculating the effect of workers' compensation on changes in the gross wage base is important to reflecting accurately the results of operation. This can be accomplished by developing a control schedule that reflects a potential retroactive liability.

Workers' compensation is controllable through education, training, and the aggressive management of claims. It is advisable to work with a qualified broker or representative to determine how an agency can decrease its workers' compensation costs. Education and training can include lifting techniques, use of rubber-soled shoes to prevent slipping in bathrooms, and implementation of safety procedures for blood, infections, and cuts. Aggressive management of claims will require establishing a reporting process for all work-related injuries; a monitoring process; and even the development of injury causes, recovery timelines, and progress outcomes.

RISK MANAGEMENT

The purpose of risk management is to reduce the HHA's exposure to accidental losses. This is usually accomplished through working with an insurance broker to determine the proper blend of insurance coverages to carry. Insurances can be purchased for director and officers' liability, malpractice, property insurance, business interruption, bonding of employees, unowned automobiles, and other related business activities.

The goal is twofold. First, there is the need to provide a safety net in the event of a loss. That is the purpose of insurance. The second goal is risk prevention. This occurs through training and proactive identification of risks. Risk identification can be accomplished by reviewing policy coverage in light of changing organizational plans, decisions, and business pursuits. Policy review is enhanced by having all policy periods coincide with the agency's fiscal year so that policy review can be considered as part of the annual planning process.

Risk management decisions consider the amount of coverage, deductibles, and timing of policies. For instance, a risk management technique to lower the cost of unowned auto premiums is to require all staff to submit copies of their personal insurance policies to make sure that they have insurance as well as the necessary insurance premiums. Another risk management practice would include making back-up copies of the HHA's database on a daily basis and storing data offsite.

PRODUCTIVITY

Productivity is a concept closely linked to the efficient use of personnel. Productivity is a measure of output for a unit of service. The unit of service could be an hour or a day. Usually, productivity is identified in relationship to the number of visits performed by field personnel on a daily basis. Productivity can also apply to administrative employees. Albeit, administrative employees present a challenge because of "thought or planning time," it is still possible to measure productivity. Productivity is a function of the output of employees' efforts and what was accomplished.

A key area for administrative employees is the reduction of cycle time. Cycle time is the length of time that a process requires. An obvious example is the amount of time that it takes to publish financial statements after the month has been closed. Figure 13–2 illustrates how multiple processes would contribute to the closing of the financial statements. Reduction of closing activities, beginning the closing process before the month has ended, and automation will reduce cycle time. Decreases in cycle time will positively affect productivity and consequently reduce cost.

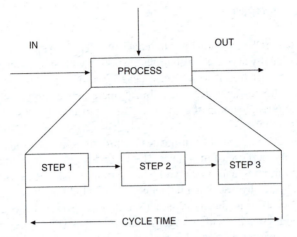

Figure 13–2 Cycle Time and Multiple Activities within a Major Process. Source: Reprinted with permission from Ligus, R.C., The Controller's Role in Reducing Cycle Time, *The Small Business Controller*, Winter 1994, pp. 36–39, © 1994, Warren, Gorham & Lamont, 31 St. James Avenue, Boston, MA 02116. All rights reserved.

PROJECT MANAGEMENT

Special projects, fiscal intermediary audits, year-end activities, increased patient census, new contracts, or myriad other factors increase the amount of activities and staff time. Serious consideration should be given to understanding the implications of volume changes and the effect that they cause on the demand for accounting resources. This requires tracking and estimating resource consumption, planning for outcome achievement and resource requirements, and identification of what combination of resources would be the most efficient and accomplish the desired outcome.

It is important to remember that temporary services can be purchased. Otherwise, the agency incurs overtime, burns out its employees, and makes staff less willing to take on additional projects. The key is being able to quantify needs in relationship to existing activities and desired outcomes. Time management is the other critical issue. Time management places accountability on the department that is requesting additional support. This prevents the additional support from becoming integrated into the existing system. If there is a need for ongoing support, then the position and reason for the temporary assistance need to be reviewed in relation to current workloads and future plans.

NOTES

1. R.H. Waterman, et al., Toward a Career—Resilient Workforce, *Harvard Business Review* (July–August 1994): 87–95.
2. J.R. Grinnell, Optimize the Human System, *Quality Progress* 27, no. 11 (November 1994): 63–67.
3. R.H. Waterman, Toward a Career—Resilient Workforce, 87–95.
4. J.R. Grinnell, Optimize the Human System, 63–67.
5. G. Eckes, Practical Alternatives to Performance Appraisals, *Quality Progress* (November 1994): 57–60.
6. R.J. Schonberger, Human Resource Management Lessons from a Decade of Total Quality Management and Reengineering, *California Management Review* (Summer 1994): 109–122.
7. *Ibid.*
8. *Ibid.*
9. *Ibid.*
10. *Ibid.*
11. *Ibid.*
12. *Ibid.*
13. *Ibid.*
14. P.J. Wendell, *Corporate Controllers Manual* (Boston: Warren, Gorham & Lamont, 1994), F2-22.
15. *Ibid.*

Chapter 14

Cash Management

Effective working capital management practices increase agency profitability and liquidity and decrease reliance on external sources of working capital. Working capital is the difference between current assets and current liabilities. Increases in assets require cash, and decreases in assets provide cash. Increases in liabilities are a source of cash, and decreases in liabilities require the use of cash. Liquidity refers to how quickly assets will convert to cash. This chapter focuses on the management of the major components of working capital, cash, accounts receivable, and disbursements before concluding with a tool for the management of working capital: the cashflow forecast.

Ultimately, the goal of working capital management is to minimize the amount of interest that is paid to external creditors for working capital loans. Therefore, the goal is to maximize the agency's use of its own resources. Resource maximization for cash can be accomplished through designing efficient banking systems, consolidating funds, and investing excess cash. Resource maximization for accounts receivable will occur through reduction of cycle time, development of credit and collection procedures, and reduction of bad-debt write-offs. Disbursements can be maximized by taking advantage of discounts, paying invoices when due, and understanding disbursement float.

Cash management is everyone's responsibility. This is because everyone is indirectly affected by cash management practices and results. Cash management problems create difficulties in paying employees, vendors and suppliers, taxes, and creditors. Agencies that have experienced these kinds of problems know how difficult it can be for all involved when cash flow is out of sync with organizational operating requirements. Therefore, proactive working capital management requires that everyone involved in the billing and collections processes, purchasing and disbursement processes, marketing, and credit functions work together. Working capital management must be treated as a number one priority; otherwise, an agency can provide as many profitable services as possible, but without sufficient cash inflows, its financial viability will be precarious and totally dependent on cash inflows from external sources.

In fact, cashflow accountability goes beyond the employees who are responsible for the billing and collection cycles. Accountability means not entering into contracts, service lines, or ventures that have undesirable service requirements, returns, and payment terms. Furthermore, working capital management should be considered as a strategic component for the evaluation of agency results over the short and long terms. By including working capital management as a key performance indicator, managers will begin to look at the agency in a holistic fashion that no longer ignores "back of the house" processes.

MANAGEMENT OF CURRENT ASSETS AND CURRENT LIABILITIES

Cash

Cash is the life blood of any business. Cash comes from different sources. Cash comes from investments of start-up capital by the owner, credit arrangements from banks and other creditors, fundraising efforts, and the collection of accounts receivable. Cash is used for many different purposes. Cash is used to pay employees, vendors, and creditors. Therefore, it is important to understand three concepts: (1) the revenue cycle, (2) the disbursement cycle, and (3) the bridge that links them or the cash cycle. Cycles are time sensitive. (See Figure 14–1.)

The revenue cycle begins with service provision. This is the point that a billable visit is performed, supplies are delivered and accepted, or private-duty services are provided. The revenue cycle is not complete until services have been paid in full. The length of time between service provision and payment, or cycle time, will vary by agency, type of service, and payor. At the agency level, factors that influence the revenue cycle are the internal policies and processes related to billing, collection of notes and data, and collection practices.

The disbursement cycle is composed of two major elements. The first element is payment for revenue-generating services. This encompasses the employees and purchased services that have provided services on behalf of the agency. Technically, the agency will recognize a liability at the time of service provision; however, the payment for services will lag behind the actual date of service. This lag is created by management in the form of payroll cycles and subcontracted vendor payment policies. The second element of the disbursement cycle is payment of the agency's administrative staff, suppliers, and creditors. Management may choose to have different payment cycles for these two groups or a common payment strategy.

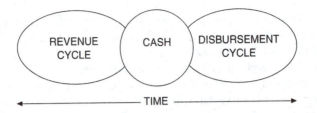

Figure 14–1 Cycle Time in Relation to the Revenue and Disbursement Cycles

The center element is cash. Cash is the net difference between collections, or the result of the revenue cycle and the disbursement cycle. If collections are insufficient, the agency needs to look to external sources for cash (financing will be addressed in Chapter 15). If the agency has excess cash, then it wants to evaluate whether the excess cash is a temporary phenomenon or a reality. The evaluation process can be accomplished through the use of cashflow forecasts and other management tools. In the event that excess cash is a reality, the agency will want to determine what course of action will offer it the greatest return. Options may include investment in business opportunities, reduction of debt, or investing.

Structuring the Cash Collection and Disbursement Process

Structuring of bank accounts will enhance the cash management process. An agency that has one bank account that handles all incoming and outgoing transactions will miss out on cash management opportunities. The use of the one bank account system is characteristic of smaller agencies (Figure 14–2).

One bank account reduces the amount of bank reconciliations that need to be performed; however, it increases the complexity of the bank reconciliation. This is because of many different types of transactions flowing through the same account. Although bank reconciliations are important from a control perspective, they have little bearing on cash management. From a cash management perspective, the agency will want to know what deposits and disbursements have cleared and what transactions are likely to clear in the next couple of days.

As the agency grows, its cash management strategies begin to change. Attention is paid to the management of disbursement float. Disbursement float is the time between a check being issued and the recipient cashing it. Disbursement float is actually made up of three parts. The first part is the length of time that it takes from when the check is mailed from the agency until it is received. The second element of disbursement float is the amount of time that it takes for the recipient to deposit the check. The final element is the amount of time that it takes for the check to clear.

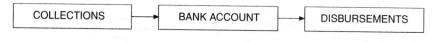

Figure 14–2 The One Bank Account Cash Management System

The first element of disbursement float is attributable to the mail system. The amount of time related to mail delivery will depend on when checks are disbursed from the agency, the day of the week of disbursement, and the disbursement's destination. Additional factors that will increase or decrease the amount of disbursement float attributable to the mail system are the time checks are picked up by the mail carrier or delivered to the post office, holidays, and use of the nine-digit ZIP code.

The second element of disbursement float will depend on the recipient. Disbursements to recipients who deposit checks immediately will have a shorter float time than those to recipients who do not deposit checks quickly. Sometimes employees do not deposit their checks immediately, thus providing float to the agency. Other factors will be the mode of deposit. A check that is cashed immediately or deposited as cash will clear quicker than a check that is deposited to an automated teller on a Friday night, which will not be recorded as deposited until Monday.

The final element of disbursement float is attributable to the banking system. The banking system is composed of different districts and banks. Deposits that are made to different banks will take longer to clear than deposits made to the agency's bank. This is also true of deposits made to banks outside of the local banking system.

Disbursement float represents money to the agency. If disbursement float is seven days, the agency would not need to cover the disbursement for seven days. Instead, the agency could choose to invest the amount of the disbursement for seven days, pay down a credit line for seven days, or not borrow money for seven days.

Assuming that on average the agency did not borrow funds the day that it made disbursements because it was managing its disbursement float, the agency would be able to realize the annualized savings shown in Table 14–1. Realizing that savings could be obtained by managing disbursement float caused agencies to change their bank accounts from single to multiple accounts.

Table 14–1 Annual Interest Expense Savings

Average float ($)	25,000	50,000	75,000	100,000
Borrowing rate (%)	7	7	7	7
Annualized savings ($)	1,750	3,500	5,250	7,000

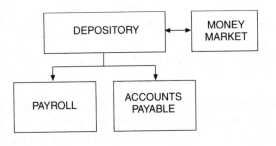

Figure 14–3 The Multiple Account Structure

The multiple account structure enabled the agency to meet its increasingly complex cash management needs (Figure 14–3). Separate accounts would be set up for payroll and accounts payable disbursements. All cash would be deposited into a separate depository, and excess funds would be transferred to a money market account. Banking regulations limit the amount of disbursements from a money market account, so a depository had to be used for the majority of disbursements to payroll and accounts payable.

The advantage of this system is that the financial players are able to determine the amount of disbursement float that they have for the payroll and accounts payable accounts. Float is the difference between checks that have been disbursed and those that have actually cleared. In the above situation, float would be managed by comparing bank account balances in relationship to book balances. A more detailed approach to determining float is to trace check disbursement dates to bank statements to determine float and deposit characteristics of employees and vendors.

Table 14–2 illustrates the monitoring of bank balances in the payroll account in relationship to book balances. Bank balances are obtained by calling the bank every morning to find out what the account's available balance is. Obtaining bank balances will depend on the sophistication of the agency's bank. Some banks will provide this information from a bank representative, others will fax you the information, and others will allow you to obtain information on-line. Tracking of bank balances in relationship to book balances will enable the agency to determine when cash transfers need to be made to cover disbursements. In Table 14–2, the agency had a net payroll of $35,000 that was disbursed on Thursday. Cash transfers were made on Friday, Monday, and Wednesday to cover checks that cleared. The process would coincide to the frequency of agency payrolls. This structure provided a vehicle to take advantage of disbursement float. Although this structure is more efficient than the single bank account structure, it still has not addressed two additional areas of inefficiency: (1) internal cash processing characteristics of the agency and (2) bank processing practices.

Table 14–2 Analysis of Average Float

Feb 95	Deposit ($)	Disbursement ($)	Book ($)	Bank ($)
1 Wed			1,000	4,350
2 Thu		35,000	(34,000)	3,500
3 Fri	10,000		(24,000)	2,250
4 Sat			(24,000)	
5 Sun			(24,000)	
6 Mon	20,000		(4,000)	5,400
7 Tue			(4,000)	8,900
8 Wed	5,000		1,000	2,000
Average float			(16,143)	

The amount of time that it takes for internal processing is analogous to the amount of time that it takes for an employee to cash his or her check. In this situation, it is the amount of time from receipt of a remittance until the check is deposited in the agency's bank. Bank processing depends on when the deposit is credited to the agency's account. This will be influenced by bank processing cut-offs.

Figure 14–4 has added a lockbox to the multiple account structure. The lockbox reduces mail float and time associated with internal and bank processing. Lockboxes are a vehicle through which remittances are processed immediately and deposited into the agency's bank account. The agency can determine how it wants to process receipts, identify different payees who may appear on the face of the check, and determine what information it wants forwarded to the agency for internal processing. For instance, the agency may want all remittance advice to be forwarded to the agency along with a photocopy of the check. The bank will also provide a summary of all items deposited on a given day.

The lockbox process enhances collections and internal controls. From a collections perspective, mail float will be reduced. The amount of float will depend on where the agency's customers are located and from where they disburse payments. Internal processing time will also be reduced. Internal processing time will be dependent on the volume of transactions, internal procedures, and the proximity of the agency's bank to the agency.

Furthermore, this has the effect of strengthening internal controls because now receipts are handled immediately, and there is external verification of the amount of money that was received by the agency on a daily basis. From the customer's perspective, it only knows that the agency has changed its remittance address. The change is from the agency's mailing address to a post office box. The post office box is the lockbox address.

There is a cost associated with the lockbox. Lockbox cost will vary based on the volume of transactions, fixed charges for monthly rental, and the amount of serv-

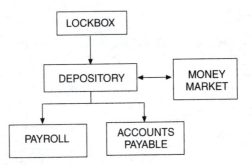

Figure 14–4 Multiple Account Structure with Lockbox

---

ices requested. Additional costs need to be weighed against the value of float reduction, improved internal controls, and efficiency. Other considerations for lockbox use may be dictated by the agency's lending institution as a requirement for secured credit lines.

Further enhancements to the cash management process can occur through the introduction of zero balance accounts (ZBAs). (See Figure 14–5.) ZBAs are accounts that have a zero balance; therefore, excess bank balances are eliminated in disbursement accounts. When checks are presented for payment, an exact amount is known. The total amount of the checks is taken from the depository or master account. ZBAs eliminate the need for estimating what checks will clear on a daily basis, enhance investment opportunities, and eliminate the potential for overdrafts because of errors in clearing estimates. ZBAs may not be available at some of the smaller local banks.

Another feature that is available at larger banks is overnight investments. Banks have the ability to sweep automatically ending bank balances into overnight investment vehicles such as money markets. This allows the agency to maximize its returns on "idle" cash. Sweeps may have minimum requirements by banks. Additionally, the possibility for being temporarily applied against credit lines may be worth investigating with banking representatives.

Other investment considerations depend on the amount of money available, senior management's and the board's stance on risk and return, and forecasted cashflow requirements. If the decision is to leave excess funds in a money market account or a depository account, an evaluation should be performed to determine whether the agency can obtain a better return by increasing compensating balances to reduce bank charges instead of leaving idle cash in a depository or money market account.

Compensating balances can be required by bankers as part of their credit extensions. Compensating balances are typically a credit that is given to a business

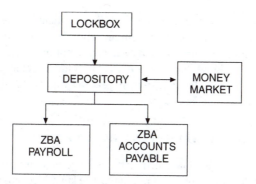

Figure 14–5 Multiple Account Structure with Zero Balance Accounts

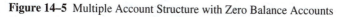

based on the average bank account balance. Compensating balance credits are based on the average collected balance, reduced for federally mandated reserve requirements, and the remainder is then multiplied by an earnings allowance. This credit is then applied against service charges. Service charges are based on the type and amount of transactions. Typical charges are for account maintenance, transactions such as deposits and disbursements, stop payments, returned items, and account reconciliations. Balances that do not cover charges would be billed to the agency, and excesses are retained by the bank. Furthermore, if compensating balances are required as part of a credit extension, this will increase the effective rate of the loan.

In Table 14–3, a 7 percent loan for $150,000 that requires $10,000 to remain in the agency's bank account as a compensating balance will effectively increase the loan rate to 7.5 percent.

Large providers may have operations that have multiple sites and several different companies to house different service lines. These providers may choose to simplify some of their operating complexities by the development of a centralized cash management structure. Figure 14–6 shows ZBAs feeding a concentration

Table 14–3 Effective Interest Rate Calculation

Loan	$150,000
Compensating balance	10,000
Net loan	140,000
Interest rate	7%
Annual interest	$ 10,500
Effective rate	7.5%

account, excess cash being invested, and disbursements being handled through ZBAs. This structure allows for maximum efficiency and optimization. The deposit ZBAs could be set up for each company, location, branch, or other criteria that reflected operations. Disbursement ZBAs would be set up by company. Furthermore, this structure allows cash managers to simplify the difficulties of intercompany loans and transfers of cash.

ACCOUNTS RECEIVABLE MANAGEMENT

Accounts receivable management is the management of assets that are due the agency for services that have been provided. The key to proactive accounts receivable management is to view the entire process known as the *revenue cycle*. Understanding the revenue cycle will allow managers to analyze the entire process, to determine whether problems are due to internal processes or external circumstances, and to develop a plan of action that corrects problems from recurring. Ultimately, the goal is to reduce cycle time to its lowest point without affecting the quality of services provided or creating customer problems.

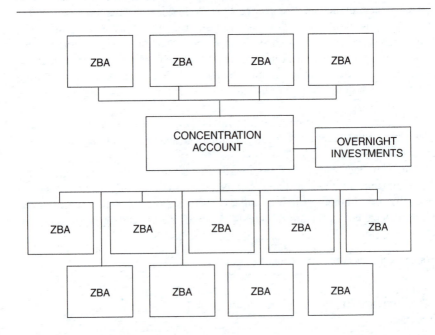

Figure 14–6 Multiple Account Structure for a Large HHA. Source: Reprinted with permission from *Corporate Cash Management Handboook* by R. Bort, p. E3, © 1994, Warren, Gorham & Lamont, 31 St. James Avenue, Boston, MA 02116. All rights reserved.

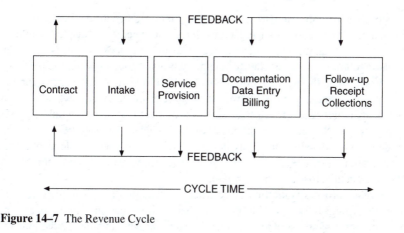

Figure 14–7 The Revenue Cycle

The revenue cycle has two primary outcomes associated with it. The first outcome has an external orientation. This outcome is from the external customer's perspective and is concerned with the output of the billing operation. From customers' perspective, they are concerned that the bills that are submitted are correct, presented in a logical fashion, and reflective of services that were provided. The second outcome is the collection of accounts receivable in a timely fashion and the reduction of cycle time.

As discussed above, increases in accounts receivable use an agency's cash. Regardless of the source of cash, the objective is to collect receivables in a timely fashion. Figure 14–7 identifies several of the components of the billing and collection process and a feedback loop. The feedback loop provides a mechanism to improve the process continuously, refine processes to meet customers' contractual requirements, and obtain the outcome of timely collections.

Contractual Requirements, Intake, and Service Provision

At the beginning of the revenue cycle are customer or contractual requirements. Contractual requirements may specify that claims are to be submitted using a specific billing form, such as the UB-92, or to contain specific documentation. Documentation may also be required to be submitted in conjunction with specific forms. Other contractual requirements may be for the agency to submit bills on a specified period, follow a predetermined format for submission, and direct all inquiries to certain individuals.

It is essential that everyone involved in the revenue cycle fully understand contractual requirements and obligations. If everyone understands the agency's responsibilities in relationship to contractual obligations, then the agency should not be penalized for noncompliance. Factors that could penalize an agency would be not obtaining preauthorization for visits, providing services in excess of policy limits, or submitting claims after the claims submission window has closed.

Contracts that the agency initiates should include favorable terms for the agency. Terms that are favorable would be short payment cycles (e.g., due in 15 days from invoice date). Terms that are not favorable to the agency would be a 75-day payment cycle beginning on receipt of the invoice. Therefore, it is important that new contracts value the timely collection of accounts receivable as much as the generation of new revenue. This is another reason why incentive systems have to be consistent across the entire organization.

The intake process is the first place where information begins to get collected on an individual basis. In addition to gathering information regarding patient problems, information should be gathered regarding what insurances the new referral has. Insurance verification should identify what coverage enrollees have, to what home health services they are entitled, whether there are any limitations or exclusions, what health benefits remain, and whether the new referral has current coverage. Depending on the type of insurance and the type of services to be provided, it may be necessary to explore whether there is secondary insurance coverage or a guarantor.

When the assessment visit is performed, the visiting nurse should verify policy numbers against the individual's insurance cards, ascertain that the insurance card is for the current period, and question whether there is any other insurance coverage available. Depending on the individual's coverage, there may be a need to bill a secondary payor. Having a photocopy of the insurance card is ideal; however, this is unrealistic in the home setting, but obtaining a signature, date, and time are realistic expectations.

The first three elements of Figure 14–7—contract or customer requirements, intake, and service provision—identify areas of input into the billing process. Proper procedures regarding insurance verification, contract compliance, preauthorization, and dollar or service unit ceilings will prevent a majority of collection problems from occurring. These types of collection problems generally result in write-offs and customer-oriented problems, both of which are undesirable.

Documentation, Data Entry, and Billing

The next element of the revenue cycle is documentation, data entry, and billing. This is the core internal process that determines the length of time between date of service and submission of claims to a payor. As identified above, the process of claim submission can be influenced by a payor determining that it only wants claims submitted once a month. However, from an internal process perspective, documentation, data entry, and the billing process are under the control of agency management. Reduction of duplicative effort, nonvalue-added activities, and manual processes will reduce cycle time.

It is important to understand that the sooner bills can be submitted to payors, the sooner accounts receivable can be converted into cash. Stated in a different fashion, the longer that it takes to submit claims and receive payment for services, the more credit has been extended to the agency's customers. Therefore, since time is money, it is important to identify ways that the billing process can be streamlined.

Elimination of manual processes is becoming one of the key ways to increase efficiency. Manual processes can include submission of handwritten documentation, data entry into a billing system, review of payor activity by a quality assurance individual, and a paper claim system. Advances in information technology and declining prices are enabling agencies to send their field personnel out with lap-top computers. Lap-top computers permit field staff to collect better documentation, review patient history to date, and determine a course of action that is consistent with previous interventions.

Not only has documentation become easier, but also the transmission of documentation into the agency's billing system has eliminated the need for data entry. Documentation can be entered directly into the billing system by downloading information via modem or by dropping off a computer disk and then transferring information.

Entry of preauthorized service limitations and patient outcome objectives will guide service provision. Linking patient problems to a customized care plan that includes service limitations and outcome objectives accomplishes several things. First, it allows the field professionals to plan and orchestrate service provision to maximize outcomes. Second, the care process can be continually improved by monitoring results against care plan objectives for each step along the clinical pathway. Finally, by educating clinicians on contract requirements, utilizing clinical pathways, and transferring ownership of the quality assurance process, the quality assurance process could also be eliminated. Instead, the focus of quality assurance would move from being retrospectively to prospectively oriented. The objectives of quality improvement would be the analysis of outcomes in relationship to care plans, tracking and monitoring variances, and continually enhancing field staff skills through ongoing training.

Manual billing processes have become more efficient as a result of advances in information technology. Directly entering nursing documentation into the billing system eliminates errors made by data entry personnel because of incorrect interpretation of long-hand notes or errors due to miskeying data. The quality assurance step that required a prebilling run in order to verify that actual service provision was consistent with plan of treatments or preauthorization can now be eliminated. In its place are documentation templates that require field personnel to document specific elements of the patient visit, automated billing validation processes, and exceptions. Investigation of exceptions instead of investigation of all activity significantly reduces cycle time.

It needs to be noted that information technology is not the answer to all internal process problems. Sound management is required to streamline processes. Information technology is purely a tool, and tools are only as good as the people using them and the systems that are in place. For instance, if the agency utilizes a great deal of nonemployee personnel to satisfy its resource needs, and these individuals or companies do not submit paperwork, adhere to agency policies for continuing education, or any number of other factors, then the best information system will not make a difference. Additionally, Figure 14–7 illustrates the need for feedback between processes. Process feedback is essential to the identification and elimination of problems. Other factors that can enhance internal processes are cross-training, common incentives, and the elimination of functional boundaries.

True process improvement will come from identifying all process inputs, determining standards for employees and suppliers, and working as a team to accomplish the objectives of the agency. In this situation, the objective is to minimize the revenue cycle from date of service until submission of the claim.

One of the methods for enhancing the billing process is utilization of electronic data interchange (EDI), commonly referred to as *electronic billing*. Electronic billing is an efficient business strategy. Use of EDI eliminates many of the repetitive tasks associated with billing. Not only are repetitive tasks eliminated, but also there is an opportunity to correct problems on line, and mail time for submission of claims is completely eliminated from the revenue cycle. Furthermore, payor processing time is eliminated, claims are entered correctly into the payors' accounts payable system, and the accounts receivable management process has a sound starting point.

Follow-up, Cash Receipts, and Collections

The final element of the revenue cycle consists of follow-up, application of receipts, and collection efforts. Follow-up is a common-sense step in the overall scheme of accounts receivable management. Follow-up is the verification that claims were received by a customer. EDI provides for on-line follow-up, and manual billing does not; therefore, for all payors that have not transitioned to an EDI environment, follow-up remains a proactive step in determining where claims are in the customer payment process.

Follow-up procedures will vary by payor, depend on payor characteristics, and utilize different approaches. An approach for a private-pay customer may be a courtesy telephone call ten days after the invoice was mailed. The purpose of the call would be to verify that the customer received the bill and to answer any questions that he or she may have regarding charges. Before hanging up, an attempt should be made to determine when payment can be expected. All communications should be documented. This enables subsequent collection efforts to reference prior conversations.

The development of a tickler file with payor characteristics, contact name, telephone number, and personal information will help the collection process. Developing a personal contact will help all future collections efforts. This process can even be enhanced by visiting the payor and having an opportunity to meet face to face. The development of a personal contact will help prevent inquiries from being treated as just another "pushy vendor." In addition to identifying a contact, the tickler file should begin to identify payor characteristics, such as length of time between claim submission and payment, determining who is the claims review individual, and documenting strategies for problem resolution. One payor may frequently lose claims. However, when claims are faxed to a specific location, they are processed immediately. This kind of information will improve cash collections and reduce cycle time.

Entry of remittance advice can be another area that has the potential for process improvement. Entry of remittance advice should be handled promptly. Otherwise, collection time will be extended if there are any claims that are not paid in full. Any claims that are partially paid, omitted, or disallowed should be investigated immediately. On investigation, if the error is attributable to internal processes, this needs to be communicated to everyone involved in the revenue cycle and used as a mechanism for learning, not for punishment. If the claim is valid, then resubmit immediately. Resubmission may require hand delivery, faxing, overnight delivery, or certified mail. It depends on the amount of the invoice and the agency's cash position.

Often, remittance advice will include overpayments. Overpayments can result from errors during payor processing. Money that does not belong to the agency represents a liability to the agency and, in the spirit of good customer relations, should be returned promptly. Medicare has instituted a quarterly reporting mechanism that all providers are required to report whether they have received any overpayments.

Collection activities are everyone's responsibility. Collection activities that are proactive have elements of the collection process identified before service is provided, employ follow-up practices, and constantly strive to collect funds using a series of techniques. Techniques involve a combination of telephone calls, balance billing, past due notices, and collection letters.

Collection efforts should focus on all payors. However, in an attempt to accelerate cash flow, there may be a need to leverage collection efforts. This approach would cause collection personnel to focus on large claims first, and then work their way down toward smaller claims. Timely collection efforts will begin several days after the due date of the claim and depend on credit arrangements that have been made with customers.

For instance, if contractual terms state that payment is due in 30 days from invoice date, then the first collection call should be initiated several days after the 30-day mark. If services have been provided to a private paying individual, there may be a need to take a different approach. The approach will depend on the agency's credit policy. The agency may require that private pay services pay in advance, use a credit card, or pay a retainer against which the agency draws. In return, the agency may offer discounted services or some other type of arrangement.

The development of a credit policy should determine what the agency's philosophy is toward the collection of deductibles and copayments. The policy should also determine whether the agency will accept insurance companies' payments as payment in full for agency charges. If the agency plans to collect 100 percent of its charges, this needs to be communicated to patients up front. They need to be notified that they are responsible for whatever their insurance does not cover. Additionally, the agency may even consider asking patients to pay them directly, bill the insurance carrier on behalf of the patient, and then remit whatever the insurance company pays to the patient. Furthermore, the agency may want to investigate an individual's credit before extending credit. This is possible with the patient's permission.

Inherent in the development of a credit policy is the agency's approach to collections. A stringent credit policy may eliminate collections problems, but it has the side effect of limiting revenue. Conversely, a loose credit policy will increase revenue but create collection problems. Tight collection policies eliminate the need for write-offs due to uncollectibility, staff hours, and the cost of services provided; therefore, in the long run, a tight collection policy is usually an efficient vehicle. Another element of the credit policy is billing for late payments. Charging patients interest on unpaid balances can offset costs associated with collection and financing activities. However, consideration needs to be given to the likelihood that interest will be paid and how interest charges will be handled in the financial statements.

In the event that internal efforts have not succeeded in collecting claims, the agency may want to consider the use of a collection agency or an attorney. Both the collection agency and the attorney will have a cost associated with their efforts, however, to realize some portion of the total claim is better than receiving none of it. Fees are normally determined by the age of the receivable and whether any other collection agency has attempted to collect the open claims. Accounts receivable that are turned over to a collection agency should be written off. In the event that anything is recovered, the recovered amount should be booked to recovery.

Write-offs occur when receivables are uncollectible. Accountants attempt to estimate the amount of uncollectible accounts receivable by setting up a provision for bad debts. The provision for bad debts is an estimate. The estimate can be more realistic if payment patterns are identified by payor groups. Estimates will then be based on time and prior experience. The total provision will reduce accounts receivable to a net realizable amount. Write-offs are then applied against the provision for bad debts.

Reduction of bad debt is an excellent indicator of how well the revenue cycle team is working together. If the collection process is efficient, this number will be low; if the team is inefficient, this number will be high. It is important to note that bad debt is very costly to the agency. It is the total of the charge that is written off, plus the carrying cost related to payment for service provision, and the cost of all follow-up and collection activities. Therefore, the reduction of bad debt expense is a prime candidate for CQI processes.

Bad debt can take many forms. Bad debt can be due to denials for services in excess of authorized amounts, policy limits being exceeded, or services being deemed not necessary by a payor's case management system. Bad debt can be attributable to not obtaining proper insurance information, patients' coverage elapsing, or a patient's death. There are many points during the revenue cycle at which incorrect inputs can cause a negative outcome; therefore, it is everyone's business to work at reducing bad debt.

Aggressive accounts receivable management begins at contract inception, integrates policies and procedures into staff training, continually seeks to develop more efficient billing and data collection processes, and links all elements of the process to team evaluations. Development of management reports such as accounts receivable agings, bad-debt analysis by payor groups, and write-offs can provide a measurement tool for outcome measurement purposes.

The aged accounts receivable report identifies the current age of the agency's accounts receivable. Various approaches can be used for aging reports. Some prefer aging reports based on date of service; others prefer aging reports based on the end of the period or when invoices were submitted. Each approach serves a different purpose. Aging by date of service is a good indicator of actual credit extension. Aging reports based on the end of an accounting period will allow reports to be reconciled to general ledger balances; however, from an actual credit extension perspective, this type of reporting tends to average results. The final approach has a positive and negative element. The positive element is it provides a truer indicator of credit extension once internal processes were completed; however, the negative side is that receivables will look better than they actually are. Running a combination of reports will identify internal processing time. Additionally, shifting the outcome measurement may reveal additional information, for instance, the composition of commercial balances. Are they primarily uncollected copayments and balance bills? If they are, consideration should be given to reclassifying, sending to a collection agency, or changing approaches.

Table 14–4 illustrates an aging based on total receivables at period end. Outstanding balances are reflected next to a provision for bad debt. The report also

Table 14–4 Accounts Receivable Aging by Payor Group

Payor	Current	30 to 60	61 to 90	91 Plus	Total	Reserve	Reserve percentage	Annualized revenue	Average revenue	DSO	Target	Variance
Medicare	85,250	43,200	14,500	2,750	145,700		0	1,023,000	2,803	52	45	(7)
Medicaid	15,320	14,895	16,325	10,632	57,172	1,595	3	183,840	504	114	90	(24)
MCOs	45,200	23,200	10,000	3,500	71,900	3,500	5	542,400	1,486	48	45	(3)
Commercial	8,500	13,450	10,000	17,359	49,309	3,472	7	102,000	279	176	90	(86)
Subcontract	23,500	24,680	800	100	49,080	100	0	282,000	773	64	60	(4)
Total	$177,770	$119,425	$41,625	$34,341	$373,161	$8,667	2	$2,133,240	$5,844	64	60	(4)

Reserve		
Actual	2	
Target	1	
Variance	−1	

measures aging and reserve targets against actual results. Use of ratios was covered in a preceding chapter. Every payor category indicates that significant improvement is required.

In this situation, the agency was not able to meet its objectives for average days service outstanding (DSO) and for its provision for bad debts. This caused the agency to incur an additional $5,700 in interest expense assuming an average annual interest rate of 9 percent, and an additional $5,568 in bad-debt expense because of not being able to meet its objectives for reducing bad-debt reserve (Table 14–5).

Accounts receivable management also includes exploration of alternative payment arrangements. This will include investigation of Medicare's periodic interim payment (PIP) system. PIP pays providers 26 payments on a regular basis. This provides an excellent tool for cash management. MCOs prepay capitated arrangements. Receipt of monthly capitated payments at the beginning of the month are more advantageous than receipt at the end of the month. Finally, requiring retainers or prepayments from private pay patients is an excellent way to stay ahead of service provision and accelerate cash collections.

PREPAYMENTS AND INVENTORY

Many insurance policies, maintenance plans, and contracts require payment for a year's worth of services in advance. Wherever possible, it is worth the time to

Table 14–5 Additional Interest Expense Caused by not Meeting Targets

	Actual	Target	Variance
Reserve	2%	1%	–1%
Medicare	$145,700	$126,123	$19,577
Medicaid	57,172	45,330	11,842
MCOs	71,900	66,871	5,029
Commercial	49,309	25,151	24,158
Subcontract	49,080	46,356	2,724
	$373,161	$309,831	$63,330
Additional interest expense	$63,330		
Average interest rate	9%		
Increased interest expense	$5,700		
Additional reserve requirement	$8,667		
Targeted reserve	$3,098		
Additional expense	$5,568		

investigate whether there are alternative payment arrangements possible. Normally, the amount of time is nothing more than a telephone call to your insurance representative. Many insurance companies offer installment payment plans for a nominal charge. The amount of financing charges will determine whether it is a financially prudent decision to request an installment payment arrangement versus a lump-sum payment.

Inventory is another area that consumes a large amount of working capital. Inventory cost is greater than the cost to purchase supplies and equipment. It is the cost of the supply, space cost for storage, interest expense for the purchased asset, cost associated with waste and obsolescence, and possibly personnel cost. Minimization of inventory items and cost can be accomplished by evaluating what supplies are used, what quantities are used on a monthly basis, and what supplies can be drop-shipped to the patient's home. Other cost-saving strategies include evaluating supplier relationships and obtaining competitive pricing. If supplies can be delivered quickly, there is no sense in carrying large inventories.

Tracking inventory usage will identify who draws supplies out of the supply closet. The challenge is to identify what supplies are used with each type of patient, what are billable versus nonbillable, and what happens to the balance. If employees are drawing excess supplies from inventory, and they are not being used but instead going bad in their trunks, this is an avoidable cost that, if managed properly, will reduce overall agency and per visit costs.

DISBURSEMENTS

Disbursements encompass payments to vendors, employees, and creditors. Payments of vendors and creditors fall into three classes: (1) vendors that offer discounts, (2) vendors that do not have specific terms, and (3) vendors that have specific terms and the ability to charge interest. Attempts should be made to take advantage of invoices that have discount offers.

Table 14–6 illustrates the approximate cost of discounts not taken. To determine the value of discounts, divide the discount percentage by 1 minus the discount percentage. This is then multiplied by the product of 360 days divided by the days that credit is outstanding less the discount period $(.01/.99) \times (360/20)$. Discounts can be taken if cash is available to take advantage of them; additionally, communication should be made to the purchasing department to try to negotiate discounts into its purchasing arrangements. If the effective discount rate is greater than the agency's cost of capital or hurdle rate, then it makes sense to take advantage of discounts.

The second class of vendors is those vendors that do not offer discounts. These vendors may have specified terms, or they may not, but they do not have the ability to charge interest. This class of vendors is typically trade vendors that can be

Table 14–6 Discounts

Terms	Discount days	Approximate cost of discounts lost (%)
1%, 10 Days, net 30	20	18.2
2%, 10 Days, net 30	20	36.7
3%, 15 Days, net 45	30	37.1

stretched in the event of cash shortages. They may attempt to charge interest but in the long run will be happy to have their main charges paid.

The final set of vendors is those that are critical to the organization and have the ability to charge interest for late payments. This group of vendors may include the landlord; the telephone and electric company; and assorted creditors, such as leasing companies. Typically, these vendors are paid on time. If they are not paid on time, they have the ability to assess an interest charge that is nonnegotiable.

Ultimately, attempts should be made at finding a balance between paying vendors when due and when they are threatening to discontinue services or ruin your credit rating. Vendors, suppliers, and the agency should work together. This may require soliciting bids for long-term suppliers that are involved in planning and distribution sessions, familiar with third-party payment problems, and willing to work with the agency in return for business. On a final note regarding vendors and suppliers, increasing the timeline between service provision and payment is a source of credit for the agency.

Payroll-related expenses are the single largest expense for any agency. Payroll-related expenses include employee gross pay, employer taxes, workers' compensation, health benefits, and any other payroll-related fringe benefit. Employees become very nervous if they are not paid on time or if they receive notices that their health insurance has been canceled for lack of payment. Therefore, health benefits and employees are included in the third group of vendors: those that are paid on a regular basis. Payroll taxes also fall into this category. If payroll taxes are not paid on a timely basis, interest and penalties are imposed and even imprisonment in severe cases.

Large Medicare providers that have transitioned to PIP can satisfy the majority of their immediate payment requirements by scheduling payments in conjunction with PIP payments. Collection efforts are still required to meet other cash disbursement requirements.

Another working capital management issue related to payroll is the issue of direct deposit. Direct deposit is a vehicle that deposits net payroll checks directly into employees' bank accounts. From an employee's perspective, this is wonderful; it eliminates the need to do banking, and it enhances cash forecasting ability. From the agency's perspective, it eliminates the ability to take advantage of employee payroll float. This is because the entire amount of net payroll must be transferred to each employee's bank accounts on the day of the payroll. In addition, there is a bank charge associated with this service. Therefore, the financial impact of transitioning to a direct deposit system must be weighed against perceived and real employee benefits and decreases in stop-payment processing time and cost.

When analyzing the cost of direct deposit, costs should be compared between the existing system and the cost of direct deposit. A paper-based payroll system has processing and bank cost associated with it. Processing cost includes the cost of printing payroll checks, preparation for mailing, distribution time, postage, envelopes, and the cost of checks. These costs will be extended by the frequency of the payroll. In addition to processing cost, there is the cost of the payroll bank account. Bank costs include monthly charges for account maintenance, deposits, disbursements, stop payments, account reconciliation, and compensating balances. In addition to these costs is the cost of lost float. In contrast, the cost for direct deposit is the cost of preparing a magnetic tape that is used to notify the bank of how much is to be credited to each employee's bank account. The bank will then handle all processing at a predetermined rate for processing. Transaction cost would be extended for the number of pay periods.

Similar to direct deposit are payments using wire transfers and preauthorized debits. Wire transfers are a vehicle to pay vendors immediately. Usually, they have a significant transaction cost associated with each transfer. Wire transfers require knowing the target bank's name, transit or routing code, and the target account number. Addresses for wire transfers can be predetermined or telephoned in on an as-needed basis. Preauthorized debits are similar to bank charges that are automatically deducted from the agency's bank account on a predefined basis. These transactions cause the agency to lose out on float and slow payment practices, but they also eliminate the need for processing because it is handled automatically.

CASHFLOW FORECAST

The cashflow forecast is an important management tool. Cashflow forecasts are used to estimate cash inflows and outflows. The net result will determine whether the agency needs to borrow funds or will have excess funds available to invest. Generally, cashflow forecasts are developed for different time spans. Practical time spans would be for a month, a quarter, or a 6-month time period, and are part of the annual budgeting process. The annual budgeting process may include a 3-year forecast as well. Attaching a cashflow forecast to the annual or 3-year forecast will help the agency determine whether current financing requirements are sufficient or whether alternative arrangements need to be made. Additionally, by looking at the entire 12-month period, credit peaks and valleys can be quantified.

Peaks and valleys could be due to seasonal fluctuations, new business growth, or the result of other transactions affecting cash.

The short-term and intermediate cashflow forecasts provide a vehicle for determining investment and borrowing strategies over a shorter time period. The cashflow forecast is composed of three major sections. The first section is receipts. Receipts can be from collections of patient accounts receivable, other accounts receivable, funding, rental payments, or other sources of operational cash. Cash receipt estimates will depend on the type of payors that the agency has, what arrangements they have negotiated for prompt payment, and the agency's collection efforts. For instance, an agency that is on PIP will be able to forecast accurately biweekly receipts. Prepayments because of capitated contracts are also easy to forecast accurately. It may be more challenging to estimate when other cash receipts will be received.

Forecasting the timing of other accounts receivable will depend on the agency's prior collection history and payor characteristics. Tracking of historic cash receipts usually will reveal a pattern. The pattern may be that 60 percent of a certain month's claims are paid within 30 days after mailing, 25 percent within 60 days, and the balance within 75 days. Identifying collection patterns by payor will provide an additional tool for cash forecasting. (See Table 14–7.)

Therefore, if revenues for a particular payor were $50,000, then $30,000 would be collected 30 days from the mailing date, $12,500 the following month, and $7,500 the following month. This technique can also be used for the annual forecasting of cash receipts on a monthly basis. It is also possible to use ratios for purposes of forecasting the annual receipts. The use of ratios tends to average seasonality and volume fluctuations unless adjusted accordingly. Furthermore, tracking collection patterns can also be used as part of continuous quality improvement efforts in the collections department.

The disbursement section will be based on net disbursements. Payroll represents the net amount exclusive of taxes that the agency will need to transfer into its payroll account to cover its biweekly payroll. If the agency is running a biweekly payroll, there will be two months every year that experience a three-payroll month. Cash planning should plan on building reserves to cover these occurrences unless they happen to fall at the same intervals as the month that the agency receives three PIP payments.

Withheld payroll taxes for federal withholding and social security can be deposited several days after the issuance of payroll. Exact deposit requirements will depend on the size of the total payroll and corresponding tax liability. In this situation, the payroll was paid out on a Thursday, and payroll taxes were not due until the following Monday.

Other disbursements include contract payments for temporary staff and therapists. Estimates for payout will depend on volume and payment terms. This will

Table 14–7 Monthly Cashflow Forecast

Receipts	Week 1	Week 2	Week 3	Week 4	Week 5	Total
Medicare		53,000		53,000		106,000
MCO	22,500					22,500
Other	8,000	3,000	12,500	7,000	400	30,900
Total receipts	$30,500	$56,000	$12,500	$60,000	$ 400	$159,400
Disbursements						
Payroll		38,500		38,500		77,000
Payroll taxes	4,320		4,320		4,320	12,960
Contract staff		12,500		12,500		25,000
Accounts payable	21,000		5,000		5,000	31,000
Lease payments		7,200				7,200
Other				2,000		2,000
Total	$25,320	$58,200	$ 9,320	$53,000	$ 9,320	$155,160
Other						
Credit line						
Intercompany						
Tax payments		(5,100)				(5,100)
Other funding						
Total other		(5,100)				(5,100)
Beginning balance	1,420	6,600	(700)	2,480	9,480	1,420
Cash requirements	5,180	(7,300)	3,180	7,000	(8,920)	(860)
Ending balance	$ 6,600	$ (700)	$2,480	$ 9,480	$ 560	$ 560

also apply to trade accounts payable. Lease payments and other are shown separately to identify disbursements that could happen on a regular basis, such as a lease payment, or on an infrequent basis, such as the purchase of equipment.

The third section is other. *Other* is where nonoperational sources of financing are listed. This can either be portrayed as net amounts or broken out separately to illustrate increases and decreases. This section would identify draws from credit lines, repayments, loan increases or payments, intercompany funds transfers, shareholder loans, tax payments, or shareholder draws.

The final section is the prior month's ending cash balance, net cash requirements, and the weekly ending cash balance. Reconciliation of the cashflow forecast to actual results will provide a vehicle for improving cashflow forecasting techniques. Also, when included as part of the annual budgeting process, the cashflow forecast helps determine accruals and changes in balance-sheet assets and liabilities in a fashion that is consistent with overall assumptions. For instance, if the assumption was that $50,000 of new computer equipment was going to be purchased in the fourth month of the fiscal year, then an amortization schedule could be developed to identify lease payments, ending current and long-term lease liability, and sales tax expense.

Other techniques analysis may require determining whether compensating balances are required or how liquid cash reserves need to be. It is not uncommon to have negative balances if cash is being properly managed.

Analysis of financing trends, purchases of equipment, and funds generated by operations can be accomplished by comparing annual results or trending on a monthly basis. Agencies that fund growth and investments in equipment from internal operations will be in healthier positions then those agencies that rely on external financing.

In summary, additional sources of working capital can be found in the following ways:

- Reduce excess inventories in nurses' trunks, supply closets, and the office.
- Accelerate the billing process by billing weekly, semimonthly, and timely.
- Actively pursue collection efforts.
- Utilize collection agencies.
- Encourage prepayment for private pay services.
- Take advantage of discounts.
- Take advantage of free credit from vendors.
- Bill electronically.
- Eliminate wasted and repetitive activities.
- Investigate electronic payment.
- Use lockboxes and controlled disbursement accounts.
- Match financing methods to the life of the asset.
- Control expenses.
- Reduce bad debt and write-offs.
- Avoid penalties and interest.

Chapter 15

Financing

Business strategy encompasses many different aspects of running a business. Strategy normally implies how one is approaching growing a business, what service lines will be developed, and how services will be marketed. Strategy also includes how one approaches financing. The concepts of financing that will be addressed in this chapter will deal with the development of the banking relationship, different types of funding strategies, and key elements in the preparation of a banking proposal, and will conclude with tools to evaluate the acquisition and expansion processes.

The previous chapter explored several concepts in the management of working capital. Working capital management is internally oriented versus financing, which has an external orientation. The reason financing has an external orientation is because funds will flow into the home health agency (HHA) from sources outside of the agency. The HHA will then be obligated to repay loans that have been made to the agency. Often, infusions of capital from owners will remain within the company. Funds are necessary for start-up, purchase of inventory and supplies, deposits for office space, and working capital.

Starting a new business is usually done with money provided by the owner. This strategy works for most business except Medicare-certified HHAs. Typically, an owner will make a loan to his or her new business, charge the business interest for the loan, and expect repayment when the new business is stable. Medicare views loans made to HHAs by related parties as capital contributions and not loans. This means that it will disallow any interest expense accrued and or paid to related parties; therefore, for finance costs to be reimbursable, interest expense accrued and payable cannot be to a related party. This approach does not make sense, especially if the owner is forced to obtain more expensive financing from a bona fide lending institution. However, this is typical of Medicare because the current program does not promote efficiency. Fortunately, this does not apply to HHAs that are not Medicare certified.

DEVELOPMENT OF THE BANKING RELATIONSHIP

The development of a banking relationship will depend on what services management is interested in obtaining. Banks provide services. This is why they are in business. Not all banks offer the same services, and each bank may have different charges for its services. Therefore, the development of a banking relationship depends on agency needs.

An agency that is able to fund its operations internally will have a different set of needs from one that must rely on external financing. An agency with operations that are simple and straightforward will have different needs from an agency with operations that are complex. Regardless of agency need and the level of services required, it is a good management practice to develop a strong relationship with banking institutions.

Banks are chosen for myriad reasons. Banks may be selected because of convenience, a referral from a board member, prior experiences, or services that meet the agency's current and future needs. Analyzing current needs and services can be done in conjunction with or independent of bankers. Needs analysis could be based on business projections that anticipate a need for a working capital loan to finance growth, transition from a traditional disbursement account to a zero balance account, a loan for the purchase of an office building or computer equipment, or transition to direct deposit. A comprehensive service analysis would consist of conducting a survey of local banks to determine what they charge for their services. A smaller analysis would consist of visiting the banker and talking to him or her about charges and service availability.

Once rates are obtained, it is fairly easy to determine what the agency's monthly bank fees would be based on historic usage or anticipated plans. The objective is twofold. The first part is to determine which bank has the most competitive pricing. This can be accomplished by using the customer account analysis illustrated in Table 15–1. Charges consist of a flat amount charged for service. The face amount of charges is one factor to consider. The other factor to consider is the effect of the bank's reserve requirement and earnings allowance. It is possible to have higher fees but less costly services because of a higher earnings allowance.

The second step is to determine whether bank fees can be paid outright or whether they must be paid through compensating balances. Compensating balances will provide the agency with a lower yield than if funds were invested elsewhere. Furthermore, if compensating balances are required as part of a loan agreement, they will increase the effective rate of the loan. Table 15–1 illustrates a hypothetical customer analysis and includes an explanation of the account analysis categories. Table 15–2 illustrates the annualized rate of return for compensating balances.

Table 15-1 Customer Account Analysis

Earnings allowance: 3.0518% (a)

Total daily ledger balance (b)	$14,867,000
Average ledger balance (c)	495,570
Less average collected funds (d)	393,570
Average collected funds (e)	102,000
Less 10.0% reserve (f)	10,200
Average balance available for services (g)	91,800
Balance required for services (h)	84,103
Balances available for additional services (i)	$ 7,697

Services provided	Units	Unit price ($)	Service charges ($)	Required balance ($)
Checks paid	407	0.14	54.95	21,200
Deposit tickets	26	0.30	7.80	3,009
Items deposited	398	0.10	39.80	15,355
Items posted	21	0.15	3.15	1,215
Redeposited item charge	1	2.00	2.00	772
Special statement cut-off	1	20.00	20.00	7,716
FDIC insurance (.16/1,000)			79.29	30,592
Maintenance fee	1	11.00	11.00	4,244
Total analyzed charges			217.99	84,103

(a) The earnings allowance represents the "interest rate" used to estimate the bank's revenues from using the business's idle funds. The earnings allowance rate normally is tied to short-term funds costs, but may contain a spread for the bank. The earnings allowance is negotiable, varying between banks and often among bank customers.

(b) The total daily ledger balance sums the ending bank ledger balance for every day in the month. The bank ledger balance reflects the full value of deposits the day they are made; therefore, the ledger balance differs from the business's general ledger by the amount of outstanding checks and deposits-in-transit. The monthly bank statement reports the bank's ledger balance.

(c) The average ledger balance (calculated by dividing the total daily ledger balance by 30 days) represents the average daily ledger balance for the month. (Banks sometimes assume all months have 30 days to simplify their calculations, and to avoid paying the annual equivalent of five days' interest.)

(d) The average uncollected funds represent the amount of uncollected deposits included in the average ledger balance amount. Because these funds were still being collected through the banking system, the depository bank cannot earn interest by investing or loaning them. In other words, to calculate an amount of idle cash the bank can use to earn revenues, the bank reduces the customer's ledger balance by the amount of uncollected deposits.

(e) The average collected balance represents the average, for the month, of each day's ending account balance that the bank could use to earn interest.

(f) The 10.0% reserve represents another amount the bank cannot earn money from and, accordingly, the bank removes this amount from the average collected balance. The Federal Reserve requires the bank to place a specified percentage (which generally varies from 7%–13%) of its collected demand deposits with the Federal Reserve. The Federal Reserve pays no interest to the bank on these reserve funds. Some banks accomplish the same adjustment by reducing the earnings allowance percentage by the 10.0%.

(g) The average balance available for services represents the company's idle cash that the bank can loan or invest.

continues

Table 15–1 continued

(h) The balances required for services represent the amount of idle cash needed for the bank's earnings to equal the business cost of services. The bank lists and prices the services used by the business in the lower portion of the customer account analysis report, and then uses the earnings allowance rate to calculate the amount of required balances ($84,103 = $217.99 ÷ 3.0518% ÷ 31 × 365).

(i) The balance available for additional services represents excess cash that earns the bank additional profits on the account. By law, the bank is prohibited from paying a commercial depositor for its excess balances. However, the business may negotiate with the bank that any balances available for additional services are carried over to the company's other accounts, carried forward to future periods, or applied to loan origination and commitment fees. If the business does not use these balances, the bank's profitability on the account increases, and the business's return on its idle funds decreases.

Source: Reprinted from *PPC's Controllership Guide* by D.A. Tolson, R.S. Ray, J.S. Purtil, et al., pp. 3–75, with permission of Practitioners Publishing Company, © 1993.

Beyond routine banking services is the need for capital. Capital requirements can be short term or long term. Generally, short-term requirements span a month or two up to a year, while long-term commitments are in excess of a year. The length of long-term commitments will depend on the nature of the loan. Obtaining short- or long-term financing will depend on the financial strength of the HHA, what type of financing the agency is interested in obtaining, the bank, and potentially the owners' credit and guarantee.

Not all banks follow the same lending criteria. Some banks are only interested in loans if they are backed by real estate, others are positioned to service specific industries, while others are only interested in loans that are short term in nature and heavily collateralized. Therefore, when considering banks, it is important to evaluate not only routine services but also whether they can meet all of the financing needs of the HHA.

Table 15–2 Return on Compensating Balances

Average collected funds	102,002
Less 10.0% reserve	10,200
Average balance available for services	91,802
Earnings allowance (3.0518% × 31 ÷ 365)	0.2592%
Subtotal	$ 237.95
Less FDIC insurance charge ($495,570 × .16 ÷ 1,000)	−79.29
Compensating balance earnings credit	$ 158.66
Annualized rate of return ($158.66 × 12 ÷ $102,002)	1.87%

Source: Reprinted from *PPC's Controllership Guide* by D.A. Tolson, R.S. Ray, J.S. Purtil, et al., pp. 3–75, with permission of Practitioners Publishing Company, © 1993.

BANK FINANCING

Credit Lines

There are several different types of bank financing available. Loans or debt financing can meet short- or long-term needs. Credit lines are typically used to meet short-term credit needs. Credit lines can be established for several months, a year, or sometimes longer. Credit lines will vary based on duration and type of credit provided. Additionally, credit lines may be renewable at the end of the term or payable in full.

There are three main types of credit lines: (1) noncommitted, (2) committed, or (3) revolving. A noncommitted line is nonbinding from the bank's perspective. Funds are available today but may not be available when needed. This may be due to changing business conditions, the overall economy, or the financial status of the HHA. Committed lines are available to be used by the agency when needed. Committed lines have a fee attached by the bank that is pledging funds availability. In fact, there is an interest fee charged for borrowed funds and the potential for a fee on the unused portion of the credit line. Interest rates typically are prime plus several points. Point range will depend on how interested the bank is in the HHA's business, the amount of the loan, and the presence of other services being provided. Additionally, committed lines will require periodic paydowns. Paydown periods range from 30 to 60 days. During this time, the borrower cannot draw any more funds from the bank.

> Committed lines require a fee to ensure availability and covenants to ensure that certain basic conditions are met. In addition to requiring a company to be solvent, such conditions and covenants may require the maintenance of a certain minimal financial profile. This might include certain financial ratio tests such as the company's ratio of debt to net worth, minimum earnings, working capital, and other limitations. When these conditions are not met, the bank may waive these requirements in consideration for past fees paid and the bank's judgment that noncompliance will not hurt its chances for repayment. While there may be no immediate need to borrow from the bank, the company may desire to put the committed line in place in anticipation of the need to borrow in the future. This approach to borrowing obviously requires the company to evaluate the commitment fee, legal requirements, severity of covenants, and interest rate before entering into an arrangement.[1]

Revolving credit lines are similar to credit cards. They do not require annual paydowns. Instead, there are monthly payments based on interest calculated on the outstanding balance and some repayment formula. Repayments will increase credit availability, and draws will decrease credit availability. Revolving lines usually require renewal and often convert to term loans.

Accounts Receivable Financing

HHAs' major assets are their receivables. Accounts receivable financing is a loan made based on a business's receivables. Generally, a bank or finance company will advance a busine's a percentage of its current receivables. Advances are calculated based on customer type, payment history, credit terms, and industry standard. Receivables that are older than a specified amount, say 75 days, would be ineligible for advances. In return, all payments must go directly to the lending institution.

There are two types of loans. One is a notification loan, and the other is a nonnotification loan. Under the notification loan, the lending institution notifies the agency's clients to submit remittances directly to the lending institution. The nonnotification loan causes this financing technique to remain blind to the HHA's customers. Obviously, this is preferable.

Normally, remittances will go directly to a lockbox controlled by the lender. The lender will deposit all remittances and return to the borrower one minus the advance rate. If the accounts receivable loan is set up in a revolving fashion, when remittances are received in the lockbox and clear the lender's bank, available credit will also increase.

Factoring

Factoring is the outright sale of receivables to a bank or factoring company. The factor will purchase receivables for a discount from face value. The discount will depend on the age and type of receivables, customers, and the frequency of receivable turnover. The discounted amount of the receivable is then advanced to the client, and the factor begins the process of collecting the receivables. This has presented a problem for Medicare receivables. Conservative factors would not purchase Medicare receivables because they are not truly owned by the agency and could not be assigned. However, entering into a three-way agreement with the bank and the factor will allow the bank to factor Medicare receipts to the factor without violating the antiassignment provision. "Medicare payments due a provider may be deposited at a financial institution as long as the check is drawn in the provider's name and the provider certifies that the following conditions have been met: (a) The financial institution is not providing financing for the provider, nor acting on behalf of another party in connection with financing, and (b) The provider has sole control of the account, and the financial institution is subject only to the provider's instructions."[2] This does not apply to other types of agency receivables.

Factors generally collect the receivables that they purchase. "Legally, a factor takes immediate title to the invoices it purchases, where the accounts receivable lender only takes title to invoices if the borrower defaults on its loan agreements."[3] Factors also will purchase receivables with or without recourse. Recourse entitles the factor to come after the client for invoice payment if the invoice becomes uncollectible. This event will take place if the invoice reaches a certain age (e.g., 120 days) and is typically handled by charging the client's account.

There are two common approaches to factoring. One approach uses a system of advances and reserves (Table 15–3). An advance rate is determined for current invoices ranging from 50 to 70 percent.[4] Then a fee is charged against the collected invoice. The longer that it takes to collect the invoice, the higher the fee will be. The other approach is a flat fee plus interest. The flat fee or commission is charged against all receivables factored. Interest is calculated against the outstanding loan balance.

"As a condition of entering into a factoring relationship, virtually all factors will insist on taking a perfected first priority security interest in client accounts receivable. Most factors prefer to take a first position on both factored and unfactored

---

Table 15–3 Advance/Reserve Factoring Schedule

Total face value of invoices $100,000
Advance paid to client (80%) $ 80,000
Reserve balance (20%) $ 20,000

Payment collected in (1)	Factoring fees/ discount rate	Reserve rebated to client	Total payment to client (2)
Day 1–15	$2,000/2%	$18,000	$98,000
Day 16–30	$4,000/4%	$16,000	$96,000
Day 31–45	$6,000/6%	$14,000	$94,000
Day 46–60	$8,000/8%	$12,000	$92,000
Day 61–75	$10,000/10%	$10,000	$90,000
Day 76–90	$12,000/12%	$8,000	$88,000

(1) The collection period begins on the day that the factor advances funds to the client (which is not always the same as the invoice date), and is normally divided into "windows" or "time bands" of equal duration. Windows most typically occur in 15-day increments, although 7-, 10-, or 30-day increments are not uncommon.

(2) When a single advance/reserve transaction covers multiple invoices, fees are usually calculated for each invoice based on its individual collection period. Accordingly, the total fees actually incurred in a given factoring transaction will reflect a blended average of aggregate invoice performance.

receivables, thereby maintaining a reasonable recovery alternative if factored invoices become uncollectible due to disputes or client fraud. On rare occasions, however, some factors have been known to restrict their security interest to factored receivables only."[5]

Term Loans

Term loans have a duration from 90 days up to several years. Repayment can be monthly or quarterly or include a balloon payment at the end. Term loans are usually used in conjunction with other types of financing, such as a credit line, and are secured by the assets of the agency and the owner. Term loans are usually for purchases of equipment, office buildings, or the result of converting a short-term working capital loan to a term loan. Interest can either be fixed or variable and is usually calculated at prime plus several points. Variable interest will fluctuate based on changes in the prime rate.

All loans will include loan covenants. Loan covenants can be positive or negative. A positive covenant states that the company will do something, for instance, maintain a certain debt-to-equity ratio. A negative covenant states that the company will not do something, for instance, will not sell any of its assets. Generally, the sole purpose of the loan document is to protect the bank's interests. It includes covenants such as making sure all taxes are paid on time, insurance polices are in force, and that the bank has the right to inspect the business premises. Other covenants could include restrictions on the amount of capital expenditures, owner compensation, and loans to affiliated or unrelated businesses, and could require notification of adverse situations.

Preparing a Bank Proposal

Bankers are nervous individuals. They have to follow prescribed formulas for lending money and can become very nervous when events do not materialize in the fashion that they were anticipating. One of the ways that the senior management team of an HHA can increase its current or prospective banker's confidence is by helping to educate him or her regarding the home health business. Most bankers will not understand the concept of cost reimbursement and businesses that have small bottom lines. However, a sound strategy pursues presenting the financial and projected operational results in a fashion that will not only enlighten current or prospective bankers about operational results but also demonstrate that the HHA is soundly managed.

This will require the development of a presentation that conveys a knowledge of exactly what financing outcome the agency is interested in achieving, how funds will be used and repaid, and a proactive management structure that is business savvy and competent. Bank proposals follow a general format of summary, senior management profile, description of the home health business, loan specifics, and projections and historical statements. Personal financial statements will probably be requested in addition to agency information.

Proposals generally begin with a summary. The summary identifies the agency, its address, the purpose of the loan, how the loan will be secured, and how it will be repaid. The next section is on the senior management team. This section expounds on the skills and managerial talent of the management team. Generally, one to two paragraphs are written for each of the key members, identifying education, skills, accomplishments, age, responsibilities, length of time at the agency, industry involvement, and experience. Portraying a strong management team helps to lend credibility to future plans and objectives.

A description of the home health business is another important element of the proposal. This section identifies how a particular agency competes, what trends are occurring within the industry, what services are being offered by the agency, what strategies are being employed for survival against competitors, and how the provider is preparing for the future. Other elements to include in this section are the HHA's legal structure, age, location(s), number of employees, customer base, identification of cyclical factors, labor issues, and agreements.

Loan specifics identify the purpose of the loan, how much funding is requested, what the mix of funding is, and how the loan will be repaid. Loan specifics should be consistent with the plans and objectives listed in the prior section; for instance, the loan is for working capital and equipment related to the expansion of an existing or new service line. The amount of the loan should be consistent with the projections identified in the following section. Therefore, asking for a different amount would be inconsistent with the rest of the presentation. Funding mix could be a combination of a credit line and a term note. The financial projections should include estimates for interest expense on the new credit instruments, repayments, and any other charges that may be incurred with the new financing.

Projections and historical statements should be presented consistently. This makes it easier for the reader. Generally, three years of historic financial statements are presented, interim statements as of the date of the bank proposal, forecasted year-end, and a projection of the upcoming year. Statements should be made in a summary fashion and include a full set of statements and notes. Supplementary information could include an accounts receivable aging, explanation of any extraordinary events, product line profitability, trend analysis, consolidations, and ratio analysis.

The banking proposal will be reviewed to determine whether historical and anticipated results fall within bank guidelines for debt-to-equity ratios, working capital, and debt repayment. Projections are reviewed for reasonableness given prior history and current management. In addition, personal financial statements will be reviewed to determine whether there is recourse against the owner in the event that the agency cannot repay its loans. Typically, the owner will become a guarantor for the agency's loan. In place of owners, the members of the board of directors could be asked to be guarantors for loans. It is important that the loans be to the HHA and not to the owner who then turns around and loans the agency the proceeds. Loans need to be directly to the agency for reimbursement purposes.

THE COST OF CAPITAL

The cost of capital is not as straightforward as using the stated amount of interest for a credit line or term note. There are other factors that will increase the stated amount to the actual effective rate:

- loan origination fee,
- points,
- appraisal cost,
- compensating balances,
- audited statements,
- legal fees,
- accounting fees,
- prepayment penalties,
- commission, and
- additional clearing time.

Table 15–4 illustrates a cost of capital calculation for a $1 million credit line of which $800,000 has been drawn. The terms of the credit line called for an annual commitment fee of 1.5 percent of the total credit line, a stated interest rate of prime plus 1.5 percent for a total of 10.5 percent, a compensating balance of 15 percent of the current outstanding balance, and an annual audit. The annual audit fee had an incremental cost of $10,000. The actual cost of capital is 16 percent and not the stated 10.5 percent. Additionally, this rate would increase if the commitment fee is paid at loan inception and not at the end of the year.

Table 15–5 illustrates how to calculate total credit requirements given a compensating balance requirement. A 20 percent compensating balance has the effect of increasing the cost of capital from 10.5 percent to 13.3 percent. This represents a 25 percent increase in the effective rate of the loan. Table 15–4 illustrated other costs associated with financing that increased the effective rate of the loan from 10.5 percent to 16 percent. In this example, loan-related costs increased the effective rate of the loan by 52 percent. Careful analysis of all loan-related costs will reveal a cost of capital that is significantly higher than the stated interest rate.

Table 15–4 Cost of Capital Calculation

Loan costs	
Loan interest @ $10.5%	$ 84,000
Commitment fee @ 1.5%	15,000
Annual audit (incremental cost)	10,000
Total loan-related costs	$109,000
Available funds	
Outstanding balance	$800,000
Less compensating balance @ 15%	120,000
Net loan	$680,000
Effective interest rate	16%

OTHER FINANCING STRATEGIES

In today's banking environment, small to middle market home health agencies, organizations billing between $500,000 to $40,000,000 per year, are underserved. The reasons are simple. The large national and regional "money center" banks are interested in providing working capital to institutional service providers such as large national public companies, academic or major hospital-based health systems. The smaller, community based banks that used to lend to small to mid-market providers have dwindled in number due to a consolidation in the banking industry. Those that remain are operating with extreme caution, particularly in the healthcare services area where the principal collateral—accounts receivable—is difficult to appreciate due to a complex reimbursement scheme. Put simply, community banks are afraid of making asset based, working capital loans to home health care agencies without alternative sources of repayment such as cash or unencumbered property.[6]

This has caused agencies to locate alternative sources of funding. An alternative source of funding, factoring, was listed above. Factoring is an option that will

Table 15–5 Calculation of Total Line Requirements with a 20 Percent Compensating Balance

Credit needed	680,000
Divide by (1 − compensating balance)	0.80
Total amount to borrow	850,000
Interest expense ($850,000 × 10.5%)	89,250
Effective rate	13.13%
Cost of capital increase	25.00%

provide additional sources of capital as receivables grow; however, there is a significant cost to factoring and potential limitations if receivables do not turn over quickly enough. Other sources of capital come from fundraising, retained earnings, personal and private sources, government agencies, equity sources, and leasing.

Fundraising is only available to not-for-profit agencies. Fundraising efforts help agencies to cover operational deficits from providing services to individuals who do not have the ability to pay for services. Fundraising activities can include $100 per plate dinners, cake sales, golf tournaments, car washes, costume balls, dances, or myriad other fundraising activities. Funds can also come from gifts, grants, endowments, or major funding agencies like the United Way. Funds can be for a specific purpose, such as for the acquisition of new equipment, or they can be general purpose funds.

Positive retained earnings or fund balance is a source of financing for the agency. Often, retained earnings are minimal or nonexistent in a Medicare-certified environment; however, related companies may have significant retained earnings. Retained earnings represent an efficient source of financing. Use of retained earnings is an internal funding concept consistent with the concepts addressed in the previous chapter. Often, customer credit falls into this category because it is usually considered in the purchase price.

Personal sources of financing would come from the owner or his or her extended family. Although this method is commonly used by most businesses, it is not practical in a Medicare-certified home health environment because of the related party concept. This does not prohibit agency principals from obtaining financing from private sources. Actually, this could be a win–win for both the agency and the lender. As noted above, the cost of capital to an agency is quite significant when one considers all of the costs related to financing. Sharing some of the spread between money market rates and the agency's cost of capital would certainly provide an attractive investment arrangement for potential investors. All loans should be thoroughly documented for clarity and the protection of the agency.

Government agencies at the state or federal level may be an additional source of funding. Federal and state governments provide a lot of money through the Small Business Administration (SBA) and other agencies for the sole purpose of helping finance small business growth. These agencies also have thresholds where they target loans that meet certain criteria (e.g., loans to businesses owned by women or other minorities). These loans will require significant lead time and may not be a vehicle for short-term working capital loans but instead a vehicle for the acquisition of equipment or other assets. Care should also be taken to make sure that the loan is to the agency and not the principals.

Equity sources of capital from public offerings of stock will not be available to the typical HHA. Large providers of intravenous (IV) therapies and services have been able to take advantage of this funding vehicle because of strong financial performance including the ability to generate significant profits.

LEASING

Leasing provides a vehicle to obtain equipment. Leasing is an alternative to acquiring assets with bank loans and/or scarce cash reserves. Leasing has gained popularity as a relatively easy mechanism to acquire assets without going through the bank loan application and approval processes. Generally, leasing companies are only interested in ascertaining whether the business has the ability to make lease payments. In the event that the financial statement of the HHA is not strong enough to support the financial requirements of the leasing company, then the leasing company will require the guarantee of the owner. If multiple companies are involved, there may be a need for cross-collateralization.

Leasing provides an agency with several advantages over traditional financing. Leasing conserves scarce cash reserves. Leasing is similar to a payment plan in that it stretches payments out over the length of the lease. Therefore, equipment can be purchased or rented over the course of the lease instead of having to make full payment on Day 1.

> Leasing usually provides 100 percent financing, requiring no down payment and allowing companies to conserve cash. In contrast, most loans for new equipment require a down payment of 20 to 30 percent of the equipment's cost. Although the payments on a lease may be higher than on a conventional loan, many expanding companies do not have the cash reserves for a substantial down payment. Leasing can be particularly attractive in periods of tight money. In addition, because leasing requires no down payment, a company can use the cash saved for investment, expansion, payroll, increased production or the reduction of current liabilities.[7]

Lease rates will depend on the length of the lease, the dollar value of the lease, who retains rights, type of equipment and residual value, buy-out options, and the lessee's credit rating. Obviously, the longer the lease, the smaller the monthly payments will be. The dollar value of the lease will also determine the rate. Placement of a small lease will have a larger interest cost than the placement of a larger lease. If the agency is in the process of expanding and knows that it will be purchasing, for example, $100,000 worth of equipment in three lots, it may be more efficient to get one lease to cover all three lots, instead of three separate leases. The aggregate purchase would put the lease into a cheaper rate category, and it would reduce administrative effort on a monthly basis.

Lease rights depend on the nature of the lease. Some leases transfer all responsibility and benefits to the lessor. These leases are referred to as *capitalized leases*. Capitalized leases require that the agency reflect the asset and corresponding liability on the agency's balance sheet, and depreciation is recognized on the income statement. A capitalized lease must meet one of the following four conditions:

1. The lease transfers ownership to the lessee at the end of the lease term.
2. The lease contains a bargain purchase option.
3. The lease is equal to or greater than 75 percent of the asset's useful life.
4. The present value of the lease payment is equal to or exceeds 90 percent of the asset's fair value.

On a monthly basis, the agency would reflect interest expense and depreciation. The principal payment would be a reduction of the liability. The bargain purchase option could be a reduction of the estimated fair market value of the equipment at lease end. This is too open-ended. It is better to have a known amount, such as $1, as the bargain purchase amount. Furthermore, for equipment that is quickly obsolete, such as computer equipment, it is advisable to get the bargain purchase option as low as possible. Operating leases, on the other hand, are rentals. At the end of the lease, the asset is returned to the lessor. These are referred to as *off balance sheet leases*.

Leasing provides a vehicle to update equipment continually. Similar to a leased automobile, one never has anything at the end of the lease; however, one has a new automobile every three years. The trade-off is a higher monthly payment for the ability to rent. "Leasing reduces the lessee's risk of equipment obsolescence by shifting that risk to the lessor, who relies on remarketing skills to ensure the highest possible resale value."[8]

Shopping for leasing prices requires that one evaluate comparable pricing. This requires that the leases being evaluated have similar assumptions regarding duration, end of the lease buy-out options, monthly payments, maintenance requirements, and executory costs.

One of the largest disadvantages of leasing is that leases do not permit termination without penalty. This feature will penalize the agency for early payoff of the lease obligation. Other disadvantages include no equity build-up, higher interest amounts, and end of the lease buy-outs for less than the fair market value of the equipment.

CAPITAL EXPENDITURES

Capital expenditures is a term used to refer to the purchase of equipment with a useful life in excess of a year. Capital expenditures are investments in the HHA's infrastructure and should be evaluated in respect to current and future needs. Most equipment acquisitions are for copiers, fax machines, telephone systems, and computer equipment. Equipment purchases need to consider current use and future requirements in relation to equipment cost and capacity. For instance, a copy machine that is purchased today for current needs but cannot handle the volume in a year from now will be replaced or supplemented. Usually, the cost of replacement or of an additional copier is greater than the incremental cost of purchasing a copier that can handle tomorrow's needs.

Needs assessment is based on current and anticipated volume, service requirements, and features. Anticipated volume analysis is directly related to business plans. Volume considerations will depend on whether visit or service volume increases, decisions are made to open or close a branch office, or changes occur in referral bases. Needs will depend on agency headcount and the effect that changes in service volume have on equipment usage.

Asset cost depends on type of equipment, options selected, warranties, service plans, and product name. Cost also depends on the amount of equipment purchased, the timing of payment, and the cost of getting the asset in-house and operational. In addition to purchase cost, there are other costs associated with insurance, maintenance, facility preparation (wiring for computer network), local and long-distance calling, supplies, and financing.

Needs assessment also requires determining whether existing equipment is enabling the agency to be as efficient as possible. For instance, a high-speed copier may reduce the amount of overall time spent making copies, or a copy machine that tracks the number of copies by individual, department, or function could enhance the cost accounting capabilities of the agency. Plain paper fax machines may reduce costs by eliminating the need to make copies of thermal paper faxes and eliminate the need to sort and uncurl fax receipts. Telephone systems that have decision trees, utilize voice mail, provide for paging, have call waiting, and have conference calling will eliminate the need for wasted time and energy.

Discounted Cash Flow

Evaluating investment decisions, capital expenditure analysis, and financing decisions can be enhanced through the use of discounted cashflow analysis. Discounted cash flow (DCF) considers the time value of money. Basically, money has a cost associated with its use. DCF analysis calculates the present value of future payment or income streams. To determine the present value of future payment or income streams requires discounting each of the future periods to determine the investment's current value.

Table 15–6 demonstrates the concept of the time value of money. In the table, $1,000 invested at 10 percent will increase the principal amount of $1,000 to $1,100 by the end of Year 1, $1,210 by the end of Year 2, and $1,331 by the end of Year 3. To determine the present value of the investment today, you would multiply the anticipated cash inflows or outflows by the present value factor. Therefore,

Table 15–6 Future and Present Value Calculations

	Year 1	Year 2	Year 3
Future value	$1,100.00	$1,210.00	$1,331.00
Present value factor	0.909091	0.826446	0.751315
Present value	$1,000.00	$1,000.00	$1,000.00

a cash inflow or outflow of $1,331 in Year 3 at 10 percent would be worth $1,000 today.

To calculate present value of an investment, a financing decision, or a cash inflow or outflow, one must determine the present value factor. The present value of a cash inflow or outflow can be calculated using the following formula where "n" represents the period in which the cash flow occurred. Cash flow is the net amount of cash that is being produced from an investment or used by a capital expenditure. It is revenues less expenses with an addback for depreciation and taxes. Depreciation represents a period expense to the agency, but it does not require an outlay of cash because the asset has already been purchased in a prior period. The effect of taxes is included to reduce net cash flows. This will not apply to not-for-profit HHAs; however, for any taxable entity, there is an economic cost attached to positive cash flow and needs to be taken into consideration. Present value can also be determined by multiplying a present value factor by the anticipated cash inflow or outflow. Table 15–7 identifies various present value factors for interest rates ranging from 6 to 15 percent and up to 10 periods.

$$\text{Present value} = \frac{\text{Amount}}{(1 + \text{Interest Rate})^n}$$

Net present value (NPV) is the sum of the present values for all cash inflows and outflows. It is the summation of all cash flows for Periods 1 through the last period, less the cost of the investment. Typically, there is a cash outflow occurring immediately (the investment) and subsequent cash inflows occurring in future periods. NPV is a measure of the present value of the investment decisions to the agency. A positive NPV indicates that the project, regardless of whether it is an investment, such as the building of a pharmacy or the acquisition of an existing business, is generating a return at least equal to the cost of capital. A negative NPV indicates that future cash inflows do not provide a return equal to the cost of capital.

This method is superior to using a payback method for evaluating investment profitability. Payback does not consider the time value of money or the cost of capital. Instead, consideration is only given to the length of time that it takes for the initial investment to be repaid.

Table 15-7 Present Value Table

Period	6%	7%	8%	9%	10%	11%	12%	13%	14%	15%
1	0.943	0.935	0.926	0.917	0.909	0.901	0.893	0.885	0.877	0.870
2	0.890	0.873	0.857	0.842	0.826	0.812	0.797	0.783	0.769	0.756
3	0.840	0.816	0.794	0.772	0.751	0.731	0.712	0.693	0.675	0.658
4	0.792	0.763	0.735	0.708	0.683	0.659	0.636	0.613	0.592	0.572
5	0.747	0.713	0.681	0.650	0.621	0.593	0.567	0.543	0.519	0.497
6	0.705	0.666	0.630	0.596	0.564	0.535	0.507	0.480	0.456	0.432
7	0.665	0.623	0.583	0.547	0.513	0.482	0.452	0.425	0.400	0.376
8	0.627	0.582	0.540	0.502	0.467	0.434	0.404	0.376	0.351	0.327
9	0.592	0.544	0.500	0.460	0.424	0.391	0.361	0.333	0.308	0.284
10	0.558	0.508	0.463	0.422	0.386	0.352	0.322	0.295	0.270	0.247

Table 15–8 evaluates the cost of building a pharmacy or purchasing an existing operation. Use of the payback method determines that both alternatives have an equal value. Using the NPV method to evaluate the two alternatives reveals that although purchasing a pharmacy has a larger outlay of cash today, the return to the HHA is greater over the five-year period. Therefore, if the NPV was the sole criterion used for investment decisions, then the choice would be to purchase a pharmacy.

The internal rate of return (IRR) is a technique that actually determines the project's rate of return. Decisions would then be based on which path yielded the highest IRR. Use of this technique would cause the agency to choose to build its own pharmacy instead of purchasing an existing pharmacy. When the IRR method is used in conjunction with NPV, investment alternatives can be ranked. Therefore, if the agency had a hurdle rate of 24 percent for all investments, it would select building over purchasing, even though purchasing had a higher NPV.

If the IRR was used in the preceding NPV calculation as the cost of capital, then the project's NPV would equal zero. The calculation of a value for the IRR requires an iterative process that begins by substituting higher interest rates into the NPV equation until NPV is less than zero. An average is developed using an interest rate that causes the NPV to be less than zero and the last interest rate that yielded a positive NPV calculation. Table 15–9 illustrates this concept using the cash flows associated with building a pharmacy.

Development of a Hurdle Rate

Earlier in the chapter, the concept of the true cost of capital was addressed. Cost of capital is more than the face amount of a debt instrument. It is the total of all

---

Table 15–8 Evaluation of Two Investment Alternatives Using a 13 Percent Cost of Capital

	Build	*Purchase*
Initial outlay	($250,000)	($500,000)
Cash-flow year 1	$50,000	$125,000
Cash-flow year 2	$75,000	$175,000
Cash-flow year 3	$125,000	$200,000
Cash-flow year 4	$125,000	$200,000
Cash-flow year 5	$150,000	$250,000
Payback period	3 years	3 years
NPV	$97,675	$144,600
Internal rate of return (IRR)	25.40%	23.10%

Table 15–9 Calculate Internal Rate of Return

	Build	Present value factor	25%	Present value factor	26%
Initial outlay	(250,000)	1.000	(250,000)	1.000	(250,000)
Cashflow year 1	50,000	0.800	40,000	0.794	39,700
Cashflow year 2	75,000	0.640	48,000	0.630	47,250
Cashflow year 3	125,000	0.512	64,000	0.500	62,500
Cashflow year 4	125,000	0.410	51,250	0.397	49,625
Cashflow year 5	150,000	0.328	49,200	0.315	47,250
		NPV	2,450		(3,675)

NPV @	26%	(3,675)
NPV @	25%	2,450
Difference	1%	6,125
IRR =	25% + ((2,450/6,125) × 1%) =	
IRR =	25.4%	

costs related to the debt instrument. The hurdle rate is the cost of capital plus adjustments for risk, investment return, and the effect of taxes.

The reason for making the tax adjustment is as follows. The value of the firm's stock, which we want to maximize, depends on after-tax income. Interest is a deductible expense. The effect of this is that the federal government pays part of the charges. Therefore, to put the costs of debt and equity on a comparable basis, we adjust the interest rate downward to take account of the preferential tax treatment of debt. It should be noted that the tax rate is zero for a firm with losses. Therefore, for a company that does not pay taxes, the cost of debt is not reduced; that is, the cost of debt is equal to zero. Note that the cost of debt is the interest rate on new debt, not the interest rate on any old, previously outstanding debt. In other words, we are interested in the cost of new debt, or the marginal cost of debt.[9]

Calculation of an investment hurdle rate would be accomplished by using the 16 percent cost of capital rate calculated earlier, adjusting it for (1–tax rate) in consideration of tax consequences, and then adjusting for risk and investment return (Table 15–10). "Management should exercise judgment when assessing the degree of risk associated with each proposed capital project. A proposal to modernize facilities may carry a low risk, but a proposal to expand into a completely new line of business may represent a moderate to high risk."[10] Risk is related to the

Table 15–10 Calculation of Investment Hurdle Rate

	Not-for-profit (%)	For-profit (%)
Cost of capital	16.00	16.00
Tax adjustment @ 27.5%		−4.40
Net cost of capital	16.00	11.60
Risk adjustment	10.00	10.00
Investment return	4.00	4.00
Hurdle rate	30.00	25.60

uncertainty of projections, the reimbursement environment, the flow of referrals, and assumptions regarding growth and return (Table 15–11). Investment return is the amount of profit that management wants to generate over and above the cost of capital.

An alternative method of incorporating risk into investment analysis is by using the expected value of the cash inflows (Table 15–12). Expected value is the process of assigning probability to an event. Probability is based on management's best guess of the likelihood of an event occurring. The expected value that would be used for the above NPV analysis would be the weighted average of cash inflows and outflows for each period. In the above example, forecasted revenues and expenses would be weighted as part of a sensitivity analysis to determine the probability of events occurring to arrive at the expected value.

The Decision Process

The decision process will evaluate capital expenditures and investments based on return (NPV, IRR), impact to cash flow, timing, the environment, and the agency's access to cash. Included in the decision process is the agency's stance on risk. Projects that are risky (e.g., starting a pharmacy) may have too much risk

Table 15–11 Investment Risk

Degree of risk	%
Little or no risk	0
Low risk	1–5
Moderate risk	6–10
High risk	11–15

Source: D.A. Tolson, R.S. Ray, J.S. Purtill, A.L. Dyer, D. Puckett, and G.W. Smith, *PPC's Controllership Guide*, pp. 7–12, Practitioners Publishing Company, 1993.

Table 15–12 Expected Value Calculation

Net cash flow	Probability	Expected value
$ 40,000	0.15	$ 6,000
60,000	0.25	15,000
80,000	0.30	24,000
100,000	0.20	20,000
$120,000	0.10	12,000
	1.00	$77,000

associated with them for the owner and the management staff to feel comfortable. However, if the risk is shared with a partner, then the project may be a viable option.

Cash flow is a major consideration. Will the agency have the available credit to complete the project and provide the working capital to grow the operation according to the projections? Is the management staff capable of pulling it off? This includes project management activities to make sure that the project will complete based on the timeline estimates included in the pro-forma, costs are managed to prevent overruns, and the organization has the technical expertise to generate sales and provide services. Additionally, what impact will the project have on overall credit availability? Will all credit be used for the new project, thus causing a financial hardship to the existing operation? If this is the case, other financing arrangements may need to be made.

Obviously, these types of questions will not apply to replacing a copier or telephone system. However, they would apply to a major strategic decision, such as starting a new service line, building a pharmacy, acquiring a new business, or changing information systems. These decisions will affect current and future operations, so it is necessary to make sure all of the elements are in place before beginning on the journey. In addition, timing becomes an important element.

Some say that timing is everything when bringing a new product or service to market. The health care marketplace is in such transition that project risk is higher than in a nontransitionary environment. This may cause an HHA to opt to invest in a new computer system that will enhance its understanding of the cost of providing care, provide better information, and improve its ability to manage patient populations. An investment in agency infrastructure such as a computer system will have a negative NPV unless the new technology eliminates cost associated with manual processes. In either case, the NPV or IRR will probably be less than expanding into a new business line. Therefore, in this situation, timing is the development of a strong base before expanding into new territory.

Once the decision has been made, then financing alternatives need to be considered. Tables 15–13, 15–14, and 15–15 represent an analysis to determine the best

Table 15–13 Lease versus Purchase Assumptions (3 @ $13,500 = $40,500 To Purchase)

	Bank loan	Lease
Down payment	$8,100.00	
Term	60 Months	60 Months
Interest	13.0%	
Monthly payment	$737.20	$963.49
Maintenance/month	$1,000.00	$1,000.00

way of financing the acquisition of three automobiles for the HHA. The analysis indicates that it is less costly for the agency to purchase the automobiles instead of leasing them. This conclusion is based on the NPV of cash outflows. The reality of the situation is that depending on the terms of the lease, how much down payment or security deposit was required under either scenario, salvage value under the purchase scenario, the HHA's tax situation, mileage limitations on the leased automobiles, and whether the HHA had the cash available for a down payment would drive the decision for which financing method was the most appropriate.

Other assumptions were that MACRS 200 percent declining balance method was used for depreciation of the automobile in Table 15–14, there would be no resale or salvage value, and maintenance and insurance costs were the same under each scenario. Taxes were also ignored. Additionally, a conversion to the straight-line method of depreciation had no effect on selection of financing method. Table 15–14 indicates a lower NPV than Table 15–5. It needs to be noted that this is actually a negative NPV because these are cash outflows.

Table 15–14 Purchase Scenario

Purchase analysis	Year 0	Year 1	Year 2	Year 3	Year 4	Year 5	Year 6	Total
Expenses								
Interest		3,926	3,246	2,473	1,594	593		11,832
Depreciation		8,100	12,960	7,776	4,666	4,666	2,333	40,501
Maintenance		1,000	1,000	1,000	1,000	1,000		5,000
Total expenses		$13,026	$17,206	$11,249	$7,260	$6,259	$2,333	$ 57,333
Cash-flow effect								
Net expense		13,026	17,206	11,249	7,260	6,259	2,333	57,333
Less depreciation		(8,100)	(12,960)	(7,776)	(4,666)	(4,666)	(2,333)	(40,501)
Down payment	8,100							8,100
Plus principal payments		4,921	5,600	6,373	7,253	8,254		32,401
Total cash outflows	$8,100	$ 9,847	$9,846	$ 9,846	$9,847	$9,847		$ 57,333
Discount rate	1	0.885	0.783	0.693	0.613	0.543	0.480	
Net present value	$8,100	$ 8,714	$7,709	$ 6,823	$6,036	$5,347		$ 42,729

Table 15–15 Lease Alternative

Lease analysis	Year 0	Year 1	Year 2	Year 3	Year 4	Year 5	Year 6	Total
Expenses								
Lease payment		11,562	11,562	11,562	11,562	11,562		57,810
Depreciation								
Maintenance		1,000	1,000	1,000	1,000	1,000		5,000
Total expenses		$12,562	$12,562	$12,562	$12,562	$12,562		$62,810
Cash-flow effect								
Net expense		12,562	12,562	12,562	12,562	12,562		62,810
Less depreciation								
Security deposit		1,927				(1,927)		
Plus principal payments								
Total cash outflows		$14,489	$12,562	$12,562	$12,562	$10,635		$62,810
Discount rate	1	0.885	0.783	0.693	0.613	0.543	0.480	
Net present value		$12,822	$ 9,838	$ 8,706	$ 7,704	$ 5,772		$44,842

NOTES

1. R. Bort, *Corporate Cash Handbook* (Boston: Warren, Gorham & Lamont, 1994), E4-19.

2. J. Huffman, Factoring Grows as a Source of Operating Revenue in Wake of Towers Debacle, *Home Health Line* (February 27, 1995): 3.

3. M. Edwards, Factoring for Cash Flow: An Option, *The Small Business Controller* (Fall 1994): 12–16.

4. J. Huffman, Factoring Grows as a Source, 3.

5. M. Edwards, Factoring for Cash Flow, 12–16.

6. E.D. Leder, Accounts Receivable Funding for Home Health Care Agencies, *The Remington Report* (August/September 1994): 29–30.

7. R.D. Wolf, Leasing: The Competitive Advantage in the 1990's, *The Small Business Controller* (Winter 1995): 42–46.

8. *Ibid.*

9. E.F. Brigham, *Financial Management: Theory and Practice* (New York: Dryden Press, 1985), 252.

10. D.A. Tolson, et al., *PPC's Controllership Guide*, 7–12.

Part VI

Strategic Management

Chapter 16

Information Systems

The home health industry is in transition. The transition is affecting all aspects of the home health delivery process. Regardless of whether the transition is referred to as the maturing of an industry or a paradigm shift, the result is that industry participants will be rewarded for cost efficiency; the ability to deliver quality; and the ability to measure, demonstrate, and manage outcomes. The other central theme is that to become cost efficient, providers must rely on information systems to streamline operations and provide economies.

A paradigm shift related to information systems is that they need to provide value to the home health agency (HHA). It is no longer acceptable to have systems that do not communicate with one another, thus requiring manual input or rekeying of data already in the system, repetitive entry of the same data, or the inability to link clinical and financial data. Systems need to reduce input time, to reduce processing time, and to facilitate ease of extracting information from within the system. Advances in hardware, software, and communication technology have transformed data processing systems into information systems. Information systems have become an integral element of agency infrastructure that enables managers to make informed decisions about the services they provide.

The concept of infrastructure is important. Infrastructure is the base of supporting systems and business applications that allow the agency to meet the regulatory, business, and competitive requirements of running a home health business. Without an automated infrastructure, there would be 100 percent reliance on manual labor and systems. The automated support structure could revolve around a central depository, or database, or the structure could link different applications using various data transfer methodologies. Advances in information technology and the development of integrated systems allow users to do more with less. Integrated information systems eliminate the need for duplicative data entry; eliminate the need for volumes of paper records; and provide for the easy transfer of information from one employee to another, from one department to another, or from the agency to a payor, a physician, or to a remote branch office. Not only have advances in information technology enabled users to accumulate information with less personnel, but also the quality of information has improved. The quality of information, and the ability of management to use information, will determine how well the agency will be able to compete in the future.

This chapter begins with the current information processing environment, identifies trends that are forcing the status quo to change, and identifies some of the changes that are beginning to take place currently and in the near future. Among the current changes are advances in hardware, software, internal communication devices, and external communication devices. Once the changing framework has been identified for information system capabilities, the chapter will transition into issues related to the management of information systems.

THE CURRENT ENVIRONMENT

Home health is a highly regulated business. The Medicare system required the submission of multiple 485s, 486s, and 487s. In addition, claims were to be submitted on UB-92s. Data processing systems were developed to meet these needs. Unfortunately, data processing systems were nothing more than the automation of a manual process, typically the billing process. Data required for the billing process are entered into a computer system by following a sequence of steps; the data are then printed out on the appropriate form; and the provider accumulates the forms and mails them to the respective payors. Enhancements to this process allowed for the electronic submission of claims to providers that accept electronic claim submission.

The collection of clinical activity required nursing professionals, therapists, and aides to submit paperwork to the HHA on a timely basis for entry into the computer system. Depending on agency protocol, field employees were either required to return to the office daily to complete paperwork, dictate results into a tape recorder and mail tapes to the office, mail paperwork, or drop off notes at a later point in time. On receipt of nursing documentation, data entry clerks transcribed data or entered information into the computer system to initiate the billing process.

The collection of clinical activity for billing is one element of the automated processes that takes place within an agency. The automation of the payroll, accounts payable, and the general ledger processes enabled managers to manage the majority of the business processes within the agency. Electronic spreadsheets such as Lotus 1-2-3 and Microsoft Excel were added to automate off-line processes, such as budgeting, forecasting, cash management, and development of support analysis for the HHA's operations. Other software packages were added to meet the growing information needs of the agency. These software packages include word processing, cost reporting, time management, tax packages, graphics packages, fixed assets, and database packages. The database packages were added as a mechanism to extract data out of the billing software to use in sophisticated analysis for responding to managed care requests. Unfortunately, the clinical and billing software were not collecting the data that managers needed to make prudent decisions regarding pricing for managed care proposals.

Table 16–1 indicates the results of a *Home Health Line* readers' survey to which 314 home health executives responded.[1] The following chart illustrates that the primary purpose of automation is for billing and that, in general, HHAs rely on automated processes for the majority of their informational needs.

Hardware purchases were dependent on the recommendations of software vendors, cash flow, agency size, and attitudes toward automation. Low-volume agencies may have initially started out with one or two personal computers. One computer housed the billing package, and the other computer was shared by personnel for word processing, analysis, and accounting-related activities. Generally, the computers and the software were supported by outside consultants or one individual who had an interest in computers and software.

Medium volume agencies were directed by their billing software vendors to invest in local area networks (LANs). LANs allowed multiple workstations to use the same billing software. This was accomplished by linking several personal computers to a file server. This step enabled several employees to be entering data into their computers at the same time and have data stored in a central repository, the file server, until it was time for billing. Accounting applications were either on the same LAN or on a separate LAN. The introduction of the LAN increased the

---

Table 16–1 How Home Care Companies Stack up on Automated Functions

	Medicare (%)	Private (%)
Creation/revision of nursing care plans	42	32
Electronic claims filing	90	31
Electronic deposit from third party	28	12
General ledger	78	70
Home care provider scheduling	32	32
In-home vital signs and other data	13	11
Interfacing with payors' MIS*	32	13
Inventory	41	37
Patient charts/records	40	31
Statistical analysis of patient satisfaction	28	24
Tracking costs versus outcomes	21	18
Other	7	6

*MIS = management information system.

sophistication of the computer system and introduced potential communication, storage, and retrieval problems, thus requiring more technical expertise to be available to support the computer system in the event of problems.

High-volume agencies were directed by their billing software vendors to invest in minicomputers. Minicomputers could support many users, provide more storage, and accommodate the needs of large HHAs. Data entry is through terminals that served one purpose only, that of data entry, and often were referred to as *dumb terminals*. Others used personal computers for both data entry into the minicomputer and for the balance of their computerized processing needs. This type of computer system is expensive to maintain because it requires investment in expensive equipment, staff to operate and maintain the system, and perpetual equipment maintenance.[2]

Regardless of the hardware selection, HHAs were still faced with multiple problems. The first problem was that they needed a vehicle to handle the automation requirements of the nonbilling processes within the agency. Some vendors provided accounting and human resource management solutions and supported various software packages but were basically unable to meet all of the financial and administrative needs of the HHA. This required investing in alternative software and additional hardware solutions. Software solutions were chosen because of prior experiences, recommendations, or the ability to accomplish a specific task. Hardware solutions were selected based on cost and need.

Beyond software solutions, manual systems had to be implemented to compensate for the inability to communicate between systems. Manual systems consisted of many steps beginning with the processing of billing data, reentry of billing data into accounting systems for purposes of financial reporting, and then reentry of financial data into electronic spreadsheets for analysis. Output from database query software added more data for purposes of analysis; however, in-depth analysis was limited because software had been designed to conform to the needs of the Medicare reporting system. Therefore, costs and clinical data were collected for purposes of billing and the filing of the cost report, not for the needs of managed care. Data beyond the scope of Medicare had to be obtained from additional data collection processes. These processes were costly, time consuming, and generally deemed unimportant until managed care organizations (MCOs) began controlling referral streams.

A second problem was related to cost. HHAs were incurring large costs in labor hours, nonproductive time, and support costs. Labor costs were related to the amount of personnel required for the data entry and billing process. Nonproductive time is the amount of time spent satisfying paperwork requirements instead of performing visits. Table 16–2 is an example of one agency's time requirements for completing Medicare documents. Nonproductive time can also be attributable to a "waiting queue" for one process to be completed before another one can begin.

Table 16–2 Time Requirements for Manual Paperwork

Document	Average time (minutes)
Intake referral	15
Initial assessment	90
Med lists (patient & chart)	90
Care plan	60
485 Form	45
Referral	40
Follow-up visit	96
Monthly 486 bill	107
Recertification	60
Updated orders	6
486 Form	30
Discharge summary	17

Source: Reprinted from Paul, L.S., Home Health Caregivers: At Their Fingertips, *Healthcare Informatics*, September 1994, pp. 35–38, with permission of Health Data Analysis, Inc., © 1994.

Support cost is an ongoing element of the cost of billing software. Software cost has three elements: (1) the initial purchase, (2) ongoing support requirements, and (3) the inability to adapt to changes or individual requirements.

Vendors lease the use of their value-added systems to home care providers and charge ongoing support fees to maintain the systems for software errors and regulatory compliance. Individual agency desires to enhance the systems they use every day are prohibited unless agreed to by the vendor as a result of determining market appeal to other customers. Innovation is discouraged, if not impossible. Individual customers are powerless to control their own systems because they don't own the software system and they may not modify it without invalidating their maintenance agreements. They cannot add data elements or modify how functions work to suit their changing business needs unless the software vendor agrees to modify "the system" to meet all customers needs, which is rarely accommodated unless mandated by regulatory requirements.[3]

PROSPECTIVE PAYMENT AND MANAGED CARE: THE CATALYSTS FOR CHANGE

The paradigm shift began with the foreshadowing of prospective payment. Under prospective payment, more is no longer better. This simple statement applies to the amount of service provided under an episodic or capitated payment structure, the amount of administrative costs under a per visit, episodic, or capitated payment system, and the length of time that patients remain on service. All of a sudden, cost analysis became a major concern, and the solution was not in the Medicare cost report. In addition to understanding whether costs were direct or indirect, costs needed to be understood in relationship to the type of services that were being provided. Service provision categories were expanded to understand costs by diagnosis-related group (DRG) classification, service line, and type of visit. Average cost per visit was no longer a good indicator of cost.

Managed care was introduced as a vehicle to reduce the outlay of health care dollars. MCOs have become middlemen whose sole purpose is to reduce spending, thereby retaining a larger amount of the health care premium for themselves. The management of the home health care delivery process is accomplished through risk-sharing payment mechanisms such as episodic and capitated payments. In addition, discount per visit payment systems utilize prior approval based on a case manager's interpretation of the amount of care a home health client will require. In addition, MCOs are demanding data regarding the quality of home health services provided, costs in relationship to client outcomes, and indicators of quality.

Success in the managed care environment requires HHAs to take a proactive stance. Successful HHAs will begin to accumulate data regarding the patients that they serve. Data regarding patient demographics, patient problems, presence of a caregiver, medical diagnoses, and nursing diagnoses must all be accumulated and analyzed. Patient problems must be dissected to determine whether increased care is because of psychosocial problems or the presence of multiple activities of daily living (ADL). Furthermore, to begin the quality and outcome measurement process, clinical pathways need to be developed that provide a standard of care but allow for customization based on patient problem, intensity, and progress. "A primary theoretical difference between traditional treatment plans and clinical paths is a data management system. Data management transforms a stagnant, regulatory tool into an evolving patient care tool that contributes to a larger, aggregate database. Data analysis will change clinical practices in the field and interventions and outcomes on the tool."[4] Evaluation against the standard will enable HHAs to improve the care delivery process, develop specialists by clinical pathway, train field employees, and evaluate team results against other team members. Additionally, this is the first step in transitioning from a quality assurance system based on retrospective review to a quality improvement system based on a prospective evaluation of care requirements.

Not only will HHAs need to develop clinical pathways and prospective care management systems, but also they will need to evaluate cost in relationship to the clinical pathway. It will be necessary to evaluate costs for the entire clinical pathway and its components and to identify the composition of costs associated with outcomes. Costs associated with an entire clinical pathway could cross organizational boundaries to include intermittent visits, private duty hours, infusion therapies, and equipment. Cost associated with the components of the clinical pathway may look at the cost of nursing only. Costs associated with outcomes will depend on how closely the patients fit within the clinical pathway, actual services provision versus planned, and milestone deviations. Exceptions should be analyzed to determine whether variances were due to internal processes, physician orders, medical complications, or patient problems.

As better data are collected, costs can be accumulated by DRG and broken down into patient problem classifications, and an evaluative tool can be developed for instantaneous pricing decisions. Classification of costs by both a medical model (e.g., DRG) and a patient problem model (e.g., nursing diagnosis) will allow HHAs to estimate prospectively how many resources a particular patient will consume. Taking this concept a step further, by linking together patient demographics, utilization, and resource consumption, the HHA would be able to bid on entire populations of potential customers.

One of the key elements of success in the managed care scenario is obtaining an information system that facilitates data collection of all elements in need of measurement and the development of a management staff that have the ability prospectively to manage costs, outcomes, and strategic direction. Without accurate data, providers will not be able to price their services accordingly. Without a sufficient return (profits), they will not be able to provide quality services, continually train and enhance employee skills, invest in information technology, and shape the evolving health care delivery system. In this new world order, information will bring a competitive advantage to those who know how to collect it, evaluate it, and market their services.

This last element is in itself a paradigm shift for many providers. Prior to managed care, referrals came freely. This will no longer be the case because other providers such as hospitals recognize that home health provides a mechanism for risk diversification and controlling another portion of the health care dollar, and offers a frontier where low costs and technological advances will ensure continued market growth. Therefore, understanding care requirements, pricing, and the relationship to acute care services places home health providers in the driver's seat. There is an opportunity to develop relationships within integrated health care systems, MCOs, or others controlling the patient population. The opportunity is that the provision of home health can save health care dollars, produce quality outcomes, and lead the way as a provider of community services. This element of the paradigm shift will reduce hospitalization to acute care and emergency situations only.

For home health providers to take advantage of these opportunities, they must have their houses in order. This means developing activity-based cost management systems, linking costs to clinical pathways, and eliminating nonvalue-added activities. All of these objectives can be advanced through the acquisition of an information system that facilitates data collection and evaluation, includes the tools for activity-based management and clinical pathway costing, and provides for the measurement of performance indicators. Without an automated process, the amount of manual labor and effort that would be required would be cost prohibitive. Additionally, without the use of an integrated database, and the flexibility to adjust and change data collection elements, providers will be no better off than they had been.

CURRENT TRENDS

Fortunately, there have been some significant advances in information technology that will provide HHAs with the tools to become winners in a prospective or managed care environment. First, the cost of personal computers continues to decline. Not only do prices continue to fall, but also the power and capabilities of the personal computer continue to grow. In fact, advances in hardware technology make personal computers as powerful as some of the minicomputers that have been recommended by software vendors, and for a fraction of the cost. From an investment perspective, purchasing computer hardware is as poor a decision as purchasing an automobile because of how quickly it depreciates. In the case of computers, this is aggravated by advances in technology causing some hardware to become obsolete.

Advances in hardware also include advances in portable computers. Portable computers provide agencies with a vehicle to collect information during the visit or immediately after the visit. Collection of data immediately provides for better data to be collected, reduces the need for the nurse or other professional to decipher notes scribbled on a piece of paper, and provides for the timely update of information into the agency's main system. Generally, portable computers enable nurses to download copies of the records of the patients whom they will visit during the course of the day. The patient record will have every aspect of prior interactions with this patient, thus providing for consistency of care and reduction of duplicative interventions and costs. During or after the visit, the professional updates his or her electronic record. Records are transferred at the end of the day or over the course of the evening to the HHA's host computer. Transmission of data is usually done over telephone lines. Telephone lines could be in the patient's home, the professional's automobile, a payphone, or the nurse's home.

Advances in telecommunications provide for additional opportunities.

Within the last few years, wireless data packet networks have been introduced in major metropolitan areas. More recently, cellular providers have announced plans to also support digital packet capabilities over their facilities. Both types of networks are designed specifically to accommodate the data communication needs of mobile workers. These wireless networks provide an additional degree of flexibility since they allow home care workers to place high-speed data calls from their homes, from their cars, from the patient's home or from anywhere in between, without the need to connect to a telephone line.[5]

Not only does this process eliminate the need for data entry back at the office, but also it enables nurses and other professionals to be more productive. Saint Mary's Home Care program in New York City estimates that the use of portable computers has reduced paperwork requirements by 75 percent, increased productivity by 36 percent, and increased cash flow by 7 to 10 days.[6] Cash flow increases because of the ability to bill payors faster instead of waiting for notes to be submitted and entered into the billing system.

Recent advances in computer technology now allow software vendors to develop solutions for the highly regulated and complex information collection, storage, retrieval, monitoring, and manipulation problems facing home health agencies. These systems improve the quality of care by reducing tedious paperwork to free nurses to practice nursing and by using computerized "expert systems" to assist in patient treatment planning and documentation. . . . The patient assessment checklist data collection facility allows for interactive data collection using a personal computer or pen-based electronic clipboard either at the agency or at remote locations (e.g., patient's home, caregiver's home, drop sites, etc.) and the computer assisted assessment can guide the caregiver through the assessment process and provide a patient-specific plan of care using master protocol libraries which reflect decisions selected by the caregiver at various "choice points." The on-line collection methodology allows for more interaction between the computer and the caregiver at the earliest point (the source) which maximizes the benefits of the system.[7]

Beyond the collection of data for clinical uses is the need to use the same data for the agency's financial and cost accounting systems. Use of patient-driven data allows for accurate costing because it is the patient's demographics, payor, and problems that will determine how data are classified within the financial statements of the agency. Moreover, by assigning costs to each unit of care at the patient level, accurate costing by clinical pathway and outcome can be accomplished.

The collection of clinical pathway costs will have two elements: (1) a direct cost and (2) an indirect cost. The direct cost is the result of labor, materials, and burden. These costs can be determined at the time of processing accounts payable or payroll by assigning their respective costs to specific patient transactions (e.g., a visit) and linking demographic, payor, and patient problem information to determine general ledger assignment. Indirect costs are the result of logistical activities, such as scheduling, delivery or transportation costs, and travel time to the patient's home.

As addressed in the activity-based costing and management section, there are additional costs that would then be assigned to the cost of the clinical pathway. These costs do not have a direct relationship to the patient; however, they are indirectly related as a result of processes that take place within the agency. There are three additional levels of cost that occur. One level is an administrative cost related to specific payors. These costs exhibit "batch-like" qualities. Batch costs cover the period between intake and discharge, and typically include billing, records management, quality assurance, and case management. The next layer of costs is business related. These costs are also process related but have less correlation to direct cost than do batch-level costs. Typically, these costs will pertain to a specific product line or to all product lines. These costs are related to human resource management, financial operations, and marketing. The last layer is enterprise costs. This is the cost of running the business that has very little correlation to per visit cost.

Capturing costs at each of these levels will provide a mechanism to transition the agency from a retrospective review of resources consumed by type of expense, to a system of prospectively managing processes that consume resources. This internal shift will enable management to understand the interrelatedness of cross-functional activities and embark on a journey of process improvement and the elimination of nonvalue-added activities. The development of a unit cost that has four elements can then be used as part of the HHA's internal benchmarking system and for proper pricing of services.

Understanding cost, clinical activities, and the relationship of costs to activities is essential for survival in risk-based contracts. Advances in information technology eliminate many of the data-entry tasks required by older systems. The effect of these advances will increase both clinical and administrative productivity. Technological advances should be quantifiable through measuring increased field productivity, improved cash flow, and the reduction of labor hours through the elimination of repetitive tasks and errors. This is possible through the use of rules-based systems and the integration of data using a common database. The new tools will also provide some less quantifiable results, such as the ability to use actual costs instead of averages.

Process improvement in accounting process will be due to the elimination of many manual processes that transferred data from one stand-alone software system to another stand-alone system. Of primary interest is being able to identify costs accurately. Integrated systems that utilize a common database provide accountants with a tool that they have only dreamed of. Not only are they able to extract data for analytical purposes, but also data will be accurate and provide sound indicators of how well the agency is performing. Furthermore, by combining clinical, financial, regulatory, and human resource applications to feed one database, the agency will have a tool available that will enable it to manage contracts centrally as well as its human assets.

The introduction of the compact disk–read only memory (CD-ROM) and multimedia applications has opened a whole new area for process improvement and the redesigning of the training function. CD-ROMs provide an inexpensive way of educating staff members using interactive formats.

> The most powerful feature of multimedia as a training tool is that the user actually hears, sees, and uses the content learned. When learning a new section, the student uses all of his or her senses to learn. The "hands-on" experience of these systems is particularly relevant when teaching software programs. Learning the concepts of Lotus 1-2-3 is one thing, but the experience and confidence gained from hands-on learning is [sic] something entirely different. A well-designed multimedia program uses self-diagnostic questions to give the student instant feedback as to whether or not they [sic] have comprehended the information. And, when a student doesn't understand, they [sic] are retrained. Self-diagnostics can be as simple as two or three multiple choice questions frequently interspersed in the material to make sure the concepts were grasped. It gives both student and teacher the tools to validate whether or not students are catching on before they go on to the next piece of information. Testing in a multimedia environment can come in several different modes: pre-test helps participants establish what knowledge they have prior to testing; post-test verifies that learning has occurred; and self-diagnostic examinations become a part of the learning experience itself.[8]

Multimedia will provide HHAs with a tool to enhance the knowledge base of all of their workers. No longer will field employees need to be pulled out of the field for day-long training sessions; instead, they can come into the office after their work has been completed to satisfy training requirements. Not only will multimedia eliminate the need for dedicated training staff (their efforts can be redirected), but also the quality of training can be enhanced and employee results tracked, monitored, and targeted as part of an organizational movement to increase the knowledge base of its workers. Training applications will include basic to advanced clinical practice procedures, updates in wound care, administrative policies and procedures, and eventually conferences. Furthermore, training becomes easy to document from an improvement and compliance perspective. Other benefits would include reduced costs for travel associated with seminars and conferences, increased productivity, and the ability to provide more training at a lower cost per employee.

The introduction of bar coding to the inventory management process has increased the ability of agency management to monitor the usage of supplies. The concept is actually quite simple and will provide a vehicle to reduce waste and obsolescence normally associated with medical supplies. All supplies would be marked with a bar code. When supplies are drawn from inventory by a nurse, he or she will run the supplies over the bar-code reader. The bar-code reader will then record the supplies that were taken. This facilitates a reconciliation of supply draws to supply usage. Variances between supply draws and usage identified in billing notes can then be investigated, thus eliminating excess bag inventories, waste, and theft.

Decreases in hardware prices and advances in connective technology have increased the efficiency of LANs. LANs have contributed to operational efficiency by permitting users to share files, thus eliminating the need to get up and go to someone's office, a file cabinet, or some other storage facility. Use of LANs also contributes to the use of common software among all members of the office staff. This makes training easier and enables employees to transfer knowledge around the office. Additional uses for office LANs include the sharing of multimedia libraries, electronic mail, and centralized back-up and security procedures.

Electronic mail is a mechanism to transfer messages to other terminals on the network. If all employees are on a common network, electronic mail provides a tool to send memos, schedule meetings, ask questions, or provide follow-up to questions. The electronic format allows users to send messages, respond, and archive. Electronic mail reduces cost associated with running around the office delivering memos or scheduling appointments. This type of communication is referred to as "sneaker-net."

Centralized back-up procedures can be initiated by the LAN administrator. This process ensures that data on individual machines are protected or "backed up" in the event of a problem. Utilization of a centralized back-up process will be accomplished using a tape back-up process. This is more efficient than backing up each machine with floppy disks or wandering around with the tape back-up to each machine on the network. Additionally, the LAN administrator can set up security levels to prevent users from accessing sensitive data.

Other LAN benefits include the ability to gain economies in peripheral devices such as printers and fax machines. LANs can be mapped so that users will send data to a designated printer or fax machine. The printer and fax machine have a waiting queue established so that data will be handled in the sequence that they arrive. Linking peripheral devices to the LAN reduces the agency's investment in hardware.

LANs provide an opportunity for transferring of data internally. Advances in communication software have enabled providers to transfer data externally. Typically, this is referred to as *electronic data interchange* (EDI). EDI encompasses the transmission of billing data to fiscal intermediaries using communication software and a modem. In fact, the economic benefits of EDI are so significant that payors such as Medicare are offering an incentive to bill payment electronically in 14 days. Payors have recognized that they reduce cost associated with the handling of paper claims through the use of EDI. It is estimated that 20 percent of the total health care expenditure is related to handling paper claims and that 70 percent of the administrative work related to paper claims is output from computers.[9]

From the provider's perspective, electronic billing is efficient because it eliminates the need to print invoices and support documentation, to package, and to mail. As discussed in the section on working capital management, invoices that are submitted to payors faster will be paid faster. Beyond turnaround is the ability to edit transmissions and correct claims that do not meet the payors' standards. Real-time correction also increases turnaround.

As payors begin to expand their EDI capabilities, HHAs will be able to inquire on-line regarding a prospective patient's service eligibility and enrollment status, thus eliminating the potential for disallowed services and bad debt. Additionally, payors will have the ability to transfer payments directly to the HHA's bank account. This is an efficient way of handling cash payments and should be chosen over traditional practices of placing a check in the mail. Advances in technology and the development of uniform standards will probably provide a vehicle for on-line posting of receipts and claim information in the future.

Other uses of EDI include the payment of vendors, placement of orders, electronic transfer of funds, and on-line inquiry to obtain information regarding patient referrals. Conversely, EDI will enable physicians, case managers, and other authorized individuals to go into the agency's database to review patient records. Linking the HHA's information system to a fax machine will enable nurse management to fax copies of patients' records to case managers or physicians while on the phone with them. This will facilitate real-time problem resolution.

Access to electronic bulletin board systems (BBSs) is another area that will benefit agencies. BBSs are databases that have been set up at sites all around the world to share information. BBSs can be accessed by using communication software and a modem. Electronic bulletin boards provide a vehicle to exchange information that is beneficial to other home health providers. Their applications are growing on a daily basis. Currently, BBSs can be used for on-line workgroups, for access to literature and research materials, for on-line journals, or as forums for education or customer focus groups. Use of electronic bulletin boards and the Internet (a series of connecting computers) will enable providers to transfer and obtain information from all around the world. Eventually, providers will be able to share costs, clinical pathway standards, and benchmarks with other providers without being threatened by how this information will be used.

THE NEAR FUTURE

According to Wendell,

> There is no doubt that the power of computers will continue to increase year after year, with little increase in price. A megabit chip is one that holds nearly one million bits; three, four, and five megabit chips have already been produced. This means that one computer chip will have the power that the largest computers had 10 years ago. Mainframe computers will virtually disappear by the end of the century, except in a few specialized situations. While the increase in computer power is impressive, the computer revolution has been powered by software. It is the availability of software that will perform every business operation and produce various analyses of sales and operations that no one ever considered doing manually that has caused the tremendous increase of computer use by business. So how will computers continue to change business operations in the last decade of this century?[10]

A few answers to that question are offered below:

- Mos\t companies will be paying their bills and receiving payments electronically using some form of EDI and electronic funds transfer. With both receivables and payables being handled by computer, cash flow should not suffer, but the days of living off the "float" will be over.
- Initial transactions, such as intake, scheduling, purchases, and payroll, will be computerized for even the smallest companies; the use of the manual bookkeeper or clerk will disappear; their efforts will be redirected.
- The computer will be able to provide financial statements, tax returns, and various analyses of operations on demand. Executives, nurse management, and team members will be able to obtain virtually any analysis of operations without going through the nursing or finance department.
- Expert systems will be able to make decisions that are now made by administrators, nurse managers, and the chief financial officer (CFO) regarding what mix of service lines to offer, what services to bundle in pricing decisions, and how to structure transactions for the maximum return to the agency with the lowest tax consequence.
- Computers will be voice-activated so that information can be inserted and withdrawn from the computer through simple English (or other language) commands.

• Computer security will be enhanced by the use of voice prints or fingerprints for identification before the computer will reveal certain files.

Additional advances in information technology will bring the ability for field personnel to access multimedia applications in the patient's home. Multimedia applications will provide answers for the optimal treatment of wounds, assessment of physical and psychological conditions, and enhancement of patient training by providing visual aides. This concept is similar to the just-in-time techniques that are employed by manufacturing processes. Access to data stored on CD-ROMs will provide a virtual library of information for the field professional or administrative employee to access.

Advances in telecommunications will provide an ability to monitor electronically patients' activities in the home. Initially, this type of equipment will be cost-prohibitive; however, like most technology, it will come down in price. "However, while video definitely has its place, electronic technology such as BBSs can offer many of the same services. Even an X-ray can be transferred with better resolution on a bulletin board than it can by a video."[11]

The electronic bulletin board system also provides a mechanism to transfer data between members of integrated delivery systems (IDSs). Information can be shared regarding prior patient history, current insurance information, current health status, a summary of all tests performed to date, and current courses of treatment. Not only does this provide significant efficiencies in the reduction of paperwork and duplicative tests, but also it provides a vehicle to optimize the care delivery process across an entire system.

In fact, through the development of a uniform approach to data collection, a longitudinal record will be possible. A longitudinal record will follow the patient, identify history, and identify current health status. Use of an electronic record would include X-rays, ultrasounds, laboratory and other test results, interventions, medication listings, and expected outcomes. A uniform approach to data collection would also facilitate the building of comprehensive clinical pathways. As attempts are made to reduce aggregate health care costs, home health care services will continue to grow.

MANAGEMENT OF THE INFORMATION SYSTEM

Management of information systems will depend on each individual HHA's strategy toward information systems. Some providers will purchase evolving systems that utilize a common database; others will use stand-alone systems and supplement their data collection needs with stand-alone software applications; some will attempt to build their own solutions; others will combine different applications and rely on data transfer protocols between applications. Strategies toward information systems also include an approach toward the development of an information system department. Small agencies may choose to have no designated information system employees and manage their systems through the use of support agreements. Others may choose to have one or two individuals who will be responsible for training and small repairs and rely on support agreements for problems beyond the scope of their expertise. Large agencies may have very technical individuals who are able to handle all of the training, software, hardware, and communication requirements. Regardless of the approach taken, there are similarities in the management of the agencies' information systems.

If the agency is paying for software support, it must be certain of what it is purchasing. Does the monthly support fee provide for regulatory updates, customer service support during business and off hours, training, and the resolution of programmatic errors? It is imperative that vendors are responsive to customer needs. If information cannot be transferred between applications, or there is some other problem with software, this will affect productivity. Decreases in productivity increase cost.

Hardware support agreements cover problems with the essential elements of the computer. Support agreements can either be purchased from the hardware manufacturer, the hardware vendor, or a third party. It is important to understand what is promised in the support contract. This includes response time, the types of parts that are covered, the type of replacement parts that will be used, the quality of the technicians used, and whether the fee is based on an hourly rate or on a monthly basis. The determination to enter into hardware contracts will depend on the quality of the agency's internal staff and the type of hardware that is being used.

Documentation of the information system is an excellent internal control procedure. Documentation is important because of employee turnover, planned maintenance, and system planning. Documentation can include recording all acquisitions of hardware and software by type, model number, and serial number. System documentation should include when software is registered, expiration date of warranties, coverage periods for service agreements, passwords, security levels, and contact names and telephone numbers for maintenance and support.

System documents should also include the steps that employees take to process different elements of business transactions, such as payroll, clinical applications, and financial applications. It is also recommended that diagnostic information be kept on file for each machine and the network and include a physical representation of how every element of the network and office communicate with one another. System documents should also include identification of controls such as passwords and authorization levels. Controls include passwords to prevent unauthorized personnel from accessing data they are not authorized to see. Authorization deals with verifying that only appropriate personnel can initiate or approve certain transactions. This concept prevents nursing personnel from issuing their own paychecks and accounting personnel from discharging patients. System authorization should be linked to internal controls for acquisition of goods and services and the system's password function.

Controls also encompass the rules that have been included in "rules-based" computer systems. A listing of rules should be included in system documentation not only to evaluate in the event that processes need to change but also to supplement other policies and procedures related to information systems. Other system-related control processes include control logs, the use of balancing algorithms, internal reference numbers, "log on" and "log off" lists, and system-generated error messages.

Management of the information system also includes developing policies and procedures related to the acquisition of equipment and software, training, maintenance, and security. Policies development could include the determination to purchase one specific brand of personal computer, to limit word processing or electronic spreadsheets to one type, or to link acquisitions to the strategic plan. Development of a uniform approach to systems development will make training and support easier, reduce costs associated with maintenance and data transfer, and reduce problems with incompatible hardware and software. Other policies may encourage company-sponsored training programs to increase employee proficiency or discourage the use of computer games (the electronic coffee break).

Policies and procedures should also consider software copyright laws. It is not uncommon for companies to purchase one package of software and transfer a copy from machine to machine. This is a violation of copyright laws. A solution to this approach is to purchase software for a file server that allows all employees to access the software or to purchase multiple registrations from the software manufacturer. Also, encouraging employees to bring in pirated copies of software is no better than stealing from someone else.

Security is a big issue with information systems. Security should include protection against software viruses, back-up procedures, disaster recovery, physical and user access, and insurance. Viruses can destroy software and are introduced to the systems data accidentally or intentionally. Virus symptoms include excessive disk access time, the appearance of hidden files and error messages, and the disappearance of programs and data files. Viruses come from software that employees bring in from home, electronic bulletin boards, and any place where a connection is made outside of a secure area. Regardless of policy, it is recommended to have the latest versions of antivirus software to check against known viruses on a daily basis. Virus-checking software is not the sole solution. Routine checks of personal computers, prevention of employees using nonagency software on office machines, right-protecting original software, and maintenance of software back-ups are preventive measures that will enhance system protection.

Back-up procedures are the process of saving data to tape or to disk. This process is designed to prevent the agency from losing data that have been entered into the system. Data can be lost because of file corruption, entry mistakes, power outages, or a combination of hardware and software problems. Use of an uninterrupted power supply (UPS) system is recommended to prevent problems from electrical failure. Surge protectors are recommended to protect systems from fluc-tuations in power coming into the system from electrical sources. Back-up proce-dures should be frequent, easy to perform, a combination of full and incremental back-ups, and back-ups stored in a fireproof vault or offsite.

Disaster recovery planning is becoming more critical as information systems become the infrastructure for business operations. Disaster can take many differ-ent forms, from natural disasters, to fire, to theft, or any unforeseen circumstance that would cause the agency to lose the use of its system. Therefore, disaster plan-ning should include a plan of how long it would take to become operational in the event of a disaster. How long would it take to get reconfigured, new hardware in place, the copy of the backed-up data loaded onto the new machines, and business functioning again? The answer to this question is the root of the disaster plan. In the event that the office were destroyed by fire, is there another location that could be used to resume operations? Is it a branch office, the owner's home, a turn-key office setup that can be rented on a moment's notice, or a suite of hotel rooms? Disaster planning needs to include peripheral equipment such as copiers, fax ma-chines, and printers. Disaster planning requires time and energy and should en-compass all aspects of the agency's operations. Hopefully, a disaster will never take place, and the disaster plan is never put into action. Furthermore, insurances should be up to date and include all acquisitions.

Another part of the management process includes determining storage require-ments, system capacity, and the replacement of inefficient components. Hard-disk storage is becoming cheaper and cheaper. Utilizing file servers with large data storage disks enables management to keep a lot of data on line. In the event that the system is producing more data than it can efficiently store, a decision needs to be made. One course of action is to invest in more hard-disk storage, another is to transfer files off line, and another is to eliminate data completely.

Investing in additional storage is practical as long as there is a need to store the data, and it does not decrease processing speed. If data are very rarely used (e.g., payroll history from two or three years ago), then it may make sense to store these data off line instead of deleting. Such data must be held to conform to Internal Revenue Service guidelines. Once data are deleted, they are gone forever. There-fore, consideration should be given before choosing this course of action.

System capacity encompasses the number of users that LAN software will sup-port, speed of machines, the amount of hard-disk storage, and RAM memory. Ca-pacity should be evaluated and included in part of the information system man-agement process. Management includes the evaluation of when upgrades will be performed, how they will be performed, and what the cost is of the upgrade. For instance, it may not be necessary to buy the latest and greatest personal computer for a secretary who only uses the machine for word processing. The minute im-provements that would be observable from a daily processing perspective would certainly not warrant the cost.

Training is a necessary element in the maximization of the agency's information systems. This may or may not be the responsibility of the information systems team. Without sufficient training, users will always have a learning curve that is counterproductive to maximum productivity. Training programs should be developed for all software selected in the agency. Additionally, there should be an opportunity for different levels of training as users become more proficient. Use of videos or multimedia or assignment of one individual as a trainer for each software package will help to accomplish this task.

PURCHASING A SYSTEM

Purchasing an information system is an investment in the future of the agency. Acquisition considerations should determine what the purpose of the information system is whether the agency possesses the expertise to run the system once it arrives, or whether staff need to be added. Determining the purpose for the system will need to include representatives from the various groups that will be using the system (e.g., nursing, finance, human resources, and information systems).

Factors to consider when purchasing a system include how flexible the software is to modifications based on agency need. Does modification include the ability to change screen design; add additional fields for data collection; create or modify reports; and attach security levels based on employee, department, or function? Does the system provide for outcome measurement, cost identification, financial reporting, and cost analysis? Will the system facilitate process redesign (e.g., the ability to eliminate a repetitive data entry task), or is the system no better than what is currently being used? Does the system have the ability to accommodate EDI requirements for both today and tomorrow? Is sufficient documentation provided with the system? Is documentation updated on a regular basis?

An additional consideration is what kind of supplier–customer relationship is the vendor willing to offer? Does the vendor provide access to support groups, share its plans for further enhancements, and have a commitment to excellence and quality that is similar to the agency's? What recourse is the vendor willing to offer in the event that the agency is not satisfied with the software it purchases, the support that it is receiving, or the evolution of the vendor's product?

There is no tried-and-true process for selection of software and hardware; however, as a practical suggestion, it makes sense to become as computer literate as possible before the process begins, determine what is wanted from the new system, and determine on what type of platform it runs. Vendors that force an agency to select a high-end hardware platform may not have its best interest at heart. This is especially true as personal computer prices continue to drop.

Furthermore, the agency should narrow the selection process down to three or four vendors. The top three or four vendors that meet the needs of the agency can then be asked to demonstrate their products. The agency should ask to enter data into their models, go to their shops and play with their equipment, or visit their existing customers. Prudent buyers will make sure that they are purchasing systems that provide value to the agency and meet current as well as future needs. Finally, the agency should make sure the vendor is financially sound, has the ability to transfer data from the existing system into the new one, and is interested in assisting the agency to accomplish its individual missions.

NOTES

1. *Home Health Line* (January 30, 1995): 7–8.
2. B. Coriaty, The Next Generation in Computer Technology Has Arrived, *The Remington Report* (June/July 1994): 24–29.
3. B. Coriaty, The Next Generation, 24–29.
4. J. Michel, Home Health Clinical Paths Produce Functional Outcome Data, *Case Management* (February 1995): 5–7.
5. N. Scalera, Home Healthcare Telecommunications Applications, *Healthcare Informatics* (August 1993): 44–48.
6. V. Torres-Suarez and J. Wong, Information Network Hits Home, *Healthcare Informatics* (September 1994): 54–56.
7. B. Coriaty, The Next Generation, 24–29.
8. S. Roden, Multimedia: The Future of Training, *Multimedia Today* 2, no. 3 (1994): 34–36.
9. G.F. Swarzman, Does Your Patient Accounting Process Pass the Test? *Health Care Financial Management* (July 1994): 27–34.
10. P.J. Wendell, *Corporate Controller's Manual* (Boston: Warren, Gorham & Lamont, 1995), A1–21.
11. R.J. Flaherty, Electronic Bulletin Board Systems Extend the Advantages of Telemedicine, *Computers in Nursing* 13, no. 1 (1995): 8–10.

Chapter 17

Strategic Management

Strategic management is a discipline that provides direction and helps to clarify intent. It is a concept that balances current and long-term requirements. Strategic management begins with the process of creating a vision, determines a mission or purpose for being, and establishes and implements the guiding values that will shape the home health agency (HHA). The management process incorporates the organizational blueprint (vision, mission, and values) with the results of the strategic planning processes to determine a course of action for the HHA. The course of action is then linked to operational plans or budgets. Strategic management goes beyond establishing an organizational blueprint and assessment to the incorporation of organizational values into daily operations. The linking of mission, vision, values, and intent to action creates strategic management.

Traditionally, this process has been referred to as *strategic planning*. However, the difference is that strategic management transitions the process from a plan that resides in the minds of several individuals to a value system that is known by all. Obviously, strategic management needs to be practiced for it to be known by all. The practicing of strategic management provides a vehicle for linking organizational values to daily operations and processes for the purpose of pursuing current and future objectives.

Inherent in the concept of strategic management are strategic choices commonly determined as part of the strategic planning process. Choices represent responses to opportunities and potential threats. Choice of direction will be influenced by the regulatory environment, the community, the presence of competition, core competencies, or myriad other factors. It is management's assessment of these factors that will influence how it chooses to position the HHA. Strategic direction will depend on the organization's mission, vision, values, and stance on risk in relationship to the assessment of opportunities and threats.

This chapter begins with the concepts of mission, vision, and values before transitioning into the development of the strategic plan. The strategic plan is an assessment tool that is used to define a course of direction. Once the strategic plan has been developed, it needs to be tested for validity and linked to operational plans and budgets. The next section develops the concept of a balanced scorecard as a mechanism to balance short- and long-term objectives. The chapter concludes with the Malcolm Baldrige criteria as an internal assessment tool to assess organizational quality and performance.

MISSION, VISION, AND VALUE

Mission is a statement of purpose. It is a statement about why the agency exists, what its purpose is, why it is in business, what its unique contribution is to society, and how it provides value.[1] Mission statements provide constancy of purpose. Mission statements often make reference to customers, employees, the community, shareholders, suppliers, and services provided. A proprietary agency may be in business solely to provide value to its shareholders. Its mission statement would focus on growth and profits. Community-based agencies may choose a reason for being that focuses on providing community services regardless of an individual's ability to pay. Hospital-based agencies may choose a mission that is complementary to the hospital's mission.

The development of an agency's mission statement is an iterative process. It requires an initial development and refinement. Refinement will occur through sharing the proposed mission statement with employees and customers. This process may create additional modifications; however, the goal is to develop a mission statement that resonates with all individuals who will be in contact with the agency.

Vision is what the organization will look like. It is a mental image of how all of the elements of the organization are working together to accomplish the entity's reason for being. "A vision is the essential element in organizational success. It provides direction and drives everything that is done in the organization. Without a vision, an organization is like a ship without a rudder."[2]

Although often used interchangeably, mission and vision statements are distinctly different, and each has its own purpose, style, criteria, and components. As shown in [Exhibit 17–1], a mission is for today's goals and the vision is for tomorrow's goals. The mission statement identifies an organization's customers and critical processes, often with a qualifier of what level of performance the organization is dedicated to delivering. The mission consists of those things that the organization concentrates on daily to survive. A vision statement, on the other hand, is a long range prospect or state of being that is worked on every day but will not

Exhibit 17–1 Mission Statement versus Vision Statement

Mission statement	*Vision statement*
Today	Tomorrow
Identifies the customers	Inspirational
Identifies the critical processes	Provides clear decision-making criteria
Level of performance	Timeless

Source: Reprinted from Latham, J.R., Visioning: The Concept, Trilogy, and Process, *Quality Progress,* April 1995, pp. 65–68, with permission of the American Society for Quality Control, © 1995.

be accomplished in the near future. The vision is that perfect state that might never be reached, but which you never stop trying to achieve. The mission–vision relationship is analogous to your personal life, in which you can categorize daily efforts into those that you do to survive today, such as going to work or fixing the car, and those you do to prepare for tomorrow, such as attending school to obtain a graduate degree or taking on a special project to prepare for higher responsibilities. For a vision to be successful, it must empower. Empowerment is a combination of motivation to act, authority to do the job, and the enablement to get it done. Enablement requires a vivid picture of the destination.[3]

Vision, like mission, should be shared. If it resides in one individual's mind, there will never be unity of purpose or the pursuit of a common vision; it will only be a personal vision. Ultimately, the goal is to develop a shared vision. Shared vision is when everyone within the organization knows what the vision is, can describe the vision, and works toward the vision.

A useful metaphor for shared vision is the hologram, the three-dimensional image created by interacting light sources. If you cut a photograph in half, each part shows only part of the whole image. But if you divide a hologram, each part shows the whole image intact. Similarly, as you continue to divide up the hologram, no matter how small the divisions, each piece still shows the whole image. Likewise, when a group of people come to share a vision for an organization, each person sees his own picture of the organization at its best. Each shares responsibility for the whole, not just for his piece. But the component "pieces" of the hologram are not identical. Each represents the whole image from a different point of view. It's as if you were to look through holes poked in a window shade; each hole would offer a unique angle for viewing the whole image. So, too, is each individual's vision of the whole unique. We each have our own way of seeing the larger vision.[4]

Values are what is important to the HHA. This is the core of strategic management. It is the linking of vision and mission to what really matters. Values represent an approach to the way business is conducted. Values are "walking the talk," they are defining what is important, and they are intrinsic to organizational success. Values could include a commitment toward quality of care for the sick and elderly, cost management, individual and organizational learning, employee and managerial accountability, and process improvement. Values provide the base for shaping the organization and creating the vision.

Values are not one-time events. They are ongoing, and they change in response to changes in organizational vision, purpose, internal circumstances, and external pressures. For instance, in a premanaged-care environment, the quantity and provision of multiple services were rarely questioned with respect to quality services. Quality and quantity seemed to go hand in hand. Now quality is demonstrated through the measurement of outcomes and relationship to cost. Both need to be quantifiable. Figure 17–1 illustrates how values change based on payment system. In a cost-reimbursed world, there was no incentive to control cost or to demonstrate quality. Service providers would be in Quadrants I or IV depending on their values, systems, and ability to measure and manage the clinical process. The initial phase of managed care is forcing prices downward. As the managed care marketplace matures, there will be increased competition for insurance premiums, forcing managed care organizations (MCOs) to reduce premium costs, provide high quality, and contract with providers that can assume increased amounts of risk, while delivering high-quality care. The provision of quality must be measur-

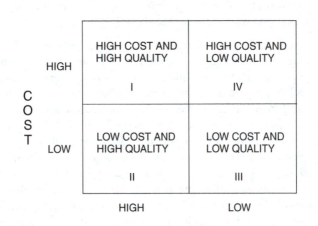

Figure 17–1 Cost/Quality Matrix. From a conversation with Donna A. Peters, Ph.D.

able and demonstrable to the patients who pay the managed care premiums and the MCOs that contract with providers.

Ultimately, the long-term winners will reside in Quadrant II. Therefore, organizational values must be consistent with what it takes to be a low-cost provider of high-quality services. High-quality services will be measurable, managed consistently by all levels of clinical staff, and supported by efficient support services. Efficient support services will be cost responsive, cost effective, and incented by the same set of values, vision, and mission as the clinical staff.

Values are reinforced through the efforts and examples of management, a continued willingness to do what is right instead of opting for shortcuts and to tell the truth. Peter Senge in his book, *The Fifth Discipline*, refers to the gap between reality and vision as creative tension. How management is able to manage the gap will ultimately determine whether vision and mission will be achievable. This is the place where core values are critical and will determine outcomes, and it is the challenge of management to hold creative tension. "The most effective people are those who can 'hold' their vision while remaining committed to seeing current reality clearly. The hallmark of a learning organization is not lovely visions floating in space, but a relentless willingness to examine 'what is' in light of our vision."[5]

STRATEGIC PLANNING

Strategic planning is an assessment of organizational strengths and weaknesses, external opportunities and threats, the determination of strategies and objectives to be pursued, and the development of an action plan to exploit opportunities or minimize threats. The planning process is usually performed by the senior members of the management team and is long term in nature, in contrast to annual budgets, which are short term.

Internal assessment consists of determining the agency's strengths and weaknesses. Strengths represent core qualities that contribute to the success of the agency and differentiate it from others. Strengths could include the ability to measure and manage outcomes, the ability to provide services within 12 hours of acceptance of a referral regardless of geographic location, financial stability, secure funding sources, highly trained employees, cutting-edge programs, or a secure relationship with multiple referral sources. The goal of strength identification is to determine how to leverage strengths to take advantage of opportunities or to minimize threats.

The internal assessment of agency weaknesses requires honesty and the willingness not to get caught up in finger pointing. The objective of weakness identification is to correct weaknesses. As identified in earlier chapters, it is important to be clear about the difference between symptoms and the root cause of the problem.

For instance, this section may identify that financial statements are never available until the 25th of the following month. This is a symptom; the actual problem may be due to the fact that there is not a tight control on note submission by field staff. Potential weaknesses that would be identified in this section could include high turnover, ineffective managers, poor controls, late financial statements, uncollectible accounts receivable, poor cash flow, an antiquated information system, or the lack of teamwork. It is important to remember that dysfunctional organizations are created from poor internal processes. Poor internal processes will affect external perceptions of quality and erode potential strengths.

Opportunity identification is based on an assessment of changes in the regulatory environment, payment mechanisms, competitors, customers, current referral bases, state initiatives, and national health care reform. Opportunities assessment can be based on analysis, hunch, intuition, or an inside tip. Opportunities can also be identified by talking with physicians, social workers, hospital and clinic administrators, MCOs, employers, civic organizations, or customers. Potential sources of opportunities include advances in technology, acquisition of complementary businesses, increased acceptance of home health care, decreasing hospital lengths of stay, alliances with competitors, joint ventures with other providers, or expansion to new markets.

Threat identification determines factors that could adversely affect the agency. Threats could include an inability to price services competitively or to provide a full range of services, the introduction of competitive products, mandated changes in service utilization, or the ability to cover a geographic area. The analysis of threats should also include an assessment of current referral sources and contracts to determine whether there is the likelihood that contracts will not be renewed or that the referral stream could be altered. An element of the threat analysis would also include determining competitors in the area, their costs in relationship to the agency's, and the scope of services that they provide. A common practice with threat identification is to estimate how threats could affect the agency if they were to materialize. This is often accomplished by a sensitivity analysis. For instance, the sensitivity analysis could quantify what would happen if a referral source was lost, prospective payment was implemented at rates lower than the average cost per visit, or the agency lost key personnel.

Once the strengths, weaknesses, opportunities, and threats have been identified, it is time to determine a course of action for the agency to pursue. The course of action or strategy may consist of building on specific strengths, planning to minimize weaknesses, or planning to take advantage of opportunities or prevent threats. Strategies will depend on the needs and wants of customers, organizational resources, the depth of management, management's stance on risk, and the status of management as reactive or proactive. Furthermore, strategies will be consistent with the agency's mission, vision, and values.

Strategies could include taking advantage of a cost-reimbursed environment to implement quality improvement initiatives, activity-based cost management, the development of clinical pathways, and outcome measures. Other strategies could include accreditation from Community Health Accreditation Program (CHAP) or the Joint Commission on Accreditation of Healthcare Organizations, investment in an information system that enables the measurement and management of outcomes, the collection of data from the field using lap-top computers or a pen-based clipboard, and multimedia education. Additionally, strategies could include forming an alliance with a pharmacist to provide high-technology infusion therapies, closing or opening a branch office, starting a hospice, or developing specialized teams to provide customized services or programs to referral sources. Strategy identification may need to be prioritized, given the agency's human, financial, and operational resources.

Not all strategies will be pursued. Strategies that are pursued become organizational objectives. It is important to evaluate objectives to determine whether they are obtainable. Inherent in the evaluative process is an objective assessment of the resources that will be required to obtain the objectives, the timeline being considered, and the ones accountable for making it happen. Resource considerations include personnel, both existing and additional, and financial resources. Consideration regarding personnel may include whether there is a sufficient number of nurses, therapists, or aides to handle new business; what the technical ability is of current management and staff; and whether the existing staff have excess capacity. If the objective is to increase the number of managed care contracts, covered lives, and geographic area, thought must be given to whether the agency have the infrastructure in place to handle the reporting and service needs of additional managed care contracts. Further consideration must be given to making sure the contract is positive for the agency, systems are in place to monitor and measure the contract on a daily basis to prevent a negative situation from occurring, and the agency has the ability to increase its debt capacity to handle the additional volume.

Financial resources may be for working capital, investment in additional office equipment, new technology, a new information system, or computer hardware. Consideration should be given to the financial feasibility of the objectives selected as part of the strategic planning processes. If an objective calls for expanding a high-technology service line through the acquisition of a pharmacy, obtaining several high-volume contracts, and recruiting additional personnel, serious attention needs to be given to working capital required for the realization of this objective. In addition to working capital, information systems, facility requirements, logistical concerns, communication requirements, personnel considerations, and changes in payment streams need to be thoroughly addressed to make sure that the objective is possible from an internal and external perspective. Financial feasibility also includes performing sensitivity analysis on growth forecasts, market potential by product, customer and geographic area, revenue streams, capital outlays, and operating costs. Often, this is accomplished by developing optimistic, average, and pessimistic forecasts. Evaluation of the extremes will determine organizational risk and the need to have additional resource availability.

The assessment process should include input from all members of the agency on how plans would change the processes that are under their control. The assessment includes financial and operational feasibility for new and existing operations. In the event of organizational resource constraints, it may be necessary to choose objectives to pursue. The use of discounted cashflow methods discussed in a previous chapter will assist in the ranking process. Once the evaluative processes have been completed, the selected objectives are listed formally as part of the strategic plan.

Everyone must be clear on who is accountable for each element of the new objectives identified in the strategic plan as well as existing operations. The development of an action plan will identify individual accountability and help to mesh current and new operations. When timelines, resource requirements, event sequence, and individual accountability are identified as part of the action plan, it serves multiple purposes. A primary purpose is it provides a methodology for incorporating into the budgeting process, thus translating strategies into tangible goals and objectives. The budgeting process includes the operating plan, capital expenditure plan, marketing plan, and plans for recruitment and staffing. A secondary purpose is that it establishes accountability.

This is where creative tension has its first test. Often, the operations people will be concerned about change, identify many reasons why things will not be able to happen, but ultimately will need to change their strategies to be consistent with the new course of action. Linking of the action plan to the budget will force consistent application of values by identifying monthly, quarterly, and annual targets, milestones, and outcomes. Reward systems need to be consistent with values and objectives. Reward systems that reward individuals for efforts that are a by-product of many individuals' efforts are also counterproductive. Furthermore, organizational and individual accountability are identified by clarifying who is responsible for the "what" and "when" of the plans.

Organizations that do not link organizational and individual accountability will always run the risk of being dysfunctional. Linking of values, vision, mission, organizational, and individual accountability to the strategic and operational plans provides a platform for the learning organization.

THE BALANCED SCORECARD

The concept of scorecards and report cards is beginning to gain acceptance as a tool to measure team or organizational performance. These vehicles have traditionally focused solely on clinical or financial results because of limitations in the design of systems and software. Traditional reporting systems were designed to meet the needs of the Medicare reporting process; however, as the home health industry changes because of managed competition, the reporting and measurement processes must also change.

Historically, performance measures were financial, visit statistics, or some other metric that was counted for external reporting purposes. These indicators or metrics are output-oriented and easy to report. However, they do very little to link day-to-day operations to the HHA's vision, mission, and values. Furthermore, because of their output orientation, these indicators tend to force a reactive management culture.

The balanced scorecard is a management measurement tool whose purpose is to link strategic vision to objective process measurement (Figure 17–2).[6] The linking of process measures to strategic objectives provides a vehicle for the integration of strategic vision to the day-to-day activities. By linking day-to-day operations and functional performance measures to strategic vision, everyone within the agency can see how his or her unique contributions fit into achieving the larger organizational objectives. "A state-of-the-art performance measurement system should do no less than monitor the vital signs of the company. At every level, it should translate an organization's highest visions into individual performance measures that focus the organization, highlight excellence, support competitive spirit, provide a foundation for continuous improvement, and support the good of the organization over the good of particular individuals or functions."[7]

The balanced scorecard is composed of four sections: (1) customers, (2) financial, (3) internal business processes, and (4) innovation and learning. Each of these

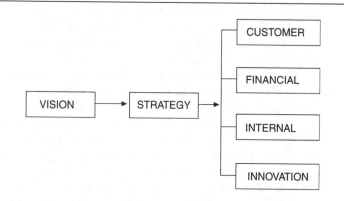

Figure 17–2 The Balanced Scorecard. Source: R.S. Kaplan and D.P. Norton, Putting the Balanced Scorecard To Work, *Harvard Business Review* (September–October 1993): 134–147.

perspectives is interrelated and when combined provides the agency with a tool that measures how well each of the areas is performing in relationship to the larger vision. Actually, the concept is quite simple. The balanced scorecard recognizes that management needs a wider variety of measurement indicators than solely financial measurements. The balanced scorecard honors this requirement by focusing on four areas that determine outcomes important to the long-term survival of any organization. There should be no more than 15 to 20 performance measures for the balanced scorecard.[8] It is also suggested that the performance measures need to be positive instead of negative indicators, based on relative terms instead of absolute; to indicate rate of change; and to be meaningful. Ultimately, "the balanced scorecard is about empowering people throughout the organization, enabling them to focus on what they should be doing to contribute to the corporate vision."[9]

The customer section of the scorecard needs to measure what is important to the agency from the customer's perspective. This information will be obtained through customer surveys conducted throughout the course of the year. Customers would include patients, referral sources, MCOs, physicians, and the patient's caregivers. A customer survey may evaluate service provision from the perspectives of responsiveness, reliability, empathy, caring, and communication. The survey could also include elements that are especially important to the customer (MCO): that new referrals are seen within 12 hours. If this were one of the indicators that was selected, then to state it in relative terms, the HHA would need to divide the number of new referrals that were seen within 12 hours by the total number of new referrals. The result represents the amount of positive events that took place. If the agency's vision was that 100 percent of referrals were seen within 12 hours, and the result indicated that only 75 percent were actually seen within 12 hours, then this metric would identify that a gap existed and that the supporting processes needed to be investigated. Analysis may indicate that the outcome was not obtainable because of weekend discharges, or geographic area; or the outcome was unrealistic and therefore should be renegotiated.

The financial section of the scorecard should measure those processes that are critical to the long-term survival of the agency. The identification of performance measures should be linked to the organizational vision. For instance, management may determine that there are three or four indicators that provide a short- and long-term measure of what is important to the agency from a financial management perspective. These indicators could be return on equity, days outstanding for accounts receivable, cash flow, and service line profitability. Return on equity would measure how well the agency is doing in the aggregate. Individual service line profitability would indicate if there was a problem with one service line. If a problem existed, further analysis would indicate what processes were out of balance. Cash flow provides the balance between the revenue and disbursement processes and financing strategies.

Internal processes measure where business processes are in relationship to strategic vision. Processes have a macro and micro element. Macro processes are the provision of patient care, logistics, business processes, human resources, and marketing. These processes will be influenced by the degree of information technology that supports the entire operation. Performance measures in this category include cycle time, cost/benefit analysis measures, and internal quality indicators. Cycle time could include metrics to measure the length of time that it takes to submit notes to the agency, collect receivables, produce financial statements, train employees, or discharge a patient. Cycle time categories can also be developed by processes that cross functional boundaries. Other process indicators could include the cost of a payroll check, vendor check, invoice, number of productive hours for field staff, cost per hour of training, advertising effectiveness, or cost per new hire. Each of these performance indicators (cost per "x") would indicate process cost. Further refinements of the scorecard process will include rate of change indicators for process improvement. It is important to measure rate of change indicators against some form of external benchmark; otherwise, an improvement rate of 5 percent is meaningless unless reported in relationship to some external criteria.

The innovation and learning section offers a perspective regarding agency growth. Without growth, the agency will slowly die. Death may be due to the inability to respond to the changing business environment or increased competition. This area is concerned with those metrics that evaluate the growth of the organization and its employees. Growth may come from spending time with customers to determine how services can be enhanced. A performance metric may be the amount of time that senior management spends with customers. Growth is also a direct result of an investment in employee training. Employee training could measure the total amount of time that is invested in each employee or group of employees. Training could include technical areas, degree-related programs, software systems, problem-solving exercises, statistics, or continuous quality improvement. This section could also include the amount of employee suggestions implemented and the resultant savings.

The balanced scorecard provides a tool to link strategy and vision to daily operations. (See Figure 17–3.) This is accomplished by developing performance measures at an individual, team, or departmental level that channel energy into the accomplishment of the larger objectives. Budgets and action plans can also be tied into the above performance measures. Specifically, vision is linked to daily operations using performance measures that everyone in the organization can understand. Performance measures help to provide the bridge between mission and vision. Performance measures could be the following:

- *Cost or Dollar Value*—Cost of a process, activity, or clinical pathway
- *Percent of a Population*—100 percent of a patient problem (e.g., surgical wounds)

- *Category*—Payor, outcome criteria (e.g., met, met early, met late, not met, or changed)
- *Time*—Elapsed time between acceptance of a referral and the first visit
- *Survey Responses*—Depends on the grading scale used

Figure 17–4 illustrates a vision wheel that can be used in conjunction with the balanced scorecard. The vision wheel has four quadrants representing each of the primary measurement groups. In the center is the vision. The vision equals 100 percent. Each spoke would represent an outcome to be measured. For instance, if 75 percent of the referrals were seen within 12 hours, then that would be identified on the vision wheel using the percent of the population that had achieved the anticipated outcome. The performance metric could be a percentage of population plotted on the vision wheel. The linking of each point will provide a graphical display of how close the agency is getting to obtaining its vision. Subsequent plottings would indicate how much progress has been made since the last measurement cycle. Subsequent plottings would also illustrate the rate of change.

Outcomes and performance measures will change as the agency's priorities change. It is important to ascertain periodically whether outcomes and performance measures are measuring critical success factors that are truly important to the agency. (See Exhibit 17–2.) Of paramount importance is determining whether the measurement tools are evaluating what is important to the agency's customers, both internal and external.

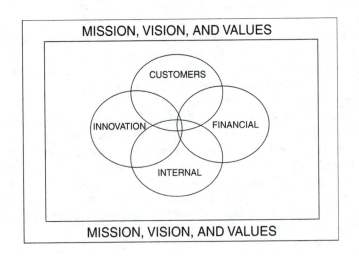

Figure 17–3 The Integration of Mission, Vision, and Values into the Balanced Scorecard

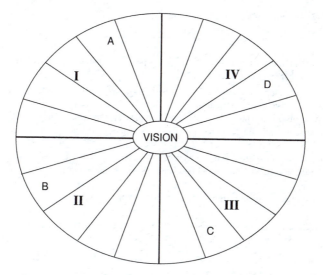

Figure 17–4 The Vision Wheel. Sample outcomes to be measured: (A) percentage of population seen within 12 hours; (B) employer training equals 3% of production time; (C) percentage of A/R collected within 45 days; (D) cash flow to debt ratio equals one. Quadrant I = Customer, Quadrant II = Innovation, Quadrant III = Internal process, Quadrant IV = Financial.

CORE VALUES AND CONCEPTS OF THE MALCOLM BALDRIGE NATIONAL QUALITY AWARD

The Malcolm Baldrige National Quality Award was designed to promote the awareness of quality and performance measurement as key elements of competitiveness. The award criteria focus on key organizational values that are deemed to be critical indicators of the ability to deliver high-quality services in the face of increasing competition. (The Malcolm Baldrige examination criteria are shown in Exhibit 17–3.) The values and scoring mechanisms have been changed to reflect the need to balance high-quality services with financial performance indicators. The award criteria identify 11 major values that potential candidates must possess. These values are integrated into the 7 categories that form the basis for organizational evaluation.

Patient-focused Quality and Value

The delivery of health care services must be patient focused. Quality and value are the key components in determining patient satisfaction. All attributes of pa-

Exhibit 17–2 Attributes of a Good Measurement System

"Regardless of which competitive priorities companies pursue, the successful measurement systems will share five characteristics."

1. Be mutually supportive and consistent with the business's operating goals, objectives, critical success factors, and programs.
2. Convey information through as few and as simple a set of measures as possible.
3. Reveal how effectively customers' needs and expectations are satisfied. Focus on measures that customers can see.
4. Provide a set of measurements for each organizational component that allows all members of the organization to understand how their decisions and activities affect the entire business.
5. Support organizational learning and continuous improvement.

Source: Reprinted from *The New Performance Challenge* by J.R. Dixon, A.J. Nanni, and T.E. Vollmann, p. 165, with permission of Business One Irwin, © 1990.

tient care delivery (including those not directly related to medical/clinical services) factor into the judgment of quality and value. Quality and value to patients are key considerations for other stakeholders, as well. Quality and value are influenced by many factors during a patient's experience in health care. These factors include a clear understanding of likely health care and functional outcomes as well as the patient's relationship with the health care provider and ancillary staff, cost, responsiveness, and continuing care and attention. For many patients, the ability to participate in making decisions on their health care is considered an important factor. This requires patient education for an informed decision. Characteristics that differentiate one provider from another also contribute to the patient's sense of quality.

Patient-focused quality and value are strategic concepts. They are directed toward obtaining and retaining patient loyalty, referral of new patients, and market share gain in competitive markets. Patient-focused quality and value demand constant sensitivity to emerging patient desires and health care marketplace requirements and measurement of the factors that drive patient satisfaction. Patient-focused quality and value also demand awareness of new technology and new modalities for delivery of health care services.

Leadership

An organization's senior administrative and health care staff leaders need to work together to set directions and create a patient focus, clear and visible values, a clear mission, and high expectations. Reinforcement of the values, mission, and

Exhibit 17–3 Malcolm Baldrige Examination Criteria

Examination categories		Point values
1 Leadership		90
a. Senior Executive Leadership	45	
b. Leadership System and Organization	25	
c. Public Responsibility and Corporate Citizenship	20	
2 Information and Analysis		75
a. Management of Information and Data	20	
b. Performance Comparisons and Benchmarking	15	
c. Analysis and Use of Organizational-Level Data	40	
3 Strategic Planning		55
a. Strategy Development	35	
b. Strategy Deployment	20	
4 Human Resource Development and Management		140
a. Human Resource Planning and Evaluation	20	
b. Employee/Health Care Staff Work Systems	45	
c. Employee/Health Care Staff Education, Training, and Development	50	
d. Employee Well-Being and Satisfaction	25	
5 Process Management		140
a. Design and Introduction of Patient Health Care Services	35	
b. Delivery of Patient Health Care	35	
c. Patient Care Support Services Design and Delivery	20	
d. Community Health Services Design and Delivery	15	
e. Administrative and Business Operations Management	20	
f. Supplier Performance Management	15	
6 Organizational Performance Results		250
a. Patient Health Care Results	80	
b. Patient Care Support Services Results	40	
c. Community Health Services Results	30	
d. Administrative, Business, and Supplier Results	90	
e. Accreditation and Assessment Results	10	
7 Focus on and Satisfaction of Patients and Other Stakeholders		250
a. Patient and Health Care Market Knowledge	30	
b. Patient/Stakeholder Relationship Management	30	
c. Patient/Stakeholder Satisfaction Determination	30	
d. Patient/Stakeholder Satisfaction Results	100	
e. Patient/Stakeholder Satisfaction Comparison	60	
Total Points		1,000

expectations requires personal commitment and involvement. The leaders need to take part in the creation of strategies, systems, and methods for achieving excellence in patient and community health care services. Senior leaders must be visible to the entire staff and must serve as role models for participation in improving the organization and its services.

Continuous Improvement and Organizational Learning

Achieving ever-higher levels of organizational performance requires a well-executed approach to continuous improvement. A well-executed, continuous improvement process has several important characteristics:

- It has clear goals regarding what to improve.
- It is fact based, incorporating measures and/or indicators.
- It is systematic, including cycles of planning, execution, and evaluation.
- It is nonjudgmental, focusing primarily on key processes as the route to better results.

The approach to improvement needs to be "embedded" in the way the organization operates. *Embedded* means improvement is a regular part of the daily work of the entire staff, improvement processes seek to eliminate problems at their source; and improvement is driven by opportunities to do better, as well as by problems that need to be corrected. Opportunities for improvement come from many sources, including staff ideas, patients' and other stakeholders' input, successful practices of other organizations, and health care research findings.

Improvements may be of several types:

- enhancing value to patients through new and improved patient care services;
- reducing errors, defects, and waste;
- improving responsiveness and cycle time performance;
- improving productivity and effectiveness in the use of all resources; and
- improving the organization's contributions and effectiveness in fulfilling its community health responsibilities.

Thus, improvement is driven not only by the objective to provide better services, but also by the need to be responsible and efficient.

Employee/Health Care Staff Participation and Development

An organization's success in improving performance depends on the capabilities, skills, and motivation of its entire staff. Staff success depends on having meaningful knowledge and skills. Organizations need to invest in the development of their staff through ongoing education, training, and opportunities for continuing growth.

For employees, development might include classroom and on-the-job training, job rotation, and pay for demonstrated skills. Increasingly, training, education, development, and work organization need to be tailored to a more diverse workforce and to more flexible, high-performance work practices.

For health care staff, development means building discipline knowledge; discipline retraining to adjust to a changing health care environment; and enhancing knowledge of measurement systems influencing outcome assessments and clinical guidelines, decision trees, or critical paths. Health care staff participation may include contributing to the development of new health care services, organizational policies, or cross-disciplinary processes that track the patient's experience (the health care delivery process); working in teams to improve the health care administrative service interface; and working in teams to improve information systems and services. Increasingly, participation enhances systems thinking, patient focus, and cross-disciplinary cooperation.

Management by Fact

An effective health care services and administrative management system needs to be built on a framework of measurement, information, data, and analysis. Measurements must derive from and support the organization's mission and strategy and encompass all key processes and services and their outputs and results. Facts and data needed for organizational improvement and assessment can be of many types, including patient, employee, community health, epidemiological, critical pathways and practice guidelines, administrative and business, payor, competitive comparisons, and customer satisfaction.

Analysis refers to extracting larger meaning from data to support evaluation and decision making at various levels within the organization. Such analysis may entail using data to reveal information—such as trends, projections, and cause and effect—that might not be evident without analysis. Facts, data, and analysis support a variety of purposes, such as planning; reviewing performance; improving operations; and comparing performance with competitors, similar health care organizations, or "best practices" benchmarks.

A major consideration in the use of data and analysis to improve performance involves the creation and use of performance measures or indicators. Performance measures or indicators are measurable characteristics of health care services, processes, and operations the organization uses to track and improve performance. The measures or indicators should be selected to represent best the factors that lead to improved health care, improved operational and financial performance, and healthier people. A system of measures or indicators tied to patient and stakeholder satisfaction and/or organizational performance requirements represents a clear and objective basis for aligning all activities with the organizational goals. Through the analysis of data from the tracking processes, the measures or indicators themselves may be evaluated and changed. For example, measures selected to track health care service quality may be judged by how well improvement in these measures correlates with improvement in patient satisfaction and health care outcomes.

Results Orientation

An organization's performance system should focus on results: reflecting and balancing the needs and interests of patients and other stakeholders. To meet the sometimes conflicting and changing aims that balance implies, organizational strategy needs to address explicitly all patient and other stakeholder requirements to ensure that actions and plans meet the differing needs and avoid adverse impact. The use of a balanced composite of performance indicators offers an effective means to communicate requirements, to monitor actual performance, and to marshal support for improving results.

From the point of view of overall organizational effectiveness and improvement, two areas of performance are particularly important: (1) patient health care results and (2) the effectiveness and efficiency of the organization's use of all its resources (financial, technological, and human).

Community Health and Public Responsibilities

A health care organization's leadership should serve as a role model in fostering improved community health and exercising public responsibility. Its leaders should stress the importance of activities in these areas. Providing public health services and supporting the general health of the community are important citizenship responsibilities of health care organizations. Playing a leadership role in carrying out these responsibilities (within limits of an organization's resources) includes influencing other organizations, private and public, to partner for these purposes. For example, individual health care organizations could lead efforts to establish free clinics or indigent care programs, to increase public health awareness programs, or to foster neighborhood services for the elderly. Leadership also could involve helping define community health service issues and delivery mechanisms for the health care industry throughout regional or national networks or associations.

A health care organization's public responsibilities include basic expectations, such as ethical practices, and protection of public safety and the environment. Ethical practices need to take into account proper use of public and private funds, nondiscriminatory hiring and patient treatment policies, and protection of patients' rights and privacy. Planning related to public safety and the environment should anticipate adverse impacts that may arise in facilities management and use and disposal of radiation, chemical, and biohazards. Plans should seek to prevent problems, to provide a forthright response if problems occur, and to make available information needed to maintain public confidence. Inclusion of public responsibility areas within a performance system means meeting all local, state, and federal laws and regulatory requirements. It also means treating these and related requirements as areas for continuous improvement "beyond mere compliance."

This requires that appropriate measures of progress be created and used in managing performance.

Partnership Development

Organizations should seek to build internal and external partnerships to accomplish their overall goals better.

Internal partnerships might include those that promote cooperation between health care staff and other employee groups, cooperation with unions, and cooperation among departments and/or work units. Agreements might be created involving staff development; cross-training; or new work organizations, such as high-performance work teams. Internal partnerships might also involve creating relationships among units to improve flexibility and responsiveness and to develop processes that better follow patient care needs.

External partnerships might include those with businesses, business associations, third-party payors, community and social service organizations, and other health care providers—all stakeholders. Partnerships with other health care organizations could result in referrals or in shared facilities that are either capital intensive or require unique and scarce expertise.

Partnerships should seek to develop longer term objectives, thereby creating a basis for mutual investments. Partners should address objectives of the partnership, key requirements for success, means of regular communications, approaches to evaluating progress, and means for adapting to changing conditions.

Design Quality and Prevention

Health care improvement needs to place very strong emphasis on enhancing health care value (addressing quality and cost factors). This places a heavy burden on the design of health care delivery systems, disease prevention programs, health promotion programs, and effective and efficient diagnostic and treatment systems. Overall design should include the opportunity to learn for continuous improvement and should value the individual needs of patients. Design also must include effective means for gauging improvement of health status—for patients and populations/communities. A central quality-related requirement of effective design is the inclusion of an assessment strategy. Such a strategy needs to include the acquisition of in-process information to allow beneficial changes in design at the earliest opportunity.

Long-range View of the Future

Pursuit of health care improvement requires a strong future orientation and a willingness to make long-term commitments to all stakeholders—patients and families, communities, employers, students, staff, and payors. Planning needs to anticipate many types of changes, including changes in health care delivery systems, resource availability, patient and other stakeholder expectations, technological developments, evolving regulatory requirements, societal expectations, and new thrusts by competitors and other health care organizations providing similar services. A major long-term investment associated with health care improvement is the investment in creating and sustaining an assessment system focused on health care outcomes. This entails becoming familiar with research findings and application of assessment methods. Education and training of staff are necessary components of developing an outcomes measurement system.

Fast Response

An increasingly important measure of organizational effectiveness is faster and more flexible response to the needs of patients and other stakeholders. Many organizations are learning that explicit focus on and measurement of response times help to drive the simplification of work organizations and work processes. There are other important benefits derived from this focus: response time improvements often drive simultaneous improvements in organization, quality, and productivity. The world's great organizations are learning to make simultaneous improvements in quality, productivity, and response time.

CONCLUSION

An HHA's strategic management process is what differentiates it from other competitors. This chapter focused on concepts of strategic planning and performance measurement before concluding with core concepts and values critical to the Malcolm Baldrige Award criteria. Regardless of the approach taken, the concepts for survival are clear. Management must evaluate how effective and efficient its services and processes are in relationship to the agency's stakeholders. Without clear processes for communication, evaluation, and implementation, survival will be threatened.

NOTES

1. P.M. Senge, *The Fifth Discipline* (New York: Doubleday/Currency, 1990), 223.
2. J.R. Latham, Visioning: The Concept, Trilogy, and Process, *Quality Progress* 28, no. 4 (April 1995): 65–68.
3. *Ibid.*
4. P.M. Senge, *The Fifth Discipline*, 212.

5. *Ibid.*, 226.

6. R.S. Kaplan and D.P. Norton, Putting the Balanced Scorecard to Work, *Harvard Business Review* (September–October 1993): 134–47.

7. J. Hoffecker and C. Goldenberg, Using the Balanced Scorecard To Develop Companywide Performance Measures, *Journal of Cost Management* 8, no. 3 (Fall 1994): 5–17.

8. R.S. Kaplan and D.P. Norton, Putting the Balanced, 134–147.

9. J. Hoffecker and C. Goldenberg, Using the Balanced Scorecard, 5–17.

Chapter 18

Differentiation Strategies

The health care delivery system is in the process of consolidation. Consolidation is causing former competitors to align and develop common strategies for survival. The consolidation process is being fueled by a growing intolerance for rising health care costs, attempts to eliminate fragmentation in the care delivery process, and managed competition. Ultimately, the consolidation process will force many smaller and financially unsound players out of the health care delivery process.

The real question is this: How can home health care providers take advantage of the many opportunities that are available as a result of an aging population, advances in technology that make care possible in the home, and a growing acceptance of the virtues of home health care? The answer is in the building of relationships. Relationships need to be built with whoever has the ability to direct the patient to take advantage of the agency's services. The development of a relationship based on common values and goals will be essential as the consolidation process evolves.

The elimination of fragmentation will be accomplished through moving to a global capitation system where large health care delivery systems are responsible for the provision of care from birth to death. Payments to these large health systems will cover all services regardless of where they are provided. It will then be up to the health system to determine the most appropriate place to provide care. Appropriateness will be based on patient need and resource consumption. Therefore, home health becomes a strategic necessity in reducing risk associated with capitation; a vehicle for risk diversification; and an integral element for successful, vertically integrated health systems.

This movement toward integrated delivery systems can either pose a threat to home health agencies (HHAs) or present an opportunity. However, the correct assessment may influence long-term financial viability. This chapter identifies

466

several of the major trends that will affect the delivery of home health care and possible strategies providers can utilize to position their agencies for continued growth.

INDUSTRY TRENDS

The first major trend is an aging population and a growing acceptance of home health care. Home health care is finally being recognized as a preferred health care delivery method from the patient's perspective.

> Home care is personalized care. Home care is tailored to the needs of each individual and is delivered on a one-to-one basis. In fact, one of the best arguments in support of home care is that it is the most humane and compassionate way to deliver health care and supportive services. Home care contributes to the emotional health and well being of the patient and family. Home care adds to the length and quality of the patient's life. The U.S. General Accounting Office has established beyond a doubt that those people receiving home care lived longer and enjoyed a better quality of life than those treated for similar ailments in institutions.[1]

This is important because "changing demographics and social patterns will greatly affect the type and number of home health care consumers. Perhaps the most significant demographic change occurring in our nation is the growth of the elderly (over 65 years) segment of the population relative to the total population. In 1940, 6.8 percent of the total population was over the age of 65; according to 1990 U.S. Census Bureau data, 12 percent of the population was more than 65 years old. Even more dramatic is the projection that by the year 2020, nearly one-fifth of the U.S. population will be over age 65. Within this market, the greatest percentage of growth has been in the over 85 segment. As medical technology finds new ways to extend life expectancy, this group will need to learn to live with more chronic illnesses, providing a significant opportunity for home health care."[2]

Furthermore, as the over-85 segment grows, there will be an increase in home health services for the chronically ill and fragile. An analysis of 1992 Health Care Financing Administration (HCFA) claims identified that approximately 10.8 percent of home health users had more than 150 visits in 1992 and 17 percent of total charges. The average for this group was 250 visits per patient and for the group of fewer than 150 visits, the average was 31 visits per patient. Patients in the over 150 visits per patient group tended to be frail and have multiple functional limitations.[3]

The second major trend is continuing advances in the sophistication of technology and services that can be provided in the home. No longer is the hospital setting the sole domain for administering intravenous (IV) therapies. Advances in the portability of pumps and the development of user-friendly equipment enable home care companies to set up the equipment, prepare the patient, and leave the patient's caregivers to monitor the process according to instructions. Technological advances make it possible to feed patients intravenously in the home; provide antibiotic, hydration, and respiratory therapies; and even provide chemotherapy. Furthermore, advances in technology have made it possible to provide home dialysis and pain management, monitor cardiac patients, and provide myriad other services. Advances in technology have broadened the spectrum of home health services to include specialized programs targeted toward pediatric populations, hospice patients, maternal–child health programs, respite services, and the human immunodeficiency virus (HIV) population. Niche market strategies can be used in these areas.

A third major trend that is occurring is the movement toward managed care. The movement toward managed care is fueling the consolidation of the marketplace. The premanaged-care health care delivery system was characterized by independent hospitals, physicians, home health agencies, and unsophisticated purchasers.[4] The introduction of managed care plans created a vehicle for rising employer health care premiums to be reduced. This was accomplished through the development of provider networks to care for their enrollees. Provider payments were typically discounted fee-for-service arrangements. As competition increased to keep premium dollars low for the employer, managed care organizations (MCOs) responded by shifting risk to providers. In turn, providers began to consolidate; develop integrated health care delivery systems; and focus on controlling resource consumption, both clinical and financial. The next evolutionary step will be the transition to managed competition where health systems bid for patient populations based on cost, quality, and outcome.[5] The progression is illustrated in Figure 18–1.

Home health care is an extremely efficient vehicle for the provision of health care services. Coupled with advances in technology and a growing preference for care, health care delivery systems are integrating the home health element into their service delivery umbrella. This accomplishes several things from their perspective and poses a potential threat to stand-alone HHAs. From an overall management perspective, the integration of home health provides a vehicle to prepare patients prior to surgery, efficiently discharge patients once surgery is completed, and follow up on their postsurgical care requirements. Additionally, home health will provide an alternative to costly hospital stays. The management of this process enables the health system to develop comprehensive clinical pathways and identify opportunities for continued streamlining and risk diversification. From the stand-alone HHA's perspective, this could mean the end of patient referrals because health system administrators want to control all aspects of the care delivery process and take advantage of incremental revenue streams.

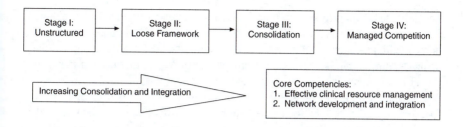

Figure 18–1 Market Framework. Source: APM, Inc., March 1993. Reprinted from Risk, R.R., and Francis, C.P., Transforming a Hospital Facility Company into an Integrated Medical Care Organization, *Managed Care Quarterly*, Vol. 2, No. 4, pp. 12–23, Aspen Publishers, Inc., © 1994.

From the MCO's perspective, this is an optimal situation because it only has one payment to the health system instead of multiple payments to providers. In addition to the elimination of multiple payments, the case management and utilization review processes become a shared process with a core group instead of multiple groups. Furthermore, by eliminating provider fragmentation, the MCO shifts the burden of elimination of duplicate tests and wasted activities to the health system provider and can begin to develop systemwide standards for care.

Managed care is also bringing the concept of consumerism back to the health care delivery process. Providers must focus on meeting the needs of the patient and the payor. From the patients' perspective, they want to return to their preepisode state or to their maximum level of independence. In addition, they are becoming increasingly educated about their rights as consumers, thus increasing their expectations. Increased expectations will require that home health providers focus on quality, technological skills, and patient–provider interactions. Expectations will mandate timely, reliable, empathetic, and compassionate service. From the managed care providers' perspective, service delivery must be reliable, be responsive, meet the needs of the MCO's home care patients and of the MCO's case managers. This may require home health care providers going beyond the call of duty.

The fourth trend is linked to the consolidation process. This trend is the development of networks to meet the home health needs of patients in the community and regionally. Network formation can be as simple as providers referring to a select number of home health agencies. Criteria for participation may be based on the HHA's ability to meet the network's service needs (e.g., provide nursing in the home, home infusion therapies, and home medical equipment). Where managed care is in its evolutionary process will dictate the arrangements that are developed with the home health provider. If the market framework (Figure 18–1) is in Stage

I or II, home health providers will provide services under a capitated or discounted fee-for-service arrangement. If the market has evolved into Stage III or IV, the home health provider may be forced to merge into the health system, become part of the health maintenance organization (HMO) or MCO, or find that it will no longer receive patients from its historical referral sources.

The final trend is the changing payment system. Medicare is moving to a prospective payment system for home health care. Prospective payment can take many possible shapes. Prospective payment utilizing a per visit amount will cap cost per visit but will not control utilization. "Payments on a per visit basis also detracts from efforts to focus clinical attention on the entire episode of care, which is essential to fostering continuity of care and to increasing emphasis on outcomes of care."[6] To control utilization and costs, the federal government will need to make providers at risk. This could take the form of episodic payments based on some medical model adapted for home health, bundling of home health payments into hospital payments, or paying capitated rates to HMOs and letting the HMO figure out how to control resource consumption. The latter two approaches are potentially more appealing because they eliminate overhead for the federal government.

Many states have been utilizing a prospective payment system based on per visit rates. Similar to the Medicare program, Medicaid programs are looking to decrease program cost, and this will probably be accomplished through some risk-sharing mechanism. State programs can contract with communities, county agencies, health systems, or select providers to provide care to Medicaid beneficiaries.

Table 18–1 indicates that only 5.5 percent of home care services are paid for through private insurance. This is probably because private insurance is characteristic of a healthier, working population. Many private insurers are transitioning to a case management approach, contracting with providers to provide care, and attempting to limit their exposure for health care expenditures. The balance of home care services is paid for privately. Private payments are for services not covered under the Medicare, Medicaid, or private insurance programs. This sector will create a niche market for providers as services are reduced under case management practices.

The trend is toward increased utilization of home care services because of an aging population, advances in technology, and the realization that home care is cost effective and preferred by customers. The fate of many HHAs will ultimately depend on what happens with state and federal health care reform. This determination will depend on what payment strategies are adopted at the federal and state levels and how programs are to be administered. Regardless of the eventual course of direction adopted by federal and state programs, the remaining providers will be part of large networks, providing traditional or specialty services. Many providers that lose out on federal and state patients will need to pursue private pay patients actively.

Table 18–1 Sources of Payment for Home Care: 1992. Source: Reprinted from *Basic Statistics about Home Care*, p. 3, with permission of the National Association for Home Care, © 1994.

Source	%
Medicare	37.8
Medicaid	24.7
Private insurance	5.5
Out of pocket	31.4
Other	0.6
Total	100.0

STRATEGIES

Identification of who controls the referral stream is a logical starting point. It is important to understand what is happening to current referral sources. If the agency's referrals are from a group of physicians, a hospital, or some other source, there may be a reason for concern. Everyone is forming new alliances and pursuing strategies for survival. Changing strategies, new alliances, and revised missions have the potential of diverting referral streams. Home health providers need to be market savvy and develop strategies for securing existing and new referral streams. Strategies for free-standing providers include pursuing managed care contracts; diversifying into other service lines; and forming relationships with hospitals, physician groups, and emerging health systems.

Obtaining managed care contracts is a vehicle to ensure a guaranteed patient stream. If contracts are properly negotiated, there will be a resulting profit. Unfortunately, profitability is directly related to the number of patient lives that the agency contracts for and the ability to control utilization within contract populations. This causes providers to contract with multiple MCOs in their geographic area or expand the range of their coverage. An alternative is to expand the scope of services that the agency provides. A full-service provider will be more appealing to an MCO's case managers because it provides an easier way to manage caseload. Full-service providers have more flexibility for pricing services and negotiating because of the ability to discount one type of service while making a profit on the others.

One drawback with contractual referral streams is that contracts expire. Contract renewal may be based on a bidding process, performance during the term of the contract, or the ability to cover a geographic area or provide a specific service. Therefore, the managed care contracting strategy needs to consist of three parts. The first part is the obtaining of contracts, the second is a continuous monitoring of results against the MCO's expectations, and the third is a strategy for the renewal of contracts. The continuous monitoring of results should be incorporated into the agency's performance measurement system, be consistent with contract requirements, and attempt to exceed expectations. The strategy for renewal should provide for no surprise when contracts come up for renewal, should be fact based, and should provide a back-up strategy in the event that the contract is lost.

Diversification into new service lines contains risk to the agency. (See Exhibit 18–1.) Risk can be minimized through developing alliances with other providers. If risk and capitalization are manageable, then diversification may be based on the agency's assessment of trends and needs. On a cautionary note, diversification that requires a large capital investment because of the needs of one contract is akin to the old story of putting all one's eggs in one basket. It should be approached with caution, allowing a sufficient timeframe to generate other business or recoup the investment. Strategies for diversification could include opening hospice, private duty, or homemaker services; starting a pharmacy; supplying medical equipment; expanding services to include pediatrics; or developing specialized programs based on referral source need. Program development could target patients with rehabilitative needs, a home monitoring program for cardiac patients, preventive programs, community outreach programs, and myriad nontraditional programs. "Expansion into non-publicly funded home care is an important option to explore. Such expansion into other areas of private pay will ensure not only survival but prosperity in the coming months and years."[7]

A second viable strategy is becoming involved with the hospitals that are currently referral sources to the agency. This strategy is one that is based on relationship building before the hospital could potentially cut off the referral stream by developing its own hospital-based agency or a relationship with another provider. Hospitals are being forced to integrate vertically. This means that they are beginning to look at controlling all aspects of care before and after hospitalization. Many hospitals begin by purchasing physician groups. The next sequence of steps is to begin to align or purchase the remaining providers.

Home health providers can approach relationship development in many different fashions. One approach would be to work with hospital administration to target specific diagnosis-related groups (DRGs) for early discharge. From the home health providers' perspective, this would be nothing more than developing specific programs to care for the targeted DRGs. For instance, if the hospital had length of stay problems with rehabilitation patients or patients with chronic obstructive pulmonary disease (COPD), the agency would be able to develop specific programs to decrease hospital length of stay. This type of situation becomes a win–win for both the hospital and the agency. The agency is helping the hospital to obtain its goals (i.e., provide care and remain profitable), and the agency is able

Exhibit 18–1 Nontraditional Home Care and Hospice Services Survey

Absentee voting assistance	High-risk obstetrics	Monitoring of health needs of
Acquired immunodeficiency	Home birthing	families separated by
syndrome (AIDS) care/	Home companion	distance
management	Home cosmetology	Nurse-staffed clinics for
Adult day care	Home equity conversion	corporations
Advanced wound care	Home financial services	Occupational health for
Art and music therapy	Home inspections and safety	corporations
Audio-visual health	Home modifications	Pediatric AIDS
education programs	Home optometry	Pediatric bereavement
Blood transfusions	Home pharmacy	Pediatric care
Cardiac care	Home phototherapy	Pediatric day care
Child abuse services	Home renal dialysis	Pediatric mental health
Chimney sweeping	Home telemetry and mobile	Pediatric residential care
Congregate housing	electrocardiograms	Pediatric respite
Day care for technology-	Immunization programs	Pet and plant house-sitting
dependent children	Information and referrals	Pet therapy
Dementia day care	In-home education for home-	Physician services
Discharge planning	bound children	Podiatry
Durable medical equipment	In-home screening	Preretirement counseling
Educational programs for	Insurance policy physicals	Prison health care
patients	Intravenous chemotherapy	Respiratory therapy
Elder abuse counseling	Job placement	Respite care
Emergency response	Legal services	Risk management
Fitness counseling	Massage therapy	School health programs
Foster care for medically	Maternal–child health care	Sexual counseling
fragile children	Meals on wheels	Shopping and errands
Foster grandparents	Medicare claims processing	Snow removal
Funeral planning and	Medication management	Speech pathology
assistance	Mental health services	Telephone reassurance
Geriatric assessment	Mobile dentistry	Transportation
Gourmet meal delivery	Mobile health screening	Wellness programs
Green thumb programs	Mobile library	Workers' compensation
Handyman services	Mobile X-ray	management

Source: Reprinted from Dittenbrenner, H., *Ensuring Survival—Expansion into Nontraditional Services*, *Caring*, June 1994, pp. 54–58, with permission of the National Association for Home Care, © 1994.

to develop a sound customer–client relationship with the hospital and the patients to whom they provide care.

HHAs may also want to consider providing management expertise to hospitals to manage their home health departments. This is a dual-edged sword approach in that the HHA could lose its referral stream and management contract. However, if the management team can develop a long-term relationship through developing cutting-edge programs and generating hospital savings, it may be viewed as an essential team member critical to the long-term survival of the institution. An alternative is the sale of the agency that includes a long-term management contract; the development of a staffing contract to provide nurses, therapists, and home health aides; or the development of start-up programs for the hospital.

Regardless of approach, if the agency is no longer receiving referrals from its traditional referral sources, it will either be forced to close its doors or generate new referral sources. Therefore, working with current referral sources provides a vehicle to manage the current environment while new referral sources are being cultivated.

Potential areas for new referral sources could include forming relationships with MCOs; workers' compensation carriers; case management companies; private insurers; county, state, or local cooperatives; or self-insured employers. Other sources of leads could come from participation in state and national home care organizations, local and state business associations, or community groups; from competitors; or from the local newspaper.

A third strategy is forming a relationship with a large employer or community that self-insures its medical coverage. Employers realize that they can save health insurance premium dollars through self-insurance. Self-insured employers negotiate with providers for rates in the event that their employees, or families of their employees, require some form of medical service. For large employers, self-insurance represents a vehicle to save money by paying for actual health insurance costs for their specific population instead of the population that an insurance company would cover. Additionally, the employer can set up its health plan to meet the needs of its employees; for instance, if the employer decides that it wants its employees to be able to stay in the hospital for three days after childbirth, then they can. Home health providers can become part of a large employer's preferred provider list and potentially participate in the case management process.

Communities, cities, and local organizations are beginning to develop their own networks to reduce the cost of their members' health care. These networks will contract with hospitals, physicians, home health agencies, and other providers to provide services to their members. The network providers are then paid according to the network guidelines. This provides another source of referrals for home health agencies. In fact, depending on the plan, there may be an opportunity to develop other community-based programs and revenue streams.

A fourth potential strategy is to partner with a competitor or a related provider. This concept is commonly referred to as *horizontal integration*, where an HHA will team up with an IV therapy company, a durable medical equipment (DME) company, and possible other HHAs. The larger group has the ability to provide more services; possibly cover a wider geographic area; and potentially meet more of the needs of a hospital, MCO, or some other potential referral source. In theory, the linking of other providers will enable the agency to capture more business; however, it also has the potential for other problems. Specifically, the other entities may have a different vision, mission, and values regarding patient care, service, and quality. These could lead to problems unless there is one strong leader or a willingness to develop a unified vision and mission with common values. Other problems could stem from operating pressures related to specific business, the inability to case manage properly, or internal power struggles.

To prevent potential problems when partnering, the agency must know its prospective partner. Does the partner have a good reputation in the community, with referral sources, and with its patients? Is this documented, or how can it be demonstrated? What is its approach to service delivery? Will it be difficult to integrate the two systems? How will combined service quality be demonstrated? Who will be accountable for what? What is the risk-reward sharing process? Is it fair to everyone? What will the new organization look like in six months, one year, three years, and so on? Investment of resources on the front end to determine a fair, equitable, and legal structure is money well spent. Furthermore, taking the time to develop a common vision and mission statement, to lithem it to a strategic plan that includes performance measures, and to determine accountability will help make the new marriage work.

Another possible strategy is to become a highly specialized provider of services. Specialized providers are extremely efficient in the delivery of a few types of service. Commonly, decisions are made to provide many services or a small subset of services and go after a highly specialized market, such as pediatrics or high-technology infusion therapy. Niche market providers have an opportunity to go after those areas that many providers have "carved out" of their management contracts because they did not have the expertise to perform or manage the service or patient population without being at risk. Niche market providers can also develop many possible revenue streams in the private pay as well as managed care sector.

A final strategy could work two ways. This is the concept of outsourcing. Outsourcing is the contracting with a third party to provide services. Common examples would be outsourcing payroll or cost reporting to a third party. Providers may want to consider outsourcing the majority of their administrative functions if they can negotiate with a third party to provide services for less money than it would cost to perform the service in-house. HHAs would be able to take advantage of economies of scale if a third party were to manage the administrative activities of multiple HHAs and only charge each respective agency based on a prenegotiated fee or even a fixed rate. This would allow clinical mangers to focus on providing efficient care, administrative costs would be known and measurable, and capitated contracts would potentially be more lucrative. The business management function would then be a function of contractual negotiations.

The other side of outsourcing is from a hospital's perspective. The hospital may decide to outsource its home health function to a local agency. The agency would provide all administrative and clinical services. The services would be managed by the hospital and billed under the hospital's name. This is another potential win–win situation. The hospital has the benefit of a knowledgeable home health provider, may be able to take advantage of cost reimbursement opportunities under current Medicare reimbursement, and can work on improving its service delivery practices. From the home health provider's perspective, its profitability will be determined at the time of contract negotiation for its service and management contracts.

THE EVOLUTION

The health care system is in the process of transitioning from institutional care to community-based care. This process will need to develop a three-way union between the needs of the customer, physicians, and nursing. The development of a three-way union that is based on the needs of the customer, and not the politics of an institution, will ultimately be how efficiency will be built into the health care delivery system.

It is possible that the home health agencies of the future will be dominated by large multiple-service providers to meet the increasingly complex medical needs of the aging communities. Professional staff will be expanded to include nurse practitioners and physicians. The inclusion of these two groups will help to develop a common base between all other health system providers. Additionally, this group of home health providers will be an integral element of a community health information network (CHIN), which will transfer patient data between providers. One of the CHIN's goals will be to develop longitudinal records; to develop comprehensive clinical pathways; and to eliminate the duplication of records, tests, and wasted activities. Furthermore, home health agencies will develop service lines that will focus on prevention and development of functional family units and will play an important role in the return to community. Home health may even include services that focus on the integration of mind, body, and spirit into the healing process.

NOTES

1. SMG Marketing Group, *Home Healthcare Agencies Report & Directory* (Chicago: December 1994), 3.
2. SMG Marketing Group, *Home Healthcare Agencies Report & Directory*, 29–30.

3. B.C. Vladeck and N.A. Miller, The Medicare Home Health Initiative, *Health Care Financing Review* 16, no. 1 (Fall 1994): 7–16.

4. R.R. Risk, and C.P. Francis, Transforming a Hospital Facility Company into an Integrated Medical Care Organization, *Managed Care Quarterly* 2, no. 4 (Autumn 1994): 12–23.

5. *Ibid.*

6. B.C. Vladeck and N.A. Miller, The Medicare Home Health Initiative, 7–16.

7. H. Dittbrenner, Ensuring Survival—Expansion into Nontraditional Services, *Caring* (June 1994): 54–58.

Glossary

Accounting Entity—Status determined by the agency's legal structure (i.e., proprietary, not for profit, corporation or partnership, department, or free-standing). The type of accounting entity will determine the nature and scope of reporting requirements.

Accounting Rate of Return (ARR)—A method of measuring investment profitability using investment cost and profit streams.

Accrual Basis of Accounting—Revenue recorded in the period when it is earned, regardless of when it is collected, and expenditures for expense and asset items recorded in the period in which they are incurred, regardless of when paid.

Accumulated Depreciation—The total amount of depreciation that has been recorded from the time the fixed asset was put into operation.

Activities—The tasks that comprise processes. Activities are performed by employees to accomplish the home health agency's mission and satisfy operational and regulatory requirements. Activities consume resources.

Activity Attributes—Additional method of activity classification. For example, activities can be classified by whether they add value or cost.

Activity-based Costing (ABC)—A costing methodology that employs multiple cost drivers to develop a causal relationship between resource consumption and cost objects (payors and product lines).

Activity-based Management—The horizontal view. Management of activities by linking cost drivers to performance measures.

Activities of Daily Living (ADL)—Limitations in a patient's ability to care for himself or herself.

Activity Drivers—Establish a casual relationship between activity pools and cost objects.

Allocable Costs—An item or group of items of cost chargeable to one or more objects, processes, or operations in accordance with cost responsibilities, benefits received, or other identifiable measure of application or consumption (also known as *general service costs*).

Allowable Costs—Costs that are reimbursable from the perspective of the Medicare program. Costs must be related to patient care or the cost of maintaining a facility.

Apportionment—The allocation or distribution of allowable cost between the beneficiaries of the Medicare program and other patients.

Assets—Something of value either of tangible or intangible form. Tangible form would be cash or equipment. Intangible would be the home health agency's reputation in the community or agency good will.

Attributes—Traits that provide additional information about activities, for instance, whether an activity provides value or cost.

Audit—A verification process that is usually conducted by a third party. Verification could include review of internally prepared financial statements for conformance with generally accepted accounting principles, payroll records to determine the appropriate workers' compensation fee, or Medicare's cost report to verify costs.

Benchmark—A measurement point against which operations are evaluated. The standard can be internally or externally developed.

Brainstorming—A creative approach to problem solving using free association.

Break-even Analysis—A determination of volume (number of units) required to cover fixed and variable cost.

Budget—A forecast of revenues, expenses, cash flow, and capital expenditure requirements for the upcoming year.

Bundling—Inclusion of multiple services under one rate that had previously been billed separately.

Calendar Quarter—Periods ending March 31, June 30, September 30, and December 31.

Capitation—A payment for services that a population may require. Rate is the total cost of estimated services for a specific population divided by the number of members in that population.

Cash Basis of Accounting—Revenues are recognized only when cash is received, and expenditures for expense and asset items are not recorded until cash is disbursed for them.

Cash Disbursement—Payment to vendors, employees, banks, or other creditors.

Cash Flow—Consists of cash receipts and cash disbursements collectively referred to as cash flow. Cash flow will be either positive or negative.

Cash Forecast—Estimate of cash receipts and cash disbursements for a specified time period. Cash forecasts are used as part of the cash management process.

Cash Management—The process of investing, borrowing, monitoring, and maximizing all cash-related activities.

Cash Receipt—Collection of cash either from receivables, prepayments, or credit source.

Charges—The published or stated rate than an agency will charge to provide a service. The following is an example of a charge structure used for the six primary disciplines:

Skilled nursing	$95
Physical therapy	$95
Occupational therapy	$95
Speech therapy	$75
Medical social services	$140
Home health aide	$50

Medicare-certified agencies traditionally have set their charges at several dollars greater than the current limits determined by the Health Care Financing Administration.

Chart of Accounts—Numeric listing of general ledger accounts.

Clinical Pathway—Identification of a series of interventions and outcomes by discipline based on patient problem. Includes medical supplies, equipment, and infusion therapies.

Continuous Quality Improvement (CQI)—A system of process improvement that focuses on internal and external customers.

Contractual Allowance—A situation that occurs when an agency enters into a contract to provide services for another provider at less than its stated charges. If an agency agrees to provide services to the Medicaid program, and the Medicaid program will only pay $65 for a skilled nursing visit, then the difference between the stated rate of $95 and Medicaid's payment rate of $65 is the contractual allowance. In this example, the contractual allowance would be $30. Contractual allowance is a discount from stated charges.

Contribution Margin—Revenue less variable cost.

Cost Accounting—An element of managerial accounting that focuses on the relationships between cost and volume.

Cost Center—An organizational unit, generally a department or its subunit, having a common functional purpose for which direct and indirect costs are accumulated, allocated, and apportioned.

Cost Driver—Explains why activities are performed.

Cost Finding—A determination of the cost of services by the use of informal procedures (i.e., without employing the regular processes of cost accounting on a continuous or formal basis). It is the determination of per visit costs for each of the disciplines provided by the assignment of direct costs and the allocation of indirect costs.

Cost Hierarchy—Process of assigning costs to cost objectives. Goal is to assign costs directly, then through the development of causal relationships using resource and activity drivers, and then finally through allocation.

Cost Objective—The target of the activity-based costing process.

Cost of Capital—The cost of borrowed funds. Cost is interest plus expenses related to the financing (i.e., accounting fees, legal costs, etc.).

Cost of Service—The cost of providing one unit of service. Cost is determined by the type of field employee utilized to make the visit and by how much he or she is paid. Home health agencies that utilize their own employees versus subcontracting can pay employees on a per visit basis, hourly, per diem, or salary. Employers are responsible for costs in addition to payment of employees. Additional cost includes payroll taxes, workers' compensation, paid time off, health insurance, and travel cost. Home health agencies utilizing a subcontractor to provide services to their patients will negotiate and pay a fixed rate.

Cost Reimbursement—A payment methodology that reimburses providers for cost incurred.

Cost Reports—Periodic reports of a provider's operations that generally cover a consecutive 12-month period of the provider's operations that the Medicare program requires each provider of services to submit.

Customary Charges—The charges for services furnished to beneficiaries and other paying patients who receive services. These charges must be recorded on all bills submitted for program reimbursement.

Customers—Internal or external recipients of an agency's services. Internal customers are coworkers and departments. External customers are patients, case managers, and payors.

Cycle Time—The amount of time a process takes from beginning to end.

Depreciation—A systematic approach to recognizing the cost of an asset over the useful life of the asset.

Depreciation Expense—Cost incurred recognizing the decline in the value of an asset.

Direct Cost—Costs directly associated with an activity, unit of service, or cost objective.

Directly Allocable Costs—Directly allocable costs are chargeable based on actual usage (e.g., metered electricity) rather than a statistical surrogate.

Downstream Costs—Cost that the home health agency will incur after the patient has been discharged. Usually associated with follow-up activities and customer satisfaction surveys.

Durable Medical Equipment (DME)—Equipment that is either rented or sold to a patient versus provided as an element of the patient visit. Examples would include walkers, wheelchairs, and commodes.

Efficiency Variance—The difference between actual cost and budgeted cost multiplied by budgeted volume.

Episodic Payment Structure—Fixed amount based on a predetermined range of services, duration, or patient problem.

Evaluation Visits—Consideration of the physical facilities available in the patient's place of residence, the homebound status, and the attitudes of family members for the purpose of evaluating the feasibility of meeting the patient's medical needs in the home health setting. Home health agencies are required by regulations to have written policies concerning the acceptance of patients by the agency. When personnel of the agency make such an initial evaluation visit, the cost of the visit is considered an administrative cost of the agency and is not chargeable as a visit since, at this point, the patient has not been accepted for care. If, however, during the course of this initial evaluation visit, the patient is determined suitable for home health care by the agency and is also furnished the first skilled service as ordered under the physician's plan of treatment, the visit would become the first billable visit. A supervisory visit made by a nurse or other appropriate personnel (as required by the conditions of participation) to evaluate the specific personal care needs of the patient or to review the manner in which the personal care needs of the patient are being met by the aide is considered an administrative function and is not chargeable to the patient as a skilled visit.

Factoring—The sale of agency receivables to a third party. Receivables are sold at a discount from face.

Fee-for-Service (FFS)—Revenue calculated on a per visit, hourly, or some other unit and charges based on each incremental unit of service provided.

Financial Ratios—A managerial tool used to evaluate a home health agency's liquidity, capitalization, activity, and profitability.

Financial Reporting—The process of reflecting the actual results of operation in a standardized format. Reports required to state financial position properly include the income statement, balance sheet, and statement of cash flows. Operational results are used for internal and external purposes, primarily for decision making.

First In, First Out (FIFO)—A method of inventory valuation that assumes the oldest inventory is used first.

Fiscal Intermediary—FI

Fiscal Year—A one-year period defined for financial reporting purposes that does not have to coincide with a calendar year.

Fixed Assets—Assets that have been capitalized with an estimated useful life in excess of one year.

Fixed Cost—Cost that does not fluctuate with volume.

Float—The amount of time between check issuance and when the check clears.

Forecast—An estimate of a future condition.

Fringe Benefits—Costs borne by an employer on behalf of an employee. These costs are in addition to salary or hourly compensation. Typical fringe benefits include paid time off, health benefits, education, auto allowances, pensions, bonus plans, and myriad other perquisites.

Full-time Equivalent (FTE)—Someone who works 2,080 hours during the year. Employees generally work less than 2,080 hours because of vacations, sick time, personal time, paid holidays, and so forth. The FTE calculation includes replacement time to compensate for the above paid time off.

General Service Cost Center—Those organizational units that are operated for the benefit of the institution as a whole. Each of these may render services to other general service areas as well as to special or patient care departments.

Generally Accepted Accounting Principles—(GAAP)

Health Care Financing Administration (HCFA)—Federal agency that administers the Medicare program.

Health Maintenance Organization (HMO)—Organization that provides health services in exchange for a fixed monthly premium.

Home Health Discipline—One of six visiting services covered under the Medicare home health benefit: (1) skilled nursing, (2) physical therapy, (3) speech pathology, (4) occupational therapy, (5) medical social services, and (6) home health aide.

Home Health Visit—A personal contact in the place of residence of a patient made for the purpose of providing a covered service by a health worker on the staff of the home health agency or by others under contract or arrangement with the home health agency; or a visit by a homebound patient on an outpatient basis to a hospital, skilled nursing facility, rehabilitation center, or outpatient department affiliated with a medical school when arrangements have been made by the home health agency for the furnishing of a covered service on an outpatient basis because it requires the use of equipment that cannot be made readily available at home.

- *Counting Visits*—If a visit is made simultaneously by two or more persons from the home health agency to provide a single service, for which one person supervises or instructs the other, it is counted as one visit (see Example 1). If one person visits the patient's home more than once during a day to provide services, each visit is recorded as a separate visit (see Example 2). If a visit is made by two or more persons from the home health agency for the purpose of providing separate and distinct types of services, each is recorded (see Example 3). If the patient is taken elsewhere for the service because the service could not be furnished in his or her residence, one visit is counted for each service he or she receives (see Example 4).
- *Example 1*—If an occupational therapist and an occupational therapy assistant visit the patient together to provide therapy, and the therapist is there to supervise the assistant, one visit is counted.
- *Example 2*—If a nurse visits the patient in the morning to dress a wound and later must return to replace a catheter, two visits are counted.
- *Example 3*—If the therapist visits the patient for treatment in the morning, and the patient is later visited by the assistant for additional treatment, two visits are counted.

- *Example 4*—If an individual is taken to a hospital to receive outpatient therapy that could not be furnished in his or her own home (e.g., hydrotherapy) and, while at the hospital, receives speech therapy and other services, two or more visits would be charged.
- *Example 5*—Many home health agencies provide home health aide services on an hourly basis (ranging from one to eight hours a day). However, in order to allocate visits properly against a patient's maximum allowable visits, home health aide services are to be counted in terms of visits. Thus, regardless of the number of continuous hours a home health aide spends in a patient's home on any given day, one visit is counted for each such day. If, in a rare situation, a home health aide visits a patient for an hour or two in the morning, and again for an hour or two in the afternoon, two visits are counted.

Independent Contractor—Individual who is not an employee of the agency.

Indirect Costs—All other costs that are not incurred in the direct provision of a unit of service.

Indirectly Allocable Costs—Costs are not chargeable based on actual usage and, thus, allocated on the basis of a statistical surrogate (e.g., square feet).

Infusion Therapies—Medicine, food, and fluids that are administered intravenously.

Inputs—Resources that go into a process.

Internal Control—A system of checks and balances designed by management to prevent errors, theft, and customer problems and to integrate ethical practices into daily activities.

Inventory—Supplies and other materials to be used in the provision of services.

Last In, First Out (LIFO)—A method of inventory valuation that assumes the newest inventory is used first.

Limits—Ceiling on provider costs determined by the Health Care Financing Administration as reasonable in determining Medicare program payments.

Lockbox—A post office address. All remittances are forwarded to the post office box and then applied against a loan balance or credited to a bank account.

Net Present Value (NPV)—The discounting of future cash inflows and outflows to the current period.

Operating Cycle—The normal amount of time that it takes to convert an asset into cash. This could be the generation and collection of receivables or the purchase and sale of inventory.

Outcome—A target or goal for a particular event or process.

Outlier—An event that is outside of a specified service range.

Output—The end result of a process.

Paid Time Off—An employee benefit, sometimes referred to as PTO. PTO can be for vacation, sick, or personal time and is determined by each home health agency. The agency may choose to have different levels of PTO depending on employee classification.

Patient Problem—Composition of factors that contribute to the patient's care requirements. Patient problem is influenced by nursing diagnoses, presence of caregivers, psychological state, presence of activities of daily living limitations, and so forth.

Payor—Anyone who is responsible for paying for services provided. A payor could be a patient or a third party such as Medicare, Medicaid, or any insurance plan.

Payor Mix—The total number of primary payors that corresponds to the activity provided for a specified period. The example listed below identifies a total of 3,615 visits were made for the period being reported. Of the 3,615 visits, 1,800 were billable to Medicare, so, therefore, Medicare is 49.79 percent of the payor mix.

	Visits	*%*
Private	1,250	34
Health maintenance organization	500	14
Medicaid	65	2
Medicare	1,800	50
Total	3,615	100

Per Diem—Daily charge.

Performance Measure—A metric used to evaluate whether activities are accomplishing their desired outcomes.

Periodic Interim Payment (PIP)—A payment vehicle provided under the Medicare program.

Preferred Provider Organization (PPO)—Managed care organizations that will contract with providers to provide services to their clients.

Process—A sequence of activities that consumes inputs and produces outputs.

Product Line—Different types of services that are offered to home health patients. Typical product lines would include continuous care, skilled intermittent, durable medical equipment, and infusion therapies.

Productivity—The level of units produced by an employee in a specified time-frame (e.g., visits, invoices, transcriptions).

Prospective Payment—Predetermined payment based on some level of service.

Quantity Variance—The difference between actual volume and budgeted volume multiplied by actual cost.

Resource Drivers—Establish a relationship between cost pools and the activities that consume resources.

Risk Corridor—Safety mechanism to protect the home health agency and managed care organization from either excessive patient care costs or excessive per member per month payments.

Seasonality—A predictable pattern of variation.

Stewardship—Management's responsibility for protecting the assets of a company. Stewardship can also include the concept of profitability, because without profit, there will be no assets.

Strategic Management—Organizational strategies that influence daily operations.

Third-party Payor—Party other than the patient that pays for services.

Upstream Cost—Cost incurred prior to the provision of direct services. Usually associated with marketing activities.

Value—Benefits that accrue to the customers of a service.

Value-added—Activity or process that increases the value of services provided from the customers' perspective.

Variable Cost—Cost that fluctuates with volume. Costs can be composed of a fixed and variable component.

Variance—The difference between actual and budget. Variance consists of two elements: efficiency and quantity.

Vendor—Supplier.

Working Capital—Current assets less current liabilities.

Zero Balance Accounts (ZBA)—Bank accounts that have zero balances. Cash is transferred in to cover the exact amount of transactions presented for payment.

Index

About the Author

Tad McKeon, MBA, CPA, is a well-respected consultant to home health agencies. Previously, he was corporate controller for a large regional home health provider, as well as a Community Health Accreditation Program surveyor. He received his MBA from Temple University. Mr. McKeon is a member of the Pennsylvania Institute of Certified Public Accountants, the American Society of Quality Control, and the Healthcare Financial Management Association. He has authored numerous articles for the *Journal of Home Health Care Practice*, and also serves as guest editor and editorial board member. His consulting practice, Creative Health and Financial Management, is located in Jeffersonville, Pennsylvania.